The Science of Self-Report
◆❖◆

Implications for Research and Practice

The Science of Self-Report
❖
Implications for Research and Practice

Edited by

Arthur A. Stone
State University of New York

Jaylan S. Turkkan
The National Institute on Drug Abuse,
The National Institutes of Health

Christine A. Bachrach
National Institute of Child Health
and Human Development

Jared B. Jobe
National Institute on Aging

Howard S. Kurtzman
National Institute of Mental Health

Virginia S. Cain
Office of Behavioral and Social Sciences Research,
The National Institutes of Health

LAWRENCE ERLBAUM ASSOCIATES, PUBLISHERS
2000   Mahwah, New Jersey   London

Lawrence Erlbaum Associates, Inc., Publishers
10 Industrial Avenue
Mahwah, NJ 07430

Cover design by Kathryn Houghtaling Lacey

Library of Congress Cataloging-in-Publication Data

The science of self-report : implications for research and practice / edited by
Arthur A. Stone . . . [et al.].
                                                                    p. cm.
      Includes bibliographical references and index.
ISBN 0-8058-2990-3 (cloth : alk. paper).—ISBN 0-8058-2991-1 (pbk : alk. paper)
Human experimentation in medicine–Congresses. 2. Human experimentation
      on psychology–Congresses. I. Stone, Arthur A.
   R853.H8S36 1999
   619—dc21   98-33155
                                                                    CIP

Printed in the United States of America
10 9 8 7 6 5 4 3 2

Contents

Preface

Peoples' reports about what they are feeling, what they are doing, what they recall happening in the past—that is, self-reported data—are essential to the health care profession and underlie many of our research endeavors. Clinicians ask their patients what their symptoms are, where they are, how long symptoms have been experienced, and under what conditions they are experienced. Researchers ask study participants similar questions, for example, about childhood experiences, use of illicit drugs or sexual practices, about recent or past stressful events, exposures to environmental toxins, appraisals of the quality of the work environment or marriage, family history, dietary intake, or adherence to medication protocols. All of this information, and much more, falls into the domain of self-report data.

This volume presents a set of chapters based on presentations given during a conference entitled "The Science of Self-Report: Implications for Research and Practice," held in the Masur Auditorium at the National Institutes of Health in Bethesda, Maryland on November 7 and 8, 1996. The goal of the conference was to present recent findings about self-report. We start out with the position that it is naive to accept all self-reports as veridical. As the chapters in the volume document, psychological and social processes influence storage and recall of self-report information. They show that there are conditions under which self-reports should be readily accepted by the clinician or researcher and that there are other conditions where healthy skepticism is required. We show that there are methods for improving the accuracy of self-reports, ranging from fine-tuning our interviews and questionnaires to employing emerging technologies to collect data in ways that minimize bias and encourage accurate reporting.

It is clear that both the limitations of self-report data as well as the new methods for improving self-report need to be known by clinicians and scientists using such data. Yet, scientists who might think themselves immune to the issues should think twice. The success of the pharmacologist or the neuroscientist developing molecular therapies to fight cancer or of the geneticist collecting family history data depend on the valid assessment of endpoints—and many of the outcomes used in research are based on self-report information. The entire scientific endeavor will be optimally productive only if self-reported outcomes are accurate.

It is our hope that this book will:

- increase general awareness of the importance of self-report in science and in practice,
- will disseminate information about innovative ways of improving reports, and
- will stimulate research about self-report.

The conference on which the book is based was planned by many dedicated individuals. Over 3 years ago, Jaylan Turkkan, Chief of the Behavioral Sciences Research Branch at the National Institute on Drug Abuse, had the idea to convene a conference about self-report, although her conceptualization of the meeting was much more specific. She discussed this idea with members of the Behavioral and Social Science Coordinating Committee of the NIH and, eventually, a planning committee was formed. Arthur Stone from the Department of Psychiatry and Behavioral Science at the State University of New York at Stony Brook was asked to chair the committee developing the conference, with Turkkan serving as co-chair. The planning committee members represented several NIH institutes and offices: Turkkan from NIDA, Christine Bachrach from the National Institute of Child Health and Human Development, Jared Jobe from the National Institute on Aging, Howard Kurtzman from the National Institute of Mental Health, and Virginia Cain from the Office of Behavioral and Social Sciences Research. Each edited a section of this book.

The conference and preparation of the book were sponsored by the Office of Behavioral and Social Science Research. Norman Anderson, the Director of OBSSR, lent his full and enthusiastic support to the endeavor.

The contributing authors are some of the finest scientists working on self-report in the world. They represent a diverse group of professions—sociology, law, psychology, medicine—and their contributions to the field have been enormous. We are very grateful to all of the authors for agreeing to present at the conference and for preparing a chapter for this volume. In addition to the chapters prepared by conference presenters, we are pleased that Anthony was able to contribute a chapter on self-report and substance abuse.

It is important to acknowledge that the research presented here is only a sampling of research being conducted on self-report. It is simply impossible to fully cover the domain of self-report research in a single volume and we point the interested reader to the references provided in the chapters. Another tangible outcome of the self-report conference is the issuance of a Program Announcement from the National Institutes of Health in February of 1998 entitled "Methodology and measurement in the behavioral sciences" (PA-98-031).

We hope that importance of this research and the creative energies of the investigators comes through in the chapters. It was a pleasure for us to be involved with such a fine group of scientists.

—Arthur A. Stone
—Jaylan S. Turkkan

PART

I

GENERAL ISSUES
IN SELF-REPORT

Jaylan S. Turkkan
The National Institute on Drug Abuse,
The National Institutes of Health

In this section, chapters by Wendy Baldwin and Donald Bersoff introduce broad issues in the use of self-report in research settings. Baldwin reminds us that even so straightforward a question as asking someone their address is fraught with potential for misunderstanding; in virtually all cases, however, we are willing to take the participant's word for where they live. In many other protocols, we feel the need to gather additional data not based on self-report. Baldwin makes the case that self-report data should not be thought of as mere proxies for other better verification methods. Indeed sometimes, as in past sexual behavior, there are no better measurement methods. In the case of past drug use also, until hair testing and other biologic verification techniques are completely validated, information on distant drug use will need to be primarily ascertained via self-report. Even where biologic or registry information is available, often it is too expensive, obtrusive, or time consuming to obtain. Consider also that biologic and other data can be as prone to false positives, false negatives, and other inaccuracies as self-report data.

Bersoff's chapter reminds us that whenever we gather information from anyone, there are special ethical considerations that we must be more mindful of. When these data are collected from children and adolescents, or from adults who may not be fully capable of understanding the research protocols, additional sensitivity and care must be provided. Although most if not all major psychological and social science organizations have published clear ethical codes of conduct, subtle instances of coercion such as the slippery slope phenomenon abound. Moreover, well-meaning researchers are understandably confused when they uncover sensitive or criminal information from minors during research protocols. Should they reveal this information to parents? If they do, will they be violating the minor's rights to privacy and confidentiality? These are questions for which there are no easy answers. Bersoff's chapter expertly leads us through the maze of ethical dilemmas that can arise when asking research participants about their experiences and opinions.

1

Information No One Else Knows: The Value of Self-Report

Wendy Baldwin
The National Institutes of Health

A volume on self-report is an opportunity to address methodological issues as well as fundamental issues of why and when we expect to use such data. I believe there is an inherent mistrust of self-report data because such data could be erroneous, not just because of measurement error with which we must always contend but because of the possibility of conscious bias in the person providing the data. Presumably, a desire to look good could distort data either intentionally or unintentionally.

However, self-report data are essential to behavioral and medical research. Also, such data are essential to medical practice, because self-report is the heart of the careful medical history that underlies so much of diagnosis and care. Therefore, it could be argued that it is an obligation of the behavioral community to help make the collection of these data the most robust that it can be.

Let me lay out two situations where we typically encounter self-report data: first, there are cases where other data exist, but they are too difficult to obtain or the costs of obtaining them are not worth the effort; then there are the cases where there is no other source for the information. The first case is one that should challenge us to clarify our underlying definitions, to consider how much error we can tolerate, to elaborate the possible incentives one might have to distort answers, and to raise our awareness about how we communicate with research participants. We routinely ask research participants or patients simple questions such as where they live. We do not follow them home and we do not usually get a verification, such as a piece of mail addressed to them. We take their word for it. Sometimes they lie. If we followed them home, we might get the wrong answer anyway; perhaps they are just staying with friends and that is not really home. Perhaps our definition of home is where they typically do live, not where their spouse still lives 100 miles away or vice versa. But, unless we are sending a bill there and fear they will not get it—and pay it—we simply ask the question and take the answer.

I am sure the readers are way ahead of me now. What about research looking at access to services? What if the hypothesis depends on measures of family and social supports? What if the environment is key to the problem of study? Then the error might be intolerable. In that case, I would suggest that it is still a case for self-report, but with better definitions and clearer questions to the participant. The correctness of the answer depends in large part on the clarity and precision of the question.

Let me take another case. There may be data that exist independent of the subject, and we would like to have them, but it is not clear that it is worth the effort to obtain them independently. This brings us to consider the distinction between what people know and may or may not tell you and what they actually do not know. Many studies of pregnancy outcome require information about birth weight of the infant. Most women, I contend, can tell you birth weight with pretty good accuracy. However, if you require great precision, this might not be enough, and if you require information about the baby's length, it probably will not do at all. Why? One piece of information—weight—is more salient to most women than the other—length. This situation, and others like it, provide interesting research opportunities to understand self-reporting. When we know we can find out some pieces of information from independent sources, we are able to compare what we get from self-report and what those other sources provide, birth weight of babies being one example. The researchers still must decide how much precision they need.

This should then position us to identify the strategies that enhance the reporting of information people already know. What are the prompts that assist recall? For example, timelines of life events and historic events can help individuals to report on activities in their own lives. We can also calibrate the level of accurate reporting needed: a category for birthweight, such as under 5½ pounds, may be very accurately reported, whereas specific pounds–ounces might not be. One wonderful example of the use of self-report data to identify a problem is the paradox of Mexican-American immigrants. Their infants have higher birth weights generally than do infants born to those who have lived in the United States for several years, even Mexican Americans born in the United States. This finding was originally based solely on self-report data but has been shown to be quite reliable and robust, with many studies and surveys (and National Center for Health

Statistics data) confirming that the phenomenon exists. Validating that certain information can be obtained through self-report is important because it opens up avenues of research where self-report data are the only data available.

We will need self-report data for items where we theoretically could get independent measures as well as where we cannot get independent measures; the former provide the research opportunities to develop our skills for the latter. What are the situations where we cannot reasonably obtain independent measures? Are they important and are they amenable to self-report? An obvious one is sexual behavior. There are numerous health issues that are confronting researchers with the need for information about their research participants, intimate behaviors that cannot be obtained in any way other than asking them: the number of partners, sexual practices, protective practices, interactions with potential partners, and more. This information may be key to understanding risk of pregnancy and sexually transmitted diseases, including those that may be lethal (such as HIV) as well as those that can have longer-term health consequences, such as human papilloma virus (HPV), which is linked to cervical cancer. These are significant pieces of relevant information. Information about what happens during sexual intercourse has no independent source; the partner is just another source of self-report. This information may be critical to understanding risk or changes in behavior or to finding opportunities for intervention.

Arguments abound over an individual's desire to present a favorable image, so we can easily hypothesize why men and women might differentially misreport data about sexual partners. Again, the necessary level of candor should be considered. If one is doing case finding in a clinical setting, missing even one partner could be a significant problem. If one is categorizing research subjects into broad categories of sexual risk taking, missing one partner could be irrelevant. In either case, we are still left with self-report data but researcher anxiety might be significantly less.

How about incentives to misreport? In the area of sexual behavior, the criticism of self-report data has included the observation that individuals are not always candid with their sexual partners; yet this observation may be largely irrelevant to the research experience. People may recall personal situations where they gave less than accurate information and therefore doubt that others will be candid about such personal information with an interviewer. However, the interview situation is fundamentally different from most personal encounters. In the interview, there is anonymity, confidentiality, and a contribution to make to science, if not to one's own welfare. The dialogue about sex in a singles' bar probably has a motive to it that does not apply to an interview. The interviewer is not going home with the respondent regardless of what is reported. The personal experiences told to an interviewer are used anonymously and, in the aggregate, are a far cry from having shared an intimacy with a family member whom one sees year after year. Because nonresearchers may be slow to make these distinctions, the research community must do so.

Sexual behavior is perhaps the most obvious arena where no independent source of data exists, but it is by no means the only one. Any process that involves a behavior over which the individual has a high degree of control is likely to require self-reporting of that information. What kinds of data would that be?

Nutrition in food consumption is difficult to measure, but short of direct observations, we need self-report. The same is true of other behaviors, such as the use of automobile seat belts, bicycle helmets, the ingestion of herbal remedies. Even where external data theoretically exist, self-report may differ significantly from information in registries because people may tell an interviewer things they may be reluctant to share with legal authorities. Motivation for behaviors is another example where the individual is the only source of information, such as what may have prompted certain criminal behaviors or sexual activities, illicit drug use, even migration.

Another area where self-report is often the only or best source of information is health behaviors. Take exercise. The questions relate not just to the effect of exercise in the lab setting but how well individuals incorporate it into their daily lives, how they cope with disruptions in their schedules. And consider health behaviors during pregnancy such as smoking, consumption of alcohol or vitamins, or other specific nutritional practices. Another example is characteristics of the environment, such as exposure to physical and psychological threats. We are beginning to look at young children's exposure to violence in their community—exposure only they can report. We know the behavioral components to many of the top diseases in the United States and we know that behavioral factors dominate the new morbidity, but the reach of health behavior issues is far wider.

Reports on global health indicate areas for research and health service attention. The concern here is not just something the United States has come to confront, but risks facing the world. What is the role for self-report there? Let me start with one high-priority area: maternal and child health. The risks here are tied not just to those associated with unsafe sexual practices (already discussed) but also the practices related to delivery (use of midwives or traditional birth attendants), use of herbal remedies or other folk practices, or specific pregnancy-related dietary practices found in some cultures. Even if there were high-tech ways to develop independent measures, health risks are greatest in geographic areas where the resources for health care and health research are the lowest. The high technology measures would be of little use and we can easily foresee the need for robust measures of self-report.

There are also risks from emerging and reemerging infections. Two noted examples are tuberculosis (TB) and malaria, each with a behavioral component. Adherence to medications for TB is a well-recognized concern. And compliance in the use of medicated mosquito nets for malaria prevention is another area of research and practical interest. As affordable interventions are developed, researchers will be dependent on self-reports of compliance as well as reports of additional risk behaviors. In addition, risks from noncommunicable diseases will be a growing threat to world health: heart disease, respiratory diseases, injury, and violence—all have some behavioral components. Injuries are a growing threat not only in the United States but in emerging economies. Our need for epidemiologic information will require self-report data about risk exposures, such as interpersonal, vehicular, and environmental. The risks from inequitable health services carry implications for research, and researchers need to understand the behavioral factors that influence people's use of services, factors that are largely visible to us only through self-report.

There is concern that use of mortality alone—a measure relatively free of self-report or measurement errors—is inadequate to assess the burden of disease or priorities for research or distribution of health services. Alternative measures frequently require attention to conditions that disable, not just conditions that kill. The measurement of disability is rather difficult and often dependent on self-report. Even where independent, technologically based measures exist, it is unlikely that they will gain widespread use in countries with emerging economies. There is an enormous need for measures that are simple and robust and many of these will be self-report measures.

In summary, the problems with self-report data are similar to those we face with other forms of data collection: clarity in underlying premises, circumstances for which and under which the data are being used, uniformity of data collection procedures, the need to estimate likely bias, and there are others. But improvements can come and they will benefit almost every disease area, in both research and practice.

I cannot give an exhaustive list of the keys to better self-report data. That is the purpose of the other chapters. However, I have tried to share my observations of health problems within the United States and around the world and the role that self-report data can play, a role that is important to our learning as much as we can about these problems as we seek information that can lead to improved interventions and, ultimately, to some solutions.

2

Ethical Issues in the Collection of Self-Report Data

David M. Bersoff
Diogenes Project

Donald N. Bersoff
Villanova University
Medical College of Pennsylvania—Hahnemann

There are very few publications that focus on the ethical issues confronting those who gather self-report data in a research context (see LaGreca, 1990). Perhaps one reason for this lack of attention is that, compared to naturalistic observation and deception-based research, self-report surveys seem rather benign. Self-report measures are usually fairly straightforward, and a willingness to fill out a survey or answer a researcher's questions implies a consent to participate in the study being conducted. In contrast, unobtrusive observations and deception studies can not, by their nature, be fully consented to without compromising the data collected, and people in such studies may not even be fully aware that they are research participants. Despite these superficial differences, self-report data collection is fraught with just as many ethical concerns, albeit of a somewhat different nature, as experimental and observational research.

Beyond the issues of privacy, confidentiality, and informed consent that are present in almost all psychological research, there are ethical issues that are somewhat unique to self-report data collection. In particular, we focus on the potential self-report research has to glean clinically sensitive data, often putting that data in the hands of nonclinicians. In addition, self-report measures can be used to collect data about third parties who have not directly or even indirectly consented to be part of the research and who may not want such information revealed to others. Of course, there is a price to be paid for adhering to sound ethical practices, and we end with a consideration of the potential costs of placing more stringent controls on the collection of self-report data.

PROTECTING BASIC RIGHTS

Informed Consent

We find many of the current practices used in the collection of self-report data to be generally inadequate in terms of protecting people's basic rights. First of all, most survey research is exempted from Human Subjects Committee (IRB) review and is not required to have a formal consent procedure (see CFR §46.101, 1996). Currently, IRB review and formal consent are mandated for survey and interview procedures only if subjects can be uniquely identified from their data and/or if disclosure of their "responses outside the research could reasonably place subjects at risk of criminal or civil liability or be damaging to the subject's financial standing, employability or reputation" (45 CFR §46.101 (b2)). There are two problems with these criteria.

The first is that risky or potentially damaging responses are not always foreseeable. Open-ended questions are quite common in self-report research and often a researcher simply cannot predict the type of information that may be gathered. A study that involves thought sampling (a technique in which subjects are beeped at random times during the day and asked to record their thoughts at that moment), for example, could just as easily yield someone's shopping list as it could a suicide ideation or a passing violent fantasy. Asking a person to relate a life-altering experience could result in a story about being lost in a shopping mall as a child as well as a date rape.

Second, these federal guidelines are less stringent than the ethical requirements of the American Psychological Association (APA), and other major social science research organizations, that mandate that researchers "inform participants of the nature of the research ... [and] of significant factors that may be expected to influence their willingness to participate ... [including] limitations on confidentiality" (APA, 1992, p. 1608). This mandate to inform potential participants about the nature of one's research still holds even if the information to be collected in a study would not necessarily put the person at risk of liability or be damaging to his or her financial standing, employability, or reputation. In addition, risk is not the only factor that can potentially and significantly influence an individual's willingness to participate in a study (Singer & Frankel, 1982), and thus, risk should not be the primary or sole basis on which to determine the necessity of having a formal consent procedure.

For these reasons, we suggest that all survey research have some sort of informed consent. At a minimum, potential respondents should be informed, even if only orally, of (a) the topic and purpose of the research, (b) the nature of the questions to be asked, (c) the time required for participation, (d) their right to skip individual questions or to withdraw from the study at any time without penalty, (e) the limits on the confidentiality of the data collected, and (f) who they can contact if they have any concerns or questions regarding the study.

Participating in research represents an investment of time and energy on the part of respondents. They are entitled to know the size of the time commitment they are being asked to make as well as the significance of the issue being examined, both of which may be key factors influencing people's willingness to take part in a given study (Singer & Frankel, 1982). If fully revealing the nature or purpose of a study, although not necessarily the particular hypotheses being tested, would compromise the data collected, then the study involves, if not a deception, at least a withholding of standard consent form information from the subject. As a consequence, assuming IRB approval of this withholding of information, respondents should at least be offered a debriefing as they would in a laboratory experiment that entailed some sort of deception (Holmes, 1976).

Some populations such as children or the mentally ill may not be considered legally competent to give informed consent. In such cases, consent will have to be obtained from a legal guardian. However, unless the potential research participant is seriously impaired either due to brain damage or extreme youth, researchers are required to obtain their assent. Needless to say, extra care needs to be used in gaining a child's assent. In particular, research has shown that children have trouble understanding the potential benefits, and even more important, the potential risks of research participation (Abramovitch, Freedman, Henry, & Brunschot, 1995). In addition, they often fail to appreciate the fact that they can end their participation at any time during the study (Abramovitch, Freedman, Henry, & Brunschot, 1995). In seeking a minor's assent, these factors need to be emphasized.

Privacy Rights

Research participants have the right not to disclose information they may feel is too personal or sensitive. This right is usually addressed in the standard consent form, when one is used, in the stipulation that participants have the right to skip, without prejudice, any questions on the survey that they may feel uncomfortable answering. Even when a consent form is not used, researchers usually operate according to this norm. But as a protection of subjects' privacy rights, permission to skip discomforting questions is not equivalent to being told the exact nature of the questions to be asked at the time of consent. Once a respondent has begun to answer a set of questions, the social psychology of the survey situation changes radically.

For example, research on the foot-in-the-door phenomenon (Freedman & Fraser, 1966) shows how easy it is to get people to accede to a larger request then they normally would have by first getting them to accede to a small and rather benign request. In the seminal foot-in-the-door study, researchers went door to door posing as volunteer workers. They asked homeowners in a residential California neighborhood if they would allow a very large and poorly lettered public-service billboard reading "Drive Carefully" to be installed on their front lawns. The request was normally and understandably refused by the great majority (83%) of the residents in the area. But among one particular group of people, a full 76% of those asked agreed to display the sign. The only difference between the highly compliant and the highly non-compliant residents was that the compliant residents had, 2 weeks earlier, been asked to make a small commitment to driver safety. A different volunteer worker had come to their doors and asked them to accept and display a little 3-inch square sign that read BE A SAFE DRIVER. It was such a trifling request that nearly all of them had agreed to it. But the effects of complying with that trivial safe-driving request were enormous. It led those homeowners to become remarkably willing to comply with another safe-driving-oriented request that was massive in size.

The implications of this research for participation in self-report studies are rather straightforward. For example, although many people may demur at taking part in a study that they are told includes questions of an explicit, sexual nature, these same people may be manipulated into answering such questions by first being led to answer some rather tame sexual inquires. Once people have made a commitment to a certain type of behavior such as answering a survey or even answering questions of a sexual nature on a survey, the desire to appear consistent and cooperative may impel them to continue answering such questions and to finish the task they have started even if doing so is ill-considered (Cialdini, 1993; Orne, 1962).

There is also the slippery slope phenomenon. Milgram's (1974) obedience experiment is an example of how a slippery slope can lead to extreme behavior. In Milgram's study, subjects began administering electrical shocks to the learner at a very innocuous level—a barely perceptible 15 volts. The shocks the participants were asked to deliver then increased only 15 volts with each error the learner made in a learning task. Although it is clear that giving someone a 450-volt shock is a very different matter from giving him a 15-volt shock, it is not so clear just where the shock level becomes inappropriately high (Sabini, 1995). As a consequence, most of the subjects did not stop shocking the learner, even when the voltage surpassed 450 volts, until they were given permission to do so (Milgram, 1974).

The implications for self-report research are again rather straightforward. If sensitive questions are ordered in a subtle gradient from tame to highly intrusive, once people have begun answering a set of such questions, it would be difficult for them to justify to themselves suddenly stopping at any one given question. After all, they just answered the only slightly less provocative question that came before it. This is not to say that such slippery slope or foot-in-the-door manipulations are common practice, but merely that the potential for their employment exists in the absence of consent forms and a complete disclosure of the nature of the questions to be asked *before* people commit to participating.

Confidentiality

Study participants have a right not to have the information that they voluntarily provide made public or used against them. This right is usually addressed in the standard consent form, again when one is used, in the stipulation that all information collected in the study will be kept strictly confidential, "except as may be required by law" (see e.g., Confidentiality Clause from the Model Consent form distributed by the University of Pennsylvania IRB). This disclaimer is quite vague and therefore problematic. It places the burden on participants to know the disclosure rules in the jurisdiction and context in which the research is being conducted in order for them to fully appreciate the limits of their confidentiality rights. But how many lay people are likely to know about mandatory reporting laws for acts such as child abuse? And how would children possibly know, unless they were explicitly told, that if they express suicidal ideation or significant levels of drug use that their parents or their school are likely to be informed?

We are not the first to suggest that researchers should be more specific about the conditions under which confidentiality may need to be broken (i.e., confidentiality limitations). In a recent edition of *Ethics & Behavior*, several authors writing about the ethical issues inherent in working with at-risk and socially disenfranchised children reminded researchers of their obligation to inform prospective subjects of reporting requirements (DHHS, 1991), including informing children that under certain circumstances their parents may be contacted (Fisher, 1994; Hoagwood, 1994; Scott-Jones, 1994).

Full disclosure of confidentiality limitations is of particular concern in self-report research, and not just that involving children, because it is a methodology that allows for the mass collection of extremely sensitive and personal information, much more so than experimental and naturalistic observation research. Ethical injunctions, for example, prevent researchers from getting subjects to commit a crime, but they are perfectly free to ask about criminal behavior. Likewise, although IRBs would, no doubt, frown on placing hidden cameras in bedrooms, sexual behavior questionnaires are quite common. In addition, as previously discussed, the gleaning of sensitive information in any particular self-report study is not always foreseeable.

Thus, even studies not originally intended to focus on touchy topics can still yield sensitive and clinically relevant information. It is for these reasons that we advocate a generally conservative stance toward the disclosure of confidentiality limitations.

ISSUES UNIQUE TO SELF-REPORT DATA COLLECTION

Competence and the Collection of Clinically Sensitive Data

Because questionnaire studies tend to be inexpensive, fast, and easy to do compared to laboratory experiments and intervention studies, much undergraduate and first-year graduate school social and clinical research involves self-report measures. It is unfortunate that the research method most capable of gathering sensitive information is also the one most accessible and commonly used.

Our special concern in this regard is whether it is really appropriate that undergraduates and untrained graduate students are gathering information from people about such things as depression, anxiety, sexuality, and traumatic life experiences. They are not, after all, allowed to administer intelligence tests, the MMPI, and a number of other personality tests. And although we are not equating the skill and training required to administer self-report measures with that required to administer sophisticated diagnostic tests, the nature of the data yielded can be equivalent in terms of its clinical sensitivity and its potential to be abused and misinterpreted. Essentially, we see this as an issue of working within one's competence, a mandate explicitly set forth in the APA ethical code (APA, 1992, p. 1600).

Although it is true that young researchers almost always have faculty advisors who have obtained doctorates (although some undergraduates are directly supervised by graduate students), the nominal presence of an advisor alone is not an adequate safeguard. Most nonclinical psychologists are trained only in research and have had little or no clinical preparation or experience (Koocher & Keith-Spiegel, 1990). In addition, advisors do not always take it on themselves to examine the raw data of individual subjects. As an advisor, the temptation is to concern oneself with only the aggregate data. Unfortunately, individual problem cases do not tend to reveal themselves in group means.

In studies in which clinical concerns are not the primary focus and a clinically sensitive inventory is only one of several measures administered, an advisor could easily miss identifying at-risk subjects, especially if that advisor is not prone to micromanaging students nor familiar enough with the measure used to know the likelihood that at least one person in a sample will produce a worrisome score. In addition, advisors, and particularly those without clinical training, may not know what to do in response to a clinically significant score on a given measure. Finally, there is the problem that many times students use their own homemade measures. In cases involving such nonnormed or standardized scales, just what qualifies as a clinically significant score may be unknown.

The issue of investigator competence is important because of a basic obligation often ignored in research involving the collection of clinically sensitive data—planning in advance what one will do if faced with the disclosure of conduct or of a frame of mind that is potentially injurious to the participant, injurious to others, and/or illegal. Of course, part of this planning must include a consideration of the psychometric properties of the instruments being used (Fisher, 1994). A relatively unreliable scale, such as one of the homemade variety, that evokes responses otherwise requiring action—for example, evidence of child abuse—may display too many false positives to serve as a justification for some sort of intervention. However, assuming that one's scales have appropriate validity and reliability, there is a responsibility to foresee and develop a course of action to respond to indications that a research participant may be in distress or jeopardy. In the one study we found that investigated whether such contingency planning is routinely done, it was quite evident that it is not.

Burbach and his colleagues (Burbach, Farha, & Thorpe, 1986) identified 30 published studies by 21 authors that assessed depressive symptomatology via self-report in community, nonclinical samples of children. They mailed each of the corresponding authors an anonymous survey asking them about various aspects of their research methodology. Twelve authors who had done 16 of the studies returned a completed survey. The authors of four of these studies reported that they did not anticipate identifying severely depressed or suicidal children. None of these authors had any contingency plans in place in the event they had, contrary to their expectations, found an at-risk child in their samples. The authors of three other studies did anticipate that they might detect at-risk children but made no decisions nor developed any plans about whether, when, and how they would intervene prior to initiating their studies. Four other researchers also anticipated identifying very depressed children but decided not to take any action in such cases for one or more of the following reasons: (a) There was little information regarding the relationship between scores on the self-report inventories and actual psychological problems; (b) their consent forms did not contain provisions for follow-up contacts with the children; and (c) they did not want to violate the confidentiality of the children.

These last two reasons help illustrate just how complicated some of the ethical issues associated with collecting clinically sensitive data can be.

Although both reasons recognize that children have a right to privacy and to be treated with fidelity by researchers, they also neglect to consider the rights of parents to the care, control, and custody their children, including the right to know about situations or events that might impair their child's safety or emotional stability. Situations such as this in which researchers are subject to contradictory ethical considerations are not uncommon nor easily negotiated (Bersoff & Koeppl, 1993). In fact, preserving participant confidentiality in this context leads to an explicit violation of the Society for Research in Child Development's ethical code which states: "When, in the course of research, information comes to the investigator's attention that may jeopardize the child's well-being, the investigator has a responsibility to discuss the information with the parents or guardians and with those expert in the field in order that they may arrange the necessary assistance for the child" (SRCD, 1990–1991). And although the APA ethical code does not directly mandate that researchers must inform parents in these situations, the code does strongly express the importance of both the principles of fidelity and beneficence, the two competing concerns in this situation.

The issue of competing obligations aside for the moment, in only five of the published studies surveyed by Burbach et al. (1986) did the researchers plan to intervene if extreme depression scores were obtained on a self-report inventory, although three of the authors did not specify on the pertinent consent form who would be contacted. Interestingly, authors in four of the five studies actually intervened. The majority of the children followed up on ultimately received appropriate professional services.

Even when working with adults, the fidelity–beneficence dilemma is not easily resolved. Although fidelity and confidentiality are certainly important, imagine how devastating it could be if someone indicated on a survey or questionnaire or in an interview that he or she had a drug problem, was involved in child abuse, or had entertained thoughts of suicide and yet received no follow-up whatsoever. Such a person could conclude that his or her problem, or perhaps that he himself or she herself, was unimportant, even if the consent form did not explicitly contain provisions for follow-up contacts.

In general, those who collect self-report data (even that of a clinical nature) may consider themselves to be researchers, but in the eyes of study participants, they may be seen as clinicians, as people in a helping profession. If investigators who seek potentially sensitive information fail to respond in a caring or concerned manner when people open up to them, that can be a very meaningful event in these people's lives.

Researchers without proper training are not qualified to intervene themselves and may not even be able to determine when intervention is actually necessary. As a result, they are probably less likely to have a plan in place in case a potentially risky situation is identified. Thus, self-report surveys and questionnaires need to be evaluated, both by primary investigators and IRBs, on the basis of their potential for ferreting out clinically sensitive data. Those questionnaires deemed highly likely to yield sensitive information should be restricted in their use to qualified, suitably trained researchers or to persons who have qualified advisors or consultants on their projects. In addition, when clinically sensitive information is being collected, someone should be directly responsible for monitoring the data gathered for potential warning signs that one or more of the research participants is at risk or is in need of intervention. This does not mean, however, that only clinical psychologists should be allowed to collect data regarding depression or violence or substance abuse, although others have suggested that all researchers who work in sensitive areas such as screening, assessment, and intervention, especially with children, should seek licensure (Scarr, 1990). What is being strongly espoused is that researchers be held responsible for assuring by some means that the individuals they study do not receive less protection or fewer safeguards due to their lack of clinical or some other specialty training.

This suggestion is offered in contrast to the practice of holding researchers with differing amounts and kinds of training to different standards, for example, only requiring licensed clinicians to monitor subjects for signs of clinical depression. This differing standards approach is often seen in the legal system. The courts tend to hold individuals with special training and experience to higher standards of care and responsibility (Liss, 1994). Only psychologists with clinical training, as a case in point, are burdened with the duty to protect third parties in Tarasoff-type situations in which threats of violence are made against third parties by clients (and perhaps research subjects; Appelbaum & Rosenbaum, 1989).

Despite this precedent, we simply do not see the training of the researcher as an ethically relevant consideration in a discussion of the rights of research participants and of others potentially affected by a research project. All participants should have the same basic rights simply by virtue of their being in a study. Appropriate ethical safeguards should be determined by the nature of the information being collected and not by what can be reasonably expected given the researcher's level of training and licensure. Doing otherwise would be to place an undue burden on research participants to be familiar with the educational history of the researchers they deal with and to understand how that history affects the level of protection that they can expect.

Our position on intervention contingency planning is predicated on the presupposition that research participants have the right to expect treatment or at least treatment referrals should they supply information to an investigator indicating that they are potentially in need of services. Although this presupposition may not be popular among research scientists, it is difficult to defend, on ethical grounds, turning a blind eye toward information that a person is potentially in psychological distress simply because the information was gathered in a research rather than a treatment setting. If a research physician involved in a medical study of bone fracture healing finds evidence on a routine x-ray taken as part of a screening exam that one of the study participants has a potentially cancerous lesion, one would hope that the physician would follow up with that participant even if it required breaking the subject number code in order to obtain that participant's name and even though the participant was not the physician's patient and even though the physician was an orthopedist and not an oncologist. There is no reason why the moral expectations should be any different when the potential problem is depression, alcohol abuse, or excessive anxiety and the primary investigator happens to be a developmental psychologist or a sociologist.

Our call for data monitoring and intervention planning also raises the issue of the ethical status of research in which participants are truly anonymous, i.e. research in which even the primary investigator does not possess the information to crack the code required to match a protocol with a name. Such research, of course, makes following up with potentially troubled or at-risk participants impossible. But because of the problem of socially desirable responding and the difficulty of getting people to discuss openly highly personal and inflammatory topics such as their AIDS status or criminal behavior, research in which participants have total anonymity (even from the research team) is sometimes necessary to increase the likelihood of collecting accurate information. To help prevent participants from expecting intervention, or from misinterpreting a lack of intervention, should they reveal clinically significant symptomatology or warning signs, the investigator's inability to respond to the data provided by individual subjects needs to be made explicit during the consent procedure. As an added safeguard, participants in anonymous studies could be invited to discuss with the investigator any concerns they may have about their well-being that arise in the course of their study participation. Concerned people who come forward could than be offered, perhaps at the completion of the study, appropriate referrals to counseling organizations. Because these recommendations are ameliorative of only some of the ethical problems associated with anonymous research, anonymous techniques should be used only when the investigator considers them vital to the collection of valid and meaningful data.

Collecting Data About Third Parties

A feature truly unique to self-report methodology is that it easily allows for the collection of information about third parties who are not present and who have not given their consent to be in the research being conducted. This information may be as simple and benign as inquiries into the professions of subjects' parents, information often used as a rough determinant of family socioeconomic status, or as potentially intrusive as the punishment practices of parents, the sexual history of subjects' partners, or the history of mental illness in subjects' families. What rights do these third parties have? If cousin Blabby agrees to be in a study, does that give the researcher the right to know anything about her family that Blabby is willing to reveal? Can cousin Blabby waive confidentiality rights regarding this information on behalf of her family members (see Bersoff & Hofer, 1990, for a discussion of the rights of parents to waive the privacy rights of their children without their consent)? This is not a situation that can be addressed simply with a new clause in the standard consent form because the person whose consent is truly required is not present.

There are three options for dealing with this problem. The first is to disallow questions regarding third parties who have not personally consented to participate in a given research study. In this regard, it is appropriate, albeit sometimes difficult, to differentiate questions that solicit facts about a third party (e.g., "Has your wife ever been unfaithful?" or "Does your best friend use illegal drugs?") from questions that solicit a participant's personal feelings about a third party (e.g., "Do you love your wife?" or "Is your best friend a good influence on you?"). Only the former type of probe entails privacy issues vis-à-vis the third party and would consequently require third party consent. The latter probes yield information more about the participant's own attitudes and opinions than about the third party as an individual and thus are covered by the participant's consent. This is the most ethically conservative alternative. Another option would be to restrict the allowable questions regarding third parties. Requiring informed consent, for example, before allowing a researcher to ask a husband about his spouse's occupation or age could be considered a bit extreme. Thus, just as IRBs act as surrogates for the interests of participants in deception experiments, perhaps they can also decide what kinds of inquiries are likely to unduly harm or compromise the privacy rights of a third party. Probes considered to represent unacceptable privacy violations would be disallowed. A third option would be to allow things to continue as they are but, at a minimum, to make clear the rights of third parties. The 1992 APA ethical guidelines germane to the performance of research, for example, do not discuss third parties as distinct entities. Are they equivalent to regular research participants in that they are entitled to be informed when data about them have been collected, to be debriefed, and to receive a copy of the study results? Do investigators have an obligation to protect the confidentiality of third parties as they do that of their primary research participants?

Of course these alternatives are not entirely orthogonal. In fact, our position encompasses aspects of all three. Specifically, we believe that researchers and IRBs should screen self-report measures for probes that could unduly harm or compromise the privacy rights of third parties. If a researcher chooses to include such questions, he or she should then be required to secure informed consent from the potentially affected people. At that point, these third parties essentially become subjects in the study, with all of the entitlements associated with that status. Although certain types of research may be more difficult to pursue under these conditions, especially that which would require someone to agree to be discussed in an unflattering context, that is not a sufficient reason to ignore the privacy rights of third parties.

THE COSTS OF STRICTER ETHICAL STANDARDS

It would be naive to think that the more stringent ethical protections suggested here for self-report research will not result in extra costs in terms of time, resources, and even the ability to address specific research questions. Because most ethical decision making is based on a costs–benefits analysis, such liabilities need to be aired in the context of any discussion of ethical regulation (Gergen, 1973).

Several studies have been done looking at the effects of informed consent and confidentiality assurances on survey responding and participation (see, e.g., Singer, 1978a, 1978b; Singer & Frankel, 1982). It was found that compared to a telegraphic description of a survey's contents and no information at all about the purpose of the interview, a full disclosure of the contents and purpose of surveys containing sensitive questions (e.g., sexual and drug use related) did not significantly affect the participation rate in studies nor the nonresponse rate to sensitive items within surveys (Singer & Frankel, 1982). This led the authors to conclude that "researchers do not pay a price by giving respondents more information ahead of time" (p. 421). Where there does seem to be a price to be paid, however, is in promises of confidentiality. In a study by Singer (1978b), respondents were told either (a) nothing at all about the confidentiality of their replies, (b) that their replies would be absolutely confidential, or (c) that the researchers would do their best to protect the confidentiality of their answers, except when disclosure was required by law. Those given an absolute assurance of confidentiality were significantly more likely to answer sensitive questions than those given a qualified assurance or no assurance at all (Singer, 1978b). Because we are advocating a more detailed explication of confidentiality limits than even the qualified assurance used in the Singer study, the result is likely to be that certain sensitive information will be more difficult to get and/or that people will be more likely to lie (Singer & Frankel, 1982). Simply put, once they are fully informed of the disclosure risks, more participants may decline to volunteer certain information.

There are remedies available, however, to this potential problem. In particular, it is possible to obtain a certificate of confidentiality from the Secretary of the U.S. Department of Health and Human Services to protect the privacy and identity of research participants (Hoagwood, 1994). Such a certificate provides the investigator with legal protection against being compelled to disclose personal, identifiable information about research participants, including possible exemption from state and local reporting requirements (Hoagwood, 1994). It also assures research participants that identifying information that they provide during a study is protected from disclosure. Such a certificate can allow researchers to study sensitive topics such as sexual practices, drug abuse, and illegal conduct with less fear of losing potential participants due to confidentiality concerns.

It should be noted, however, that the protection offered by these certificates has never been tested in court; and that in research involving minors, these certificates do not protect children against the disclosure of information to their parents (Hoagwood, 1994). This caveat, however, may not necessarily be problematic. When adolescents were asked about the importance of confidentiality over the need to intervene when children are at risk, most of the respondents felt that in cases involving what they perceived to be seriously dangerous behavior, attending to the needs of the child was more important than honoring confidentiality promises (Fisher, Higgins-D'Alessandro, Rau, Kuther, & Belanger, 1996). If adolescents actually approve of and expect intervention when information about severe problems comes to light, there might not be a large chilling effect on their participation in research resulting from a full disclosure of the fact that their parents or guardians may be informed if they reveal certain information.

There also seems to be a price to pay for having contingency plans in place in case at-risk participants are identified during a research investigation. In one study (Stanton, Burker, & Kershaw, 1991), undergraduates' responses on a depression measure were examined to see if they changed as a function of the level of follow-up students could expect to receive if they manifested depressive symptoms. The manipulation information was communicated via the consent form. The results indicated that subjects who potentially could receive the most intrusive intervention, that is, experimenter contact with the subject and a significant other, were less likely to report depressive symptoms than were subjects who were led to anticipate a less intrusive potential follow-up (Stanton, Burker, & Kershaw, 1991). This cost of ethical practice may be reduced, however, by having intervention contingencies in place, but allowing people to self-refer. Participants could be given the choice of treatment, of referral to an appropriate professional or agency, or of refusing all follow-up intervention.

The price of acknowledging the rights of third parties can only be speculated on, as we could not find any research on this matter. The implications seem rather straightforward, however. The more stringent the requirements are regarding what can and cannot be asked without third party consent, the more difficult it will be to do certain types of research from a practical standpoint. Where, exactly, the line should be drawn is a matter requiring debate.

Ultimately, all of the costs just discussed manifest themselves in a single, ethically relevant consideration: what the final sample of a study will look like if the greater protections suggested here are implemented in some form. This is not to deny that there would also be consequences in terms of greater expenditures of time, effort, and money to collect certain types of data, but these costs are not generally recognized as legitimate reasons to circumscribe the rights of research participants. In addition, the fact that more stringent ethical precautions might lead to a greater refusal rate among potential respondents is not problematic from a psychometric point of view in and of itself. A problem will exist only if the potential participants in the refuse group differ in some systematic and psychologically important way from those who still consent after the suggested procedures are instituted. Such a group difference would mean that the generalizability of the research would be compromised. This is not a trivial or even an entirely scientific concern, as social science data are often used in making social policy decisions and to evaluate the efficacy of social and educational programs. Such decisions and evaluations will be unsound or meaningless if they are not based on data that faithfully reflect the attitudes and behaviors of the relevant populations likely to be affected by those policies and programs. These considerations do carry moral weight and may legitimate some degree of compromise regarding the protection of subjects' rights.

Unfortunately, generalizability problems due to volunteer bias already occur even without the onus of the additional ethical protections being advocated. In sexuality research, for example, people who volunteer to participate in studies involving explicit sexual content tend to report a more positive attitude toward sexuality, less sexual guilt, and more sexual experiences than nonvolunteers (Strassberg & Lowe, 1995). Clearly, the validity of the results, for the population as a whole, of sexuality research involving explicit content must be questioned given the characteristics of the typical subject sample. Research into other sensitive areas is also likely to be prone to volunteer bias, a bias that may become more pronounced if consent forms become more detailed and explicit about survey content and about the limits of confidentiality.

Although the ethical concerns raised here possess a certain *prima facie* validity and importance, their resolutions are not as readily apparent. In fact, we believe that the specifics of their proper resolutions are, to a significant extent, an empirical matter. Although ethics is not usually considered to be an empirically driven field of endeavor, we believe that solutions to ethical problems should be informed by data (Gergen, 1973). This is in large part because of the cost–benefit analysis that comprises most moral decision making. Whereas rights do not generally require empirical legitimation, costs can often be empirical matters. The costs that the ethical safeguards suggested here would engender only become ethically meaningful liabilities at the point where these safeguards result in study samples that no longer allow researchers to generalize their results to the relevant populations being studied. Hard data would give some indication of the point at which our recommendations start significantly to bias research samples. The cost-benefit debate would then revolve around a discussion of how much generalizability social scientists and consumers of social science data are willing to sacrifice in deference to the rights of research participants to fidelity, justice, autonomy, and beneficence. But until these data are generated, we believe that, at a minimum, self-report, survey-based data collection should receive ethical scrutiny at least as critical as that accorded to deception and manipulation research.

ACKNOWLEDGMENTS

This chapter was written under the auspices of the Diogenes Project. We would like to thank Carol Ripple and three anonymous reviewers for their helpful comments on an earlier draft of this manuscript.

REFERENCES

Abramovitch, R., Freedman, J. L., Henry, K., & Brunschot, M. V. (1995). Children's capacity to agree to psychological research: Knowledge of risks and benefits and voluntariness. *Ethics & Behavior, 5*(1), 25–48.

American Psychological Association. (1992). Ethical principles and code of conduct. *American Psychologist, 47*, 1597–1611.

Appelbaum, P. S., & Rosenbaum, A. (1989). *Tarasoff* and the researcher: Does the duty to protect apply in the research setting? *American Psychologist, 44*, 885–894.

Bersoff, D. N., & Hofer, P. T. (1990). The legal regulation of school psychology. In C. R. Reynolds & T. B. Gutkin (Eds.), *Handbook of school psychology* (2nd ed.; pp. 939–963). New York: Wiley.

Bersoff, D. N., & Koeppl, P. M. (1993). The relation between ethical codes and moral principles. *Ethics and Behavior, 3*, 345–357.

Burbach, D. J., Farha, J. G., & Thorpe, J. S. (1986). Assessing depression in community samples of children using self-report inventories: Ethical considerations. *Journal of Abnormal Child Psychology, 14*, 579–589.

Cialdini, R. B. (1993). *Influence: The psychology of persuasion*. New York: Morrow.

Fisher, C. B. (1994). Reporting and referring research participants: Ethical challenges for investigators studying children and youth. *Ethics & Behavior, 4(2)*, 87–95.

Fisher, C. B., Higgins-D'Alessandro, A., Rau, J. B., Kuther, T. L., & Belanger, S. (1996). Referring and reporting research participants at risk: Views from urban adolescents. *Child Development, 67*, 2086–2100.

Freedman, J. L., & Fraser, S. C. (1966). Compliance without pressure: The foot-in-the-door technique. *Journal of Personality and Social Psychology, 4*, 195–202.

Gergen, K. J. (1973). The codification of research ethics: Views of a Doubting Thomas. *American Psychologist, 28*, 907–912.

Hoagwood, K. (1994). The certificate of confidentiality at the National Institute of Mental Health: Discretionary considerations in its applicability in research on child and adolescent mental disorders. *Ethics & Behavior, 4(2)*, 123–131.

Holmes, D. S. (1976). Debriefing after psychological experiments. I. Effectiveness of postdeception dehoaxing. *American Psychologist, 31*, 858–867.

Koocher, G. P., & Keith-Spiegel, P. C. (1990). *Children, ethics and the law*. Lincoln: University of Nebraska Press.

La Greca, A. M. (Ed.). (1990). *Through the eyes of the child: Obtaining self-reports from children and adolescents*. Boston: Allyn and Bacon.

Liss, M. B. (1994). Child abuse: Is there a mandate for researchers to report? *Ethics & Behavior, 4(2)*, 133–146.

Milgram, S. (1974). *Obedience to authority*. New York: Harper & Row.

Orne, M. T. (1962). On the social psychology of the psychological experiment: With particular reference to demand characteristics and their implications. *American Psychologist, 17*, 776–783.

Sabini, J. (1995). *Social psychology* (2nd ed.). New York: Norton.

Scarr, S. (1990). Ethical dilemmas in recent research: A personal saga. In C. B. Fisher & W. W. Tryon (Eds.), *Ethics in applied developmental psychology: Emerging issues in an emerging field* (pp. 29–42). Norwood, NJ: Ablex.

Scott-Jones, D. (1994). Ethical issues in reporting and referring in research with low-income minority children. *Ethics & Behavior, 4(2)*, 97–108.

Singer, E. (1978a). The effect of informed consent procedure on respondents' reactions to surveys. *Journal of Consumer Research, 5*, 49–57.

Singer, E. (1978b, April). Informed consent: Consequences for response rate and response quality in social surveys. *American Sociological Review, 43*, 144–162.

Singer, E., & Frankel, M. R. (1982, June). Informed consent procedures in telephone interviews. *American Sociological Review, 47*, 416–427.

Society for Research in Child Development. (1990–1991). Ethical standards for research with children. *Directory of the Society for Research in Child Development*, 337–339.

Stanton, A. L., Burker, E. J., & Kershaw, D. (1991). Effects of researcher follow-up of distressed subjects: Tradeoff between validity and ethical responsibility? *Ethics & Behavior, 1(2)*, 105–112.

Strassberg, D. S., & Lowe, K. (1995). Volunteer bias in sexuality research. *Archives of Sexual Behavior, 24(4)*, 369–382.

U.S. Department of Health and Human Services. (1991, August). Title 45 Public Welfare, Part 46, *Code of Federal Regulations, Protection of Human Subjects*. Subpart A Federal Policy for the Protection of Human Subjects 56 FR 28003.

II

COGNITIVE PROCESSES
IN SELF-REPORT

Jared B. Jobe
National Institute on Aging

When a respondent answers a question about his or her health care visits, past diet, or health history, the interviewer (survey researcher, epidemiologist, and health care professional) usually assumes that the information reported is accurate. This information about the respondent is usually about his or her own experiences; this information is stored in a system called autobiographical memory. According to researchers (e.g., Tourangeau, 1984), for a respondent to provide accurate information, the respondent must, at a minimum, comprehend the question being asked, recall information from memory, make decisions about the accuracy of the information recalled, and format an answer (for a review of respondent models, see Jobe & Herrmann, 1996). Errors are possible at each of these tasks.

Self-report questions used in surveys, epidemiologic studies, and health care interviews can pose considerable autobiographical memory challenges for respondents. Many questions ask about the frequencies with which certain events occurred within a reference period: How many health care visits were made, how many times certain foods were eaten, and so forth. These items require that respondents remember whether relevant events occurred, how often, and when each event took place. The accuracy of the responses to these questions is important for public health, in as much as self-report data are used to determine the relationship between behaviors and disease. For example, the accuracy of self-reports of past diet are used by nutritional epidemiologists to understand the relationship between dietary fat and certain cancers.

Moreover, many variables affect the accuracy of the kind of autobiographical events that are the foci of surveys, epidemiologic studies, and interviews with health care professionals. Some of these variables include recall strategies, instructions, mood, time elapsed since the target event, and response formats (for reviews, see Jobe, Tourangeau, & Smith, 1993; Sudman, Bradburn, & Schwarz, 1995). Although some research on these variables has been conducted since the 1940s, research in the survey arena did not begin in earnest until the mid-to-late 1980s following a series of conferences in the United States, Germany, and England (see Jobe & Mingay, 1991 for a history of this enterprise). Interest by epidemiologists has been more recent (see e.g., Friedenreich, 1994).

Although cognitive laboratory research methods, theories, and findings are very relevant to self-report data obtained in surveys and other settings, there are several important distinctions between the reporting conditions of a survey, epidemiologic, or health care interview and those of cognitive laboratory research.

First, the time period between the acquisition of the information and the reporting of it is typically much longer in interviews than in laboratory studies. The reference period of self-report questions is often the last 2 weeks, the last month, the last quarter, or even the last year. Only recently has cognitive psychology begun to investigate retrieval over such long intervals.

Second, the retrieval cues provided by self-report questions to respondents are often poorly defined compared to those used in laboratory studies. In laboratory research on memory, the experimenter presents the to-be-recalled information and thus can present specific cues to prompt recall. Interviewers will not have been present at the events about which they ask and can provide only general cues.

Third, self-reports are based typically on incidental, rather than intentional, learning. The respondent is unaware that events such as dietary intake or prior health care visits will have to be reported. Thus, the target events likely have not been encoded for subsequent reporting. However, in the laboratory, the nature of learning may be controlled.

Finally, self-report interviews often focus on recurring events that may blend together in memory and be especially difficult to report individually. Generally, such events have not been the focus of much laboratory research.

The chapters in this section concern several of the most critical aspects of the cognitive factors underlying self-reports: Remembering what events occurred, remembering when the events occurred, reporting the frequency with which events occurred, and the influence of emotion on remembering. Roger Tourangeau's chapter 3 describes the critical role that memory plays in the ability of respondents to accurately report autobiographical information. He describes models of autobiographical memory including key processes such as: encoding what occurred, storage of the memory of the event, retrieving the event from memory, and reconstructing the event. He then describes the memory aids that have been developed to facilitate the memory processes at each of these four stages of memory.

In chapter 4, Norman Bradburn describes the important role of event dating in self-reports. The accuracy of event dating is critical to many epidemiologic studies and surveys in order for researchers to determine whether an event occurred during a particular reference period. However, as Bradburn states, calendar time is not a good retrieval cue and most events are not encoded with their calendar dates. He describes features of memory that relate to time, how time is represented in memory, and how dates are retrieved from memory. Finally, he describes eight generalizations about the accuracy of dating events.

In chapter 5 of this section, Geeta Menon and Eric Yorkston describe another important cognitive process in self-reports: the accuracy of reporting the frequency with which people engage in behaviors, such as how many times per week green beans were eaten in the past month or year. They describe the two sources of information that respondents use to make frequency judgments: memory-based information and context-based information. They then describe the different methods used to report frequencies and rates of occurrence, such as recall and count and estimation strategies. They describe the variables that affect the accuracy of frequency reports such as the actual frequency of occurrence and the regularity of the behavior. They make recommendations about ways to improve the accuracy of frequency reports, including the manipulation of context. All of these factors are tied together in an integrative theory of frequency reports.

Chapter 6, by John F. Kihlstrom, Eric Eich, Deborah Sandbrand, and Betsy A. Tobias, describes an important relationship often overlooked by cognitive researchers: the relationship between mood and memory. They begin by discussing the effects of the emotional valence of the to-be-recalled information and the retrieval cues. The next topic is equally important: the affective state of the respondent at the time of encoding and retrieval. Finally, they discuss the practical issues of the possible emotional distortion of memory from anxiety and depression. This is especially relevant to early childhood retrospective reports. Their chapter indicates the dangers of relying too heavily on early childhood memory in clinical situations.

REFERENCES

Friedenreich, C. M. (1994). Improving long-term recall in epidemiologic studies. *Epidemiology*, 5, 1–4.

Jobe, J. B., & Herrmann, D. J. (1996). Implications of models of survey cognition for memory theory. In D. Herrmann, M. Johnson, C. McEvoy, C. Hertzog, & P. Hertel (Eds.), *Basic and applied memory: Research on practical aspects of memory* (pp. 193–205). Hillsdale, NJ: Lawrence Erlbaum Associates.

Jobe, J. B., & Mingay, D. J. (1991). Cognition and survey measurement: History and overview. *Applied Cognitive Psychology, 5*, 175–192.

Jobe, J. B., Tourangeau, R., & Smith, A. F. (1993). Contributions of survey research to the understanding of memory. *Applied Cognitive Psychology, 7*, 567–584.

Tourangeau, R. (1984). Cognitive sciences and survey methods. In T. B. Jabine, M. L. Straf, J. M. Tanur, & R. Tourangeau (Eds.), *Cognitive aspects of survey methodology: Building a bridge between disciplines* (pp. 73–101). Washington, DC: National Academy Press.

Sudman, S., Bradburn, N., & Schwarz, N. (1995). *Thinking about answers: The application of cognitive processes to survey methodology.* San Francisco: Jossey-Bass.

3

Remembering What Happened: Memory Errors and Survey Reports

Roger Tourangeau
The Gallup Organization, Rockville, MD

A central tool of social science research—perhaps *the* central tool—is asking people questions about what happened. Because of the critical role of retrospective reports, a major source of error in social science data is memory error. This chapter presents a brief overview of memory and its contribution to error in self-reports. It begins by examining models of autobiographical memory and then explores the processes responsible for forgetting and other memory errors.

AUTOBIOGRAPHICAL MEMORY

Perhaps the most elementary question we can ask about memory is what gets remembered. What sort of thing do we store in memory? It is immediately apparent that are at least three distinct types of material in memory— facts culled from books or oral descriptions, personal experiences, and knowledge about how to do things. What most of us think of as memory consists largely of memories for personal experiences, and it is this sort of memory—autobiographical memory—that is usually at issue when we gather self-report data. There is general agreement that the basic format in which events or personal experiences are encoded is that of the story. We experience our lives as organized around actors who have intentions and carry out plans that succeed or fail; these mini-narratives are the stuff of which autobiographical memory is composed.

Memory Structure

If the unit of autobiographical memory is the experience or event, then the next issue is how they are represented and structured. There are two basic models of the structure of autobiographical memory. According to one, memories form an associative network (e.g., Anderson, 1983; see Collins & Quillian, 1969, for an early version); according to the other, memories form a hierarchy (Barsalou, 1988; Kolodner, 1985). Network models represent concepts or ideas as nodes in the network, and the relationship between concepts as links. These links reflect basic semantic relations between concepts such as the subset–superset relation. Network models typically assume that we search memory by tracing the links between concepts. Retrieval is the process of activating a concept—bringing it to consciousness—and activation is thought to spread from one concept to another along the links of the memory network.

According to the hierarchical model of memory, similar events are organized into categories. The categories may encompass both subtypes and individual experiences. For example, in Kolodner's (1985) hierarchical model, the category-level representations are called event memory organization packages (EMOPs, for short). New EMOPs are formed when a sufficient number of memories—several events of the same type—are stored under an existing EMOP. Memory search begins with the relevant category (the EMOP) and proceeds downward as indices (distinguishing particulars) are generated that define ever finer categories until individual experiences are found. The Kolodner model is an example of a schema-plus-tag theory, in which memories are seen as consisting of a general pattern stored at the category level (the schema) plus one or more individuating details (the tags). The general pattern for a class of events (say, doctor visits) might include information about the usual participants (doctors, nurses, patients, receptionists, and so on), the typical location (the doctor's office or HMO), the larger sequence to which the event might be linked (the treatment of a chronic condition), the superordinate category to which this one belongs, and the subcategories of this class of experiences (visits to different types of doctors).

These ideas—that a memory for an experience includes both generic and unique information, that retrieval encompasses both automatic and controlled processes (e.g., spreading activation and the generation of retrieval cues), and that memory search consists of generating progressively more specific cues—are widely shared, even by memory researchers who do not subscribe to other assumptions of the Anderson or Kolodner models.

Sources of Forgetting

Within this framework, we can distinguish at least four major classes of memory problems. The first involves encoding. We may never form a representation of an event in the first place or the representation that we do form may be so sketchy as to render retrieval difficult or impossible. When there are serious encoding problems, little or no information ever reaches long-term memory. A second class of problems involves errors introduced *after* the original encoding; things that happen after the original experience can be woven into the representation of the experience and distort our memory of it. Another class of memory problems involves retrieval failure. We may have encoded the experience adequately in the first place and have preserved this representation intact, but when it is time to recall the event, we may simply be unable to remember it. A final class of errors involves reconstruction. When we fill in details missing from the memory, based on our general knowledge of a class of events or our expectations about change over time, we may introduce inaccuracies. In some cases, retrospective reports are not based on specific recollections at all, but represent estimates or other types of inferences (Bradburn, Rips, & Shevell, 1987; Burton & Blair, 1991; Menon & Yorkston, chapter 5, this volume).

ENCODING PROBLEMS

The most extreme encoding problems involve cases in which the relevant information is never noticed in the first place and so never enters memory, but there can be less extreme encoding problems as well. To the extent that the initial encoding of the information is superficial, the information will be hard to remember later on. The principle that deeper encoding leads to better recall was initially established for passages of text (Craik & Lockhart, 1972); subjects remembered a passage better when their task required them to process it deeply (e.g., to summarize the passage) than when it required them to process it only superficially (to count the number of words in it). Later work suggests that the more elaborated the initial representation, the more likely the experience can be retrieved later on (Anderson & Reder, 1978). According to a network model, elaborative encoding establishes multiple links to the experience, each of which can serve as a path for retrieving it; similarly, in a hierarchical model, elaborative encoding produces multiple indices that can be used to search memory for the experience.

Aside from the problems resulting from insufficient or superficial encoding of an experience, the initial representation of an event can give rise to a second type of memory problem—it may fail to match the retrieval cue provided later on (Tulving & Thomson, 1973). When the experience is stored in one category (or EMOP) but the retrieval cue triggers the search of a different one, we are unlikely to recall the experience. In fact, as Tulving and Thomson demonstrated, if the retrieval cue makes us think of the wrong category, we may not even recognize the relevant experience.

We recently carried out a study in which encoding problems appeared to be the main culprit in producing reporting errors in a survey (Brittingham, Lee, Tourangeau, & Willis, in press). The study examined parents' reports about their children's vaccinations. Two national surveys monitor rates of vaccination coverage among children. Both surveys ask parents about their children's vaccinations, encouraging them to consult the "shot cards" that many pediatricians provide; these cards record information about each vaccination the child has received. Unfortunately, many parents do not have the cards and are forced to rely on unaided recall instead. Such reports are known to be error-prone (e.g., Goldstein, Kviz, & Daum, 1993). Our study investigated whether parents take in the information about which shots their children got in the first place. Parents may dutifully take their children for their scheduled shots without paying too much attention to which ones were administered on any specific occasion.

We interviewed a sample of parents as they were leaving an HMO, just after their child had received one or more vaccinations. The questionnaire asked parents to describe what happened during the visit and probed them specifically about any immunizations the child received. Table 3.1 shows the main results from the study, displaying several measures of the accuracy of the parents' reports. The results can be summarized very simply: Even as the parents were leaving the doctor's office, their reports were close to chance levels of accuracy. The overall correlations between the reports and the records were significant for only three of the five immunizations and

TABLE 3.1
Immunization Study Results

	Accuracy Measure			
Vaccine	False Negative Rate	False Positive Rate	Phi	Net Bias
Hepatitis B	51.7%	20.0%	.20	−41.4
	(60)	(10)	(70)	(70)
DTP (Diphtheria-Tetanus-Pertussis)	41.4%	16.7%	.32*	−31.4
	(58)	(12)	(70)	(70)
Polio	33.9%	14.3%	.42*	−24.3
	(56)	(14)	(70)	(70)
Hib (Haemophilus Influenzae b)	86.5%	0.0%	.20	−64.3
	(52)	(18)	(70)	(70)
MMR (Mumps-Measles-Rubella)	33.3%	19.4%	.23*	17.1
	(3)	(67)	(70)	(70)

Note. Parenthetical entries are cell sizes; asterisks indicate a *phi* correlation significant at $p < .05$. The false negative rate is the percentage of parents who failed to report a vaccination the child received that day. The false positive rate is percentage who reported a vaccination the child had not received that day. *Phi* is the overall correlation between the parent's report and the clinic's records about whether the child had received a given vaccine. Net bias refers to the difference between the percentage of parents reporting the vaccination and the percentage of children actually receiving it.

Source: Brittingham et al. (in press).

these three correlations were none too impressive. We also conducted a follow-up interview with parents 10 weeks later. Performance after 10 weeks was not much worse than it was after a few minutes. If they took in the information at all, the parents were, for most part, able remember it over the 10-week interval.

Why was accuracy so low? As a general rule, the depth and elaboration of the encoding of an event reflects such variables as its distinctiveness, emotional impact, and duration. Unusual or dramatic events, or those that unfold over a long period of time, tend to grab our attention and hold it long enough to ensure that a rich representation is created and stored in long-term memory. Childhood vaccinations have none of these characteristics; to the contrary, they are frequent, routine, and quick. When we did our study, children were supposed to have received at least 14 doses of five different vaccines by their second birthday. (Since then, a sixth vaccine has been added to the recommended list.) The long and technical names of the vaccines (Haemophilus influenzae b), the relative unfamiliarity of the illnesses they prevent, and the administration of multiple vaccines during a single visit may also inhibit accurate encoding.

So, one potential source of error in retrospective reports is that the respondent never really knew the answer in the first place. We may fail to encode enough information to produce an accurate account of the experience later—even when later is only a few minutes after the event took place.

STORAGE PROBLEMS: THE INCORPORATION OF POST-EVENT INFORMATION

A second class of memory problems arises after the initial encoding of the event; it involves what happens to the memory while it is being stored in long-term memory. Rehearsal—time spent thinking or talking about the event—is thought to play a key role in maintaining the accessibility of a memory. Take flashbulb memories as an example. These are the peculiarly vivid memories left by events like the assassination of President Kennedy or the explosion of the space shuttle *Challenger* (Brown & Kulik, 1977; see also Conway, 1995). The literature on such memories singles out two major groups of variables believed to affect their level of detail—the amount of rehearsal and the degree of surprise or other emotion initially engendered by the event (e.g., Pillemer, 1984; Rubin & Kozin, 1984; Winograd & Killinger, 1983). The level of emotional impact probably affects the elaboration of the encoding of the experience, but rehearsal probably affects its long-term accessibility to retrieval. Although some studies of flashbulb memories indicate that the importance of rehearsal may have been overstated, the consensus is that rehearsal plays a key role in maintaining detailed and vivid memories over long spans of time.

Of course, as Neisser and Harsch (1992) demonstrated, the presence of a detailed memory is no guarantee of its accuracy. In fact, the process of recounting an event may not only preserve the memory but add details to it, often inaccurate ones (e.g., Loftus & Kaufman, 1992). Our recollection of an experience may change every time we recount it. Details of the event may be elaborated or abbreviated depending on the context in which the event is described, and any errors introduced in the telling may become part of the memory for the event. Rehearsal may produce greater error when the memory is vague or nonexistent to begin with. Perhaps no researcher has demonstrated the difficulties we face in distinguishing what we actually experienced from what we heard, thought, or learned later on than Loftus (see chapter 12, this volume). These difficulties derive from our tendency to incorporate "postevent" information into our representation of the event without distinguishing its source. What we experienced firsthand may differ in vividness or detail from what we said or heard later on, but the differences between the two types of information may fade as time passes.

The same mechanisms that account for the distorting effects of postevent information (including self-generated postevent information) may also explain another common type of memory error—reporting something that did not happen. In studies of memory, such errors are referred to as false alarms or intrusion errors. Once again, the problem is in distinguishing what actually happened from what sounds good, seems to fit, or was merely imagined. These reporting errors are all the more likely when memories for what did occur are indistinct, reducing the difference between events that were actually experienced and those that were merely heard about or imagined. Two studies reported by Johnson, Foley, Suengas, and Raye (1988) illustrate these problems; the studies found very few differences between subjects' memories for actual childhood events and their memories for dreams and fantasies from childhood. By contrast, there were many differences between memories for actual and imagined adult experiences. By adding detail and increasing the apparent familiarity of an event, repeated rehearsal or visualization can further reduce the difference between memories for actual and imagined events.

Three factors affect whether a memory is accepted as genuine (i.e., based on an actual experience rather than a fantasy or secondhand report)—the qualities of the memory itself, its overall plausibility, and the strictness of the standard used in judging the memory's genuineness.

The Qualities of the Memory

Memories seen as arising from direct experience differ from those seen as originating in other sources (e.g., reading or imagination) in several ways. Memories judged to be based on direct experience include more perceptual detail than those thought to be derived from other sources (Johnson, Hashtroudi, & Lindsay, 1993); similarly, results from the flashbulb memory literature suggest that the vividness of the memory (presumably reflecting the presence of perceptual details) is related to confidence in the accuracy of the memory (Neisser & Harsch, 1992). Memories judged to be based on actual experience are also more likely to include peripheral details of the event and less likely to include information about cognitive processes (Johnson et al., 1993; Schooler, Gerhard, & Loftus, 1986). A final variable that may affect judgments about the source of a memory is the ease of retrieving it (Jacoby, Kelley, & Dywan, 1989). Unfortunately, none of these variables are infallible guides to the source of a memory. Repeated rehearsal can affect ease of retrieval; visualization can add perceptual detail. Techniques used to make recall easier may simultaneously make it harder to distinguish real from imagined incidents (cf. Lindsay & Read, 1994).

Relative Plausibility

At least some of the time, judgments about the accuracy of a memory reflect information beyond that contained in the memory itself. The presence of conflicting (or corroborating) evidence clearly affects judgments about whether a memory is genuine. For example, the literature on eyewitness accuracy indicates that delay between the event and the recall attempt can affect the acceptance of misleading postevent information (Lindsay, 1990; Loftus & Hoffman, 1989), a finding that may reflect the diminished accessibility of conflicting information in memory derived from the original experience. Supporting evidence from other witnesses can also increase acceptance of false postevent information, even of information that implicates oneself as the guilty party (Kassin & Kiechel, 1996).

Decision Criteria

Some tasks may require only a relatively low threshold for deciding to accept a memory; others may demand a more careful sifting of the evidence. It is one thing to claim to recognize someone who seems to know us, quite another to identify a potential criminal in a lineup (cf. Lindsay & Johnson, 1989). External pressures (such as fatigue or social pressure) or characteristics of the person making the judgment (such as his or her youth or suggestibility) may bias the judgment as to whether the memory is real (Johnson, Kounios, & Reeder, 1994).

In short, memory is not judgment-free. What we retrieve from memory often consists of our current beliefs about an incident, beliefs that reflect what we actually experienced (and remember), what we did not experience but infer, and what we learned later on. The problem is that it can be difficult to distinguish between beliefs acquired through direct experience and those acquired through other means.

RETRIEVAL FAILURE

Retrieval failure is often cited as the most common source of forgetting. It occurs when information is stored in long-term memory but we are unable to get it out. Problems with retrieval loom large as a source of forgetting because it is clear that memory often contains far more information than we think it does. Unaided or free recall is likely to yield fewer memories than recall aided by retrieval cues or hints, and cued recall generally yields fewer memories than recognition. The more help we give the retrieval process, the more information it seems to turn up, including some things we thought were quite beyond its reach. In addition, since Ebbinghaus' (1885) initial explorations of the phenomenon, it has been known that even when we seem to have completely forgotten a topic, we often demonstrate savings in learning the material over again. Something has been retained in memory that makes it easier to acquire the information a second time than to learn it initially. Finally, even severely amnesic patients may show implicit memory; for example, they are more likely to complete a word missing one or more letters (HO_S_) with a word they had seen earlier (HORSE), even though they cannot recall the earlier word itself (Warrington & Weiskrantz, 1968). These patients stored *something* in memory even if it was beyond the reach of retrieval and could no longer be made conscious. (See Schacter, 1987, for a more thorough discussion of implicit memory). All of these findings suggest that a major source of forgetting is failure to retrieve information that is still there.

One of the most obvious facts about forgetting is its relation to the passage of time. No single variable seems to have such a profound impact on the accessibility of a memory than its age. Most theories of memory attribute this loss of accessibility over time to the interfering effects of later experiences. The problem is that the characteristics that made the experience unique initially are shared with later experiences; as a result, the original event may get lost among the similar events experienced afterwards. It is easy to recall our only trip to a doctor; it is far more difficult to pick out a particular trip when we have made dozens of similar ones.

Both the network and hierarchical models of the structure of long-term memory offer ready accounts for the interfering effects of later experiences. Both types of models assume that when similar events are experienced, a "generic" memory is formed, which leaves out the details of the individual incidents but records their overall pattern. These generic memories—EMOPs in Kolodner's model—explain why it so much easier to recall what usually happens than to recall the specific details that distinguish one incident of a given type from another (see also Means & Loftus, 1991; and Smith, Jobe, & Mingay, 1991).

According to the network model, multiple incidents of the same type (such as doctor visits) are likely to be linked to a single node (the node representing our concept of doctor visits). As we try to recall an individual event by thinking about the general concept, activation spreads along the links leading from that concept to the nodes representing individual experiences. Unfortunately, the more links leading away from the node where retrieval begins, the more that activation is dissipated across these links and the less likely that the memory we seek will receive enough activation to be retrieved (see Fig. 3.1). Anderson (1983) referred to this as the "fan effect." According to the hierarchical model, as we experience similar events, we form new subcategories (in the Kolodner model, new EMOPs) that capture finer distinctions among the events. The creation of these subcategories can impose an added burden on the retrieval process, requiring ever more detailed indices to be generated in order to locate the specific memory.

Retention Curves

The effects of the passage of time on recall accuracy have been demonstrated with almost every kind of event (e.g., Rubin & Wetzel, 1996). For example, a recent review of the survey literature found reduced levels of reporting or reduced reporting accuracy for hospital stays, health care visits, medical conditions, dietary intake, smoking, car accidents, hunting and

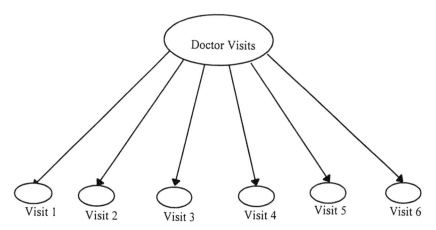

FIG. 3.1. Network representation of the general concept of doctor visits and of memories for individual visits. Activation may not reach the nodes representing the individual visits because of the large number of links leading away from the node for the general concept of doctor visits.

fishing trips, consumer purchases, and home repairs as the length of the retention interval increased (Jobe, Tourangeau, & Smith, 1993). Given the importance of these effects, it is hardly surprising that there have been a number of attempts to find the empirical function that best relates the amount of information retained in memory to the length of the retention interval. At least four functional forms have been proposed (Rubin & Wetzel, 1996).

Exponential Decay

Suppose we retain a fixed proportion of the information we learned originally over each unit of time that passes. For example, we may remember 90% of the items we purchased a month ago. After 2 months, we remember 81% of them (90% of 90%), and so on. If p denotes the fixed proportion retained each month, then after t months we will remember p^t. Under this model, the proportion retained (r) after t units of time have passed is:

$$r = ap^t$$
$$= ae^{bt}$$

in which a reflects the level of initial learning (the percent retained at time zero) and b is the natural logarithm of p (cf. Sudman & Bradburn, 1973). The parameter a is useful for situations (like the immunization study) in which the initial encoding of the memory is not perfect.

Hyperbolic Decay

If the factor responsible for the decline of memory over time is the accumulation of similar events, then a different functional form may capture the impact of the passage of time more accurately. Suppose events accumulate at a rate of b events per unit of time; for example, we might purchase three or four items during the average month. The proportion of events retained in memory over a time period of length t would be inversely related to the total number of similar events that occurred over that period:

$$r = \frac{1}{a + bt},$$

in which a again reflects performance at time zero.

Logarithmic Decay

A third functional form has been suggested, based on the idea that equal ratios of elapsed time should produce equal amounts of memory loss. As Rubin and Wetzel (1996) observed:

There is an easy way to arrive at the logarithmic function if in psychological terms equal ratios of time, not equal intervals, are important. Assume that the psychological difference between the 3 to 4 ratio of 3 and 4 seconds is the same psychological difference as that between 30 and 40 minutes, or 18 and 24 hr, or 3 and 4 decades ... The simplest function to describe retention is the linear function, $y = -m \cdot x + b$. If one uses the logarithm of time, as suggested by the equal ratios observation, instead of time for x, this equation becomes the logarithmic equation. (p. 749)

Expressing the logarithmic equation in the same format as the exponential and hyperbolic functions yields:

$$r = a - b \ln(t).$$

It is sometimes easier to work with $\ln(t + 1)$, which again makes a the level of initial performance.

Power Function

The final family of curves is based on the power function:

$$r = \frac{a}{(t+1)^b} \, .$$

(Again, $t + 1$ is used in the denominator instead of t for the sake of mathematical convenience.) This model implies equal ratios of retention with equal ratios of time (i.e., the ratio between the proportion retained at 5 and 10 years will be the same as the ratio between retention at 1 and 2 days). The power function has received some empirical support from work by Anderson and Schooler (1991), and Rubin and Wetzel's (1996) meta-analysis suggests that, of the four functions, it provides the best fit to the autobiographical memory data.

Still, all four functional forms share several basic predictions—that forgetting increases monotonically over time, but that it occurs rapidly at first and then slows down. In addition, it is not too difficult to find values for b so that the different models yield similar quantitative predictions. In Fig. 3.2, the value of a has been set to 1 for all four models (that is, performance is perfect at the outset) and values of b were found that yielded nearly identical predictions for Time 1. As the figure illustrates, the shape of the four curves is quite similar and the divergence among them is not very noticeable until a relatively long time has passed. It can, then, be quite difficult to distinguish the different models empirically (but see Bradburn et al., 1987, for a somewhat different view on this issue).

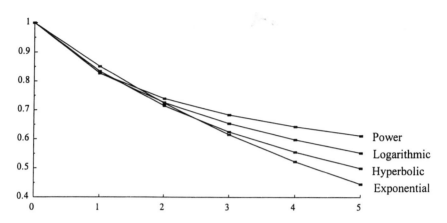

FIG. 3.2. Theoretical retention curves. The four curves demonstrate the similar shapes of the four functions when the key parameters are deliberately set to produce similar predictions.

Aiding Retrieval

Researchers have investigated a number of methods for improving recall. For example, it is apparent that simply taking more time to remember can help. Although there is doubtless some upper bound on this strategy, in one study (Williams & Hollan, 1981), subjects continued to recall new items even after nine previous sessions, each lasting an hour. Even a little extra time can produce benefits (Cannell, Miller, & Oksenberg, 1981).

Other methods thought to increase the amount of information retrieved include:

- Decomposition, a strategy that breaks a class of events down into subclasses, each of which is then recalled separately;
- Recalling events in reverse chronological order (that is, beginning with the most recent event and working backwards in time), a strategy that seems to help sometimes (Loftus & Fathi, 1985; Loftus, Smith, Klinger, & Fiedler, 1992) but not always (Jobe et al., 1990; Smith, 1991);
- Listing temporal boundaries or landmarks, such as major life transitions, to aid in the recall of events near those landmark events (Means & Loftus, 1991).

The decomposition strategy converts a free recall task into a cued recall task with the subclasses serving as additional retrieval cues. For example, it is probably easier to recall all of our doctor visits if we are cued to think about each of the major specialties. The findings about the usefulness of temporal boundaries (such as moving to a new city or starting a job) suggest that autobiographical memories are organized not only into categories based on the type of event, but also by periods in a person's life. Other results also indicate that we think of our lives as organized into major phases or chapters bounded by temporal landmarks—graduations, weddings, new jobs. Events near these landmarks seem to be remembered more easily than those occurring farther from the boundaries between periods (e.g., Robinson, 1986).

Number and Types of Cues

We do not remember every aspect of an event equally well. It is often difficult to remember names, and exact dates are notoriously difficult to remember. By contrast, we recognize faces quite readily. Several careful studies of autobiographical memory confirm these everyday observations. Perhaps the best of these is the monumental study by Wagenaar (1986), who recorded some 2,400 events from his daily life over the course of 6 years. Wagenaar noted what happened ("had dinner with friends"), who took part, and when and where the event took place. He tested his memory for each type of fact about the events later on. The results indicated that the different aspects of the events were not equally memorable. Regardless of the initial cue Wagenaar used to jog his memory, he had the most difficulty recalling the date of the event (to within a week of the actual date). On the other hand, there were no real differences among the levels of recall for the participants, activities, and locations of the events. In addition, the different aspects of the events were not equally effective as retrieval cues; information about the nature of the event was the best cue for retrieving other facts about the event and information about when an event occurred was the worst cue.

The effectiveness of a given type of cue will depend on several variables, including the nature of the memory task and the encoding of the event. If the task is to retrieve a particular event, then the best cue will be the one that most successfully distinguishes that event from similar events—given that the cue is consistent with the initial encoding of the event. In the extreme case, some representation of the event or information itself will be the best cue; it is, for example, far easier to recognize someone's name than to recall that name with the aid of some other cue. In Wagenaar's study, the description of what happened was probably the most effective at distinguishing the event in question; persons and places can be linked to many experiences and so are less helpful in picking out any specific one. Although time cues are potentially quite distinctive to the target event, it appears that we rarely encode our experiences with exact dates (see Bradburn, chapter 4, this volume); as a result, time cues do not help us very much. Different considerations apply when the task is to retrieve as many events as possible. In that case, cues linked to many incidents may have the advantage. Barsalou's (1988) results suggest that, with this task, locations may prompt the recall of more events than activities or times and that activities and times may outperform persons as retrieval cues.

RECONSTRUCTION ERRORS

As Wagenaar's (1986) results illustrate, retrieval often yields only partial results, turning up some details of an experience but not others. When this happens, we often attempt to fill in or reconstruct the missing pieces. Unfortunately, as Bartlett (1932) first demonstrated nearly 70 years ago, the details we add are not always an accurate representation of what actually happened.

A major source of the details added during this reconstruction process is our general knowledge about what is typical for events of a given type. Thus, the reconstructed event may deviate from the original in a systematic direction—that of resembling too closely the typical pattern for events of its type. Bartlett's subjects tended to drop particularly odd details from the Indian folk tales they were trying to remember and to add things that made the stories a little more sensible. In interpreting stories, we often supply the unstated connections between events (e.g., Bower, Black, & Turner, 1979); it seems clear that we do the same sort of filling in the gaps in memories for firsthand experiences as well. Because the details we add conform to the pattern for the situation, individual peculiarities are lost and the representation of the individual events comes to resemble the generic representation for events of that type. Inferences that fill in missing or implicit details may be made at the time of encoding, later on during subsequent rehearsal, or at the time of retrieval, but regardless of when they are made, the inferences are likely to be similar in content.

There may also be relatively subtle differences among the processes of generating retrieval cues that bring back memories of actual experiences, making reasonable inferences about details missing from partial memories, and imagining plausible scenarios that never really took place. In each case, we are likely to imagine what might have occurred based on our general knowledge. The result is sometimes an accurate recollection of a real experience, sometimes a plausible reconstruction of what might have occurred, and sometimes a complete fabrication. With distant or poorly recalled events, it may be difficult to tell these three situations apart.

Retrospective Biases

Numerous studies have examined situations in which respondents are asked to report on some personal characteristic—such as their views about an attitude issue—and then are asked at some later time to report both the current value of that characteristic and their earlier answers as well. The results often suggest that the current value is used as an anchor on which the "memory" of the past value is based. In an early demonstration, Bem and McConnell (1970) assessed subjects' attitudes, exposed them to a procedure that produced large changes in their attitudes, and then asked some of the subjects whose attitudes had changed to report their current views and others to recall their earlier reports about their attitudes. The group reporting their initial attitudes gave answers that closely paralleled those who reported their current views; in fact, as Bem and McConnell observed, "The figures are so similar . . . that it would appear that we had asked subjects for their current attitudes rather than their initial attitudes" (p. 28). The phenomenon has been replicated several times since Bem and McConnell's initial demonstration (e.g., Smith, 1984; see Ross, 1988, for a review of the findings). The impact of our current state on our recollection of the past is apparent for other types of memory as well—such as our recall of pain, past use of illicit substances, or income in the last year (see Pearson, Ross, & Dawes, 1992, for further examples).

These results suggest that we may reconstruct the past by consulting the present and projecting it backwards, assuming more stability in the characteristic or behavior in question than it actually exhibits. There are, on the other hand, times when we seem to exaggerate the amount of change we have undergone. Conway and Ross (1984) reported that persons who completed a self-help program rated their preprogram skills lower after they completed the program than they had beforehand; persons on a waiting list showed no comparable changes in recalling their initial level of skill. Believing they had changed, those who completed the program apparently exaggerated the amount of improvement they had experienced.

The exaggeration of both consistency and change may reflect a single underlying process—the attempt to reconstruct the past using the present as an anchor. We may adjust this anchor but we seem to underadjust when we expect the characteristic to be stable and to overadjust when we expect it to change. Either way, what we "recall" is, in fact, a kind of estimate:

Estimation Versus Recall

Other findings also suggest that inference and estimation processes can supplant retrieval as the basis for retrospective reports. Burton and Blair (1991) identified two main strategies for answering behavior frequency questions (e.g., questions about the number of doctor visits in the past 6 months). One strategy, which they call episode enumeration, is to recall and count individual incidents; the other, rate-based estimation, is to project the typical rate over the length of the recall period. Burton and Blair found that respondents were less likely to use episode enumeration as the period covered by the questions grew longer, as there were more episodes to recall, and as the respondents were more rushed for time. As it becomes more difficult to recall each incident, we reconstruct the total by estimating it. (See Menon & Yorkston, chapter 5, this volume, for additional findings on the role of estimation in answers to questions about behavioral frequencies.)

Estimation and inference are likely to have an impact with other memory tasks as well. For example, a study by Huttenlocher, Hedges, and Bradburn (1990) examined answers to a question about how long ago an event had taken place. The further back in time the event was, the more likely the answers were to be reported as round numbers (such as "40 days ago"). These results suggest that, as it became harder to remember exactly when the event occurred, respondents switched to estimation strategies that yielded only approximate answers. Similarly, in a recognition task, we may judge whether we encountered an item before based on its overall plausibility rather than its familiarity (Reder, 1987). Such inferential processes may be especially important in helping us to distinguish events we have experienced but forgotten from those we never experienced at all. Our judgment about whether we experienced the event may hinge on whether it is the sort of thing we think we would remember (Gentner & Collins, 1981).

CONCLUSIONS

Several processes can make it hard for us to remember what happened. We do not notice everything that happens; as a result, some experiences are never stored in memory at all and the ones that are stored may lack key details, such as information about exact dates. Once a representation of the experience does enter memory, it does not necessarily remain static over time. New information, including inferences we draw about the experience or embellishments we add in recounting it, can become part of the memory. Even when a memory has been preserved intact, it may be difficult or impossible to retrieve it. The accumulation of similar experiences over time seems to be the chief source of difficulties in retrieval, producing a rapid drop in our chances of retrieving the item over the short run and slower drops as further time passes (see Fig. 3.1). The best cues to help us recall an experience are ones that most clearly distinguish the experience from all the others with which it might be confused, but even a cue that uniquely picks out the experience will not trigger the retrieval of the memory if it does not match the event's representation in memory. We often try to fill in what we cannot retrieve, using inferential processes or estimation strategies based on our general assumptions about different types of events. These reconstruction processes are a final source of memory errors.

There can be a fine line between retrieving a memory and inferring what might have happened. Autobiographical memory seems designed to record our current beliefs about the past; one aspect of those beliefs that does not seem particularly well represented in memory is their source. As memories fade, we lose our ability to distinguish those parts of our picture of the past that were derived from direct experience from those added through inference, secondhand reports, or imagination. The fact that we can remember something—even have vivid and detailed memories for it—carries no guarantee that we remember it accurately.

REFERENCES

Anderson, J. R. (1983). *The architecture of cognition.* Cambridge, MA: Harvard University Press.

Anderson, J. R., & Reder, L. (1978). An elaborative processing explanation of depth of processing. In L. Cermak & F. I. M. Craik (Ed.), *Levels of processing and human memory* (pp. 385–403). Hillsdale, NJ: Lawrence Erlbaum Associates.

Anderson, J. R., & Schooler, L. J. (1991). Reflections of the environment in memory. *Psychological Science, 2,* 396–408.

Barsalou, L. W. (1988). The content and organization of autobiographical memories. In U. Neisser & E. Winograd (Eds.), *Remembering reconsidered: Ecological and traditional approaches to the study of memory* (pp. 193–243). Cambridge, England: Cambridge University Press.

Bartlett, F. (1932). *Remembering—A study in experimental and social psychology.* Cambridge, England: Cambridge University Press.

Bem, D. J., & McConnell, H. K. (1970). Testing the self-perception explanation of dissonance phenomena: On the salience of premanipulation attitudes. *Journal of Personality and Social Psychology, 14,* 23–31.

Bower, G. H., Black, J. B., & Turner, T. J. (1979). Scripts in memory for text. *Cognitive Psychology, 11,* 177–220.

Bradburn, N. M., Rips, L. J., & Shevell, S. K. (1987). Answering autobiographical questions: The impact of memory and inference on surveys. *Science, 236,* 157–161.

Brittingham, A., Lee, L., Tourangeau, R., & Willis, G. (in press). Errors in parents' reports of children's immunizations. *Vital & Health Statistics.* Series 6.

Brown, R., & Kulik, J. (1977). Flashbulb memories. *Cognition, 5,* 73–99.

Burton, S., & Blair, E. (1991). Task conditions, response formulation processes, and response accuracy for behavioral frequency questions in surveys. *Public Opinion Quarterly, 55,* 50–79.

Cannell, C. F., Miller, P. V., & Oksenberg, L. (1981). Research on interviewing techniques. In S. Leinhardt (Ed.), *Sociological methodology 1981* (pp. 389–437). San Francisco: Jossey-Bass.

Collins, A. M., & Quillian, M. R. (1969). Retrieval time from semantic memory. *Journal of Verbal Learning and Verbal Behavior, 8,* 240–247.

Conway, M. A. (1995). *Flashbulb memories.* Hove, UK: Lawrence Erlbaum Associates.

Conway, M. A., & Ross, M. (1984). Getting what you want by revising what you had. *Journal of Personality and Social Psychology, 47,* 738–748.

Craik, F. I. M., & Lockhart, R. (1972). Levels of processing: A framework for memory research. *Journal of Verbal Learning and Verbal Behavior, 11,* 671–684.

Ebbinghaus, H. (1885). *Uber das Gedächtnis.* Leipzig: Duncker and Humblot.

Gentner, D., & Collins, A. (1981). Studies of inference from lack of knowledge. *Memory and Cognition, 9,* 434–443.

Goldstein, K. P., Kviz, F. J., & Daum, R. S. (1993). Accuracy of immunization histories provided by adults accompanying preschool children to a pediatric emergency department. *Journal of the American Medical Association, 270,* 2190–2194.

Huttenlocher, J., Hedges, L., & Bradburn, N. M. (1990). Reports of elapsed time: Bounding and rounding processes in estimation. *Journal of Experimental Psychology: Learning, Memory, and Cognition, 16,* 196–213.

Jacoby, L. L., Kelley, C. M., & Dywan, J. (1989). Memory attributions. In H. L. Roediger & F. I. M. Craik (Eds.), *Varieties of memory and consciousness: Essays in honour of Endel Tulving* (pp. 391–422). Hillsdale, NJ: Lawrence Erlbaum Associates.

Jobe, J. B., Tourangeau, R., & Smith, A. F. (1993). Contributions of survey research to the understanding of memory. *Applied Cognitive Psychology, 7,* 567–584.

Jobe, J. B., White, A. A., Kelley, C. L., Mingay, D. J., Sanchez, M. J., & Loftus, E. F. (1990). Recall strategies and memory for health care visits. *The Milbank Quarterly, 68,* 171–189.

Johnson, M. K., Foley, M., Suengas, A., & Raye, C. (1988). Phenomenal characteristics of memories for perceived and imagined autobiographical events. *Journal of Experimental Psychology: General, 117,* 371–376.

Johnson, M. K., Hashtroudi, S., & Lindsay, D. S. (1993). Source monitoring. *Psychological Bulletin, 144,* 3–28.

Johnson, M. K., Kounios, J., & Reeder, J. A. (1994). Time-course studies of reality monitoring and recognition. *Journal of Experimental Psychology: Learning, Memory, and Cognition, 20,* 1409–1419.

Kassin, S. M., & Kiechel, K. L. (1996). The social psychology of false confessions: Compliance, internalization, and confabulation. *Psychological Science, 7,* 125–128.

Kolodner, J. (1985). Memory for experience. In G. H. Bower (Ed.), *The psychology of learning and motivation* (vol. 19, pp. 1–57). Orlando, FL: Academic Press.

Lindsay, D. S. (1990). Misleading suggestions can impair eyewitnesses' ability to remember event details. *Journal of Experimental Psychology: Learning, Memory, and Cognition, 16,* 1077–1083.

Lindsay, D. S., & Johnson, M. (1989). The eyewitness suggestibility effect and memory for source. *Memory and Cognition, 17,* 349–358.

Lindsay, D. S., & Read, J. D. (1994). Psychotherapy and memories of childhood sexual abuse: A cognitive perspective. *Applied Cognitive Psychology, 8,* 281–338.

Loftus, E. F., & Fathi, D. C. (1985). Retrieving multiple autobiographical memories. *Social Cognition, 3,* 280–295.

Loftus, E. F., & Hoffman, H. G. (1989). Misinformation and memory: The creation of new memories. *Journal of Experimental Psychology: General, 118,* 100–104.

Loftus, E. F., & Kaufman, L. (1992). Why do traumatic experiences sometimes produce good memory (flashbulbs) and sometimes no memory (repression)? In E. Winograd & U. Neisser (Eds.), *Affect and accuracy in recall: Studies of "flashbulb" memories* (pp. 212–223). New York: Cambridge University Press.

Loftus, E. F., Smith, K. D., Klinger, M. R., & Fiedler, J. (1992). Memory and mismemory for health events. In J. M. Tanur (Ed.), *Questions about questions: Inquiries into the cognitive bases of surveys* (pp. 102–137). New York: Sage.

Means, B., & Loftus, E. (1991). When personal history repeats itself: Decomposing memories for recurring events. *Applied Cognitive Psychology, 5,* 297–318.

Neisser, U., & Harsch, N. (1992). Phantom flashbulbs: False recollections of hearing the news about *Challenger.* In E. Winograd & U. Neisser (Eds.), *Affect and accuracy in recall: Studies of "flashbulb" memories* (pp. 9–31). Cambridge, England: Cambridge University Press.

Pearson, R. W., Ross, M., & Dawes, R. M. (1992). Personal recall and the limits of retrospective questions in surveys. J. M. Tanur (Ed.), *Questions about questions: Inquiries into the cognitive basis of surveys* (pp. 65–94). New York: Sage.

Pillemer, D. B. (1984). Flashbulb memories of the assassination attempt on President Reagan. *Cognition, 16,* 63–80.

Reder, L. (1987). Strategy selection in question answering. *Cognitive Psychology, 19,* 90–138.

Robinson, J. A. (1986). Temporal reference systems and autobiographical memory. In D. C. Rubin (Ed.), *Autobiographical memory* (pp. 159–188). Cambridge, England: Cambridge University Press.

Ross, M. (1988). The relation of implicit theories to the construction of personal histories. *Psychological Review, 96,* 341–357.

Rubin, D. C., & Kozin, M. (1984). Vivid memories. *Cognition, 16,* 81–95.

Rubin, D. C., & Wetzel, A. E. (1996). One hundred years of forgetting: A quantitative description of retention. *Psychological Review, 103,* 734–760.

Schacter, D. L. (1987). Implicit memory: History and current status. *Journal of Experimental Psychology: Learning, Memory, and Cognition, 13,* 501–518.

Schooler, J. W., Gerhard, D., & Loftus, E. F. (1986). Qualities of the unreal. *Journal of Experimental Psychology: Learning, Memory, and Cognition, 12,* 171–181.

Smith, A. F. (1991). Cognitive processes in long-term dietary recall. *Vital and Health Statistics,* Series 6, No. 4 (DHHS Publication No. PHS 92-1079). Washington, DC: U.S. Government Printing Office.

Smith, A. F., Jobe, J., & Mingay, D. (1991). Retrieval from memory of dietary information. *Applied Cognitive Psychology, 5,* 269–296.

Smith, T. W. (1984). Recalling attitudes: An analysis of retrospective questions on the 1982 General Social Survey. *Public Opinion Quarterly, 48,* 639–649.

Sudman, S., & Bradburn, N. M. (1973). Effects of time and memory factors on response in surveys. *Journal of the American Statistical Association, 68,* 805–815.

Tulving, E., & Thomson, D. M. (1973). Encoding specificity and retrieval processes in episodic memory. *Psychological Review, 80,* 352–373.

Wagenaar, W. (1986). My memory: A study of autobiographical memory over six years. *Cognitive Psychology, 18,* 225–252.

Warrington, E. K., & Weiskrantz, L. (1968). New method of testing long-term retention with special reference to amnesic patients. *Nature, 217,* 972–974.

Williams, M. D., & Hollan, J. D. (1981). The process of retrieval from very long-term memory. *Cognitive Science, 5,* 87–119.

Winograd, E., & Killinger, W. A. (1983). Relating age at encoding in early childhood to adult recall: Development of flashbulb memories. *Journal of Experimental Psychology: General, 112,* 413–422.

4

Temporal Representation and Event Dating

Norman M. Bradburn
University of Chicago/NORC

Many studies ask respondents to remember not only that certain events happened, but also to place them in real time. To perform this task, respondents must depend on their memories for both these events and the time at which they took place. Thus, to understand how people arrive at their responses, and the degree of error in such self-reports, we need to know about the organization of what is called autobiographical memory and how time is represented in that memory.

Event dating may be important by itself in epidemiologic studies, but it also plays an important role in more common questions in health surveys in which respondents are asked to report the number of times they have done something within a specified reference period, for example, "How many times have you gone to the doctor in the past 3 months?" For such frequency questions, respondents must search their memories for the occurrence of the requested events and then place them in the referenced time period. This latter cognitive task requires them to place the events in calendar time. Thus, the accuracy of frequency reports of behavior partially depends on the accuracy of event dating.

This chapter begins with several empirical observations about autobiographical memory, then discusses how events and time are represented in memory, looks at how dates are retrieved, and concludes with a short review of what we know about errors in the dating of events.

SOME EMPIRICAL OBSERVATIONS ABOUT
AUTOBIOGRAPHICAL MEMORY

Studies of memory often distinguish between autobiographical memory and semantic memory. Autobiographical memory is memory about things that take place in space and time, whereas semantic memory is about facts that are not experienced in time or place.

The first observation about autobiographical memory is that events in people's lives are experienced as a temporal flow; that is, we are conscious that things are happening now or they happened then or at some past time, or that they are going to happen or will happen in some future time. In spite of the ubiquity of this temporal experience, however, calendar time is not a good retrieval cue for most events for most people (Barsalou, 1988; Wagenaar, 1986).

The second observation will surprise no one, namely that our memory for dates is bad. Although there is considerable individual variation in people's ability to remember dates of significant events, and even greater variability for trivial ones, most people are acutely aware of the limitations of their memory when it comes to the calendar dates of events. In one event-dating study, subjects occasionally misdated an event that actually occurred within the previous 4 months by as much as 3 months (Thompson, 1982). In another study, subjects reported that 20% of their dating attempts for autobiographical events were pure guesses (Thompson, Skowronski, & Lee, 1988).

The third observation, somewhat paradoxically, is that time is related to the accuracy of recall. The longer ago an event occurred, the more difficulty we have in recalling it. The functional form of the relationship between time and forgetting has been classically studied by Ebbinghaus (1894/1964) who showed that, at least for nonsense syllables, it was a negatively accelerating curve. More recent work, however, suggests that it may be nearly linear for some types of knowledge (Bradburn, Rips, & Shevell, 1987). The data displayed in Fig. 4.1 suggest that the shape of the forgetting curve is more nearly linear for high school classmates' and teachers' names but that it looks more like the classic Ebbinghaus curve for street names in the town where respondents went to college or for the critical details of events that were rated, in an experimental situation, as certain to be recalled. These data are from studies of long-term recall. Note that the absolute level of recall is still fairly high for discrete knowledge like names even after 10 years. (For a more complete description of forgetting curves in self-report research, see Jobe, Tourangeau, & Smith, 1993).

Whereas accuracy declines with time, variation in reports around the true date increases with time; that is, not only do we make more mistakes about dates of events that are further in the past, but we do so in systematic ways.

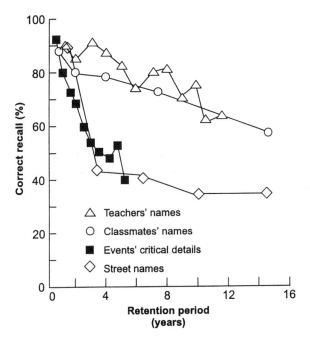

FIG. 4.1.   Rate of forgetting for common types of autobiographical information.

Although this increase in variability has not been studied to a great extent, Baddeley, Lewis, and Nimmo-Smith (1978) estimated that the size of the absolute error in reports about previous visits to a laboratory increases by 19 days for each 100 days of elapsed time between the visit and the report of the visit.

Putting these three observations together—personal events are experienced as a temporal flow, memory for dates is poor, and accuracy of dating declines with time—we start with a guiding hypothesis: Although events are experienced in temporal sequence, calendar dates are rarely coded, and rarely stored, as part of the experience. Thus, the dating of past events is largely reconstructive. Most calendar dates have to be estimated from other memories coded with an event.

HOW ARE EVENTS REPRESENTED IN MEMORY?

A useful device is to think of memory as a large storehouse of drawers full of files of information. What is commonly referred to as memory is long-term memory (as distinct from short-term memory), and retrieval from long-term memory is what we ordinarily call remembering. Remembering is a process in which long-term memory is searched for the requested information. If we think of memory as a big storehouse, it is clear that it must be organized in some fashion so that material can be retrieved. Just as we label files that we put in our filing cabinets, we must label information that is stored in memory. The labeling process is often called encoding and refers to the various aspects of information or experience that are attached to the item when it is stored in memory so that we can retrieve it.

A useful framework for thinking about autobiographical memory was proposed by Barsalou (1988). In studies of free recall, he found that memories were hierarchically organized. Their highest level of organization was chronological order. What was ordered, however, were not specific events but rather sequences of events, what Barsalou called extended events such as a trip, a stay in the hospital, or working at a job. This finding suggests that people do not store in memory a stream of isolated events, but rather they store them as temporal–causal sequences. For example, a person might remember a stay in the hospital as beginning with a pain and a visit to a doctor, followed by admittance to a hospital and various treatments while there, followed by discharge and return home, and finally by follow-up doctor visits. Recall of specific events, such as an X-ray or particular tests (a detail in a sequence file), would take place within the sequence (a file in a drawer), rather than be treated as isolated events (a whole drawer of files on, say, unrelated doctor visits). Giving cues to remind respondents about the sequence might be more effective than attempting to get directly at the specific events, although this strategy has not been tested.

In addition to being chronologically organized, event sequences are hierarchically organized along meaningfully clustered lines, such as cause–effect relationships, goal attainment, or primary socially defined roles such as work, school, family, or social relationships. Specific events themselves are nested within large categories of event sequences. Thus, health might be the superordinate category that is subdivided into a chronologically organized health history that includes drawer labels such as childhood diseases, episodes of acute illness, important encounters with health providers, onset of chronic illnesses or disabilities, and so on. Within each of these categories, further subdivisions are likely, down to the most recent illnesses and doctor visits.

HOW IS TIME REPRESENTED IN MEMORY?

In order for people to have a memory for when things happened, events must be associated in memory with some representation of time. Events may be represented in memory by their place in a commonly shared calendar, such as an hour, a day, month and year, or in quasi-calendar units such as seasons; or socially defined time periods, for example, during the fall semester; or idiosyncratic reference points, for example, 2 days before the NIH Conference on Self-Reports. Events may also be represented by reference to elapsed time, for example, 5 days ago (Sudman, Bradburn, & Schwarz, 1996).

The categories for the representation of time are hierarchically organized. For example, in recalling on what day of the week an event occurred, very few errors are made between weekdays and weekend days. Errors occur within the two categories, rather than between them. Larger categories such as seasons, holidays, work-related calendars, and school terms—which themselves can be related to the common calendar—provide first-level coding for the time of events.

The social patterning of time—that is, coding the time of events in terms of socially shared events—is an interesting phenomenon that has implications for the accurate recall of dates of events. Not all autobiographical sequences are useful as temporal reference points. In one clever experiment, Brown, Shevell, and Rips (1986) recorded the reaction time of college students as they decided whether each of a series of news events took place during an earlier period (1978–1980) or a later period (1981–1983). These periods were described in different ways. For half of the subjects, the earlier period was described as "President Carter's term of office" and the later period was described as "President Reagan's term of office." For the other half, the earlier period was described as "the time you were in high school," whereas the later period was described as "the time you were in college." Because the subjects were all seniors in college at the time of the experiment, the two sets of descriptors covered the same time periods. The events that were dated were also of two types: either obviously political events (e.g., Mitterrand's election as President of France) or nonpolitical, but still public, events (e.g., the Three Mile Island reactor accident). On average, the subjects were able to date political events faster than nonpolitical events within the presidential terms, but the nonpolitical events were dated more quickly within the autobiographical period (Fig. 4.2).

The encoding of time as elapsed time (e.g., 10 days ago) has several features of note. The first is that there is a constantly changing reference point (right now) so that the value for the code is always changing rather than being a stable value as in the case of categories that have a fixed relationship to a calendar (e.g., Dec. 15, 1997). The second is that people use different groupings and rounding algorithms as the elapsed time increases. When asked how many days ago an event happened, respondents will answer in terms of discrete days—for example, last Monday—for periods up to about a week or, at most, 10 days. After that, the number of days gets rounded into conventional categories such as 10 days ago, 2 weeks ago, a month ago, and so forth (Huttenlocher, Hedges, & Bradburn, 1990). In the frequency distribution of reports of elapsed time between an original inter-

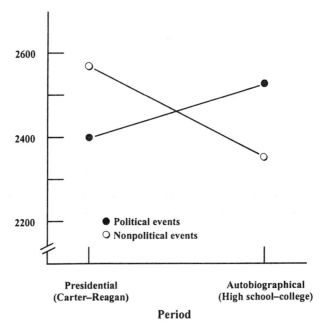

FIG. 4.2. Mean time to decide whether a target event occurred during an earlier or later interval.

view and reinterview in which respondents were asked how long ago the first interview took place, results show (Fig. 4.3) an enormous piling up of reports at canonical rounding values such as 2 weeks (14 days), a month (30 days), and 2 months (60 days). There is also a smaller tendency to round to the nearest value ending in 5 or zero.

HOW ARE DATES RETRIEVED?

Exact dates for a few events are rehearsed sufficiently to be easily recalled; for example, the date of our own birthday (because it is called for on so many forms), or significant public holidays such as Christmas or Independence Day. Similarly, dates of events that are important in our own lives, such as a wedding day or the birthdates of our own children, may be (although we know too well that they are not always) recalled with ease. The dates for most events, however, are retrieved through reconstruction by using characteristics of the events in the autobiographical temporal–causal sequence (that drawer of files, again) as cues to when they happened.

For example, in trying to recall the last time I was at NIH, I tried to recall what I was doing (being on a review panel), what were the topics of the

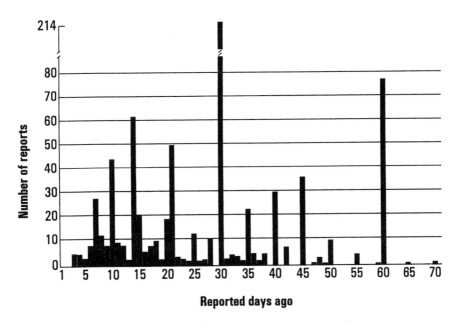

FIG. 4.3. Reported elapsed days since event occurred.

papers we were to review (surveys related to mental health), how did that relate to what I was working on at the time (similar methodological problems). I also tried to recall other events in my own life that I can date and that I can connect with that trip. In order to narrow down the range of likely dates, I had to recall something about the event that would allow me to connect it to some other event that I can date in time with reasonable accuracy. The accuracy of the final self-report will depend on how well I can connect the event whose date is to be recalled with some other events that I can date, either autobiographical or public events, such as who was President or, perhaps more relevant for this example, who else was on the panel.

When dates are being used to compute frequencies of events within a time period, the cognitive processes are somewhat more complex. If there are very many events within the time period, it is clear that people do not directly recall events and then sum them up. People give up trying to enumerate individual events when the number of occurrences within the time period is more than 7 +/- 2, the magic number of bits of information that we can hold in consciousness at one time (Burton & Blair, 1991; Miller, 1956). When people were asked what method they used to come up with their answers to the question, "How many times have you eaten out in a restaurant in the past 6 months?" most respondents who reported 5 or less times used individual enumeration of the events as the method to come up with an answer (see Table 4.1). When the frequency became higher than 5,

TABLE 4.1
Effect on Response Processes

Frequency of Dining at a Restaurant[a]	Response Formulation Process				
	n	Enumeration %	Rate	Other	Total %
1	12	100	0	0	100
2	28	68	32	0	100
3	29	93	7	0	100
4–5	40	63	35	2	100
6–10	53	15	59	26	100
11–25	58	0	66	34	100
26–100	86	0	77	23	100
>100[b]	26	0	100	0	100

[a]Chi-square = 231. Df = 14; p < 0.001; with enumeration versus all other processes (i.e., rate and other categories combined) = 211, df = 7, p < 0.001.
[b]To 9 respondents at 183; 1 at 366.

a majority shifted over to making an estimation based on a frequency rate, such as "once a week." With more than 10 events, no one reported trying to enumerate the events. Thus what looks on the surface like a question that involves extensive searching of memory for dated events may, in fact, be answered by using an estimation rule. (For a more complete discussion of judgment strategies for behavioral frequencies see Menon, 1994.)

WHAT DO WE KNOW ABOUT ERRORS IN DATING?

With our present state of knowledge, there are eight generalizations about the accuracy of dating events that we can make with some confidence:

1. The better an event is remembered, the greater the likelihood of being able to date it (Brewer, 1988; Linton, 1978). But even here, the direction of errors is related to knowledge of the event. In one experiment (Brown, Rips, & Shevell, 1985), public events of differing degrees of publicity were dated. Events that were judged by the experimenters as being less well known were more likely to be judged as having happened longer ago than they actually happened, whereas more well-known events were judged as having occurred more recently than actual. When subjects were asked to do their own ratings of their knowledge of the events, the same pattern was observed but the frequencies were moved over (Fig. 4.4).

2. A frequent time error is misplacing a date by some systematic calendar related factor, for example making a 7-day or a 1-year error; that is, being

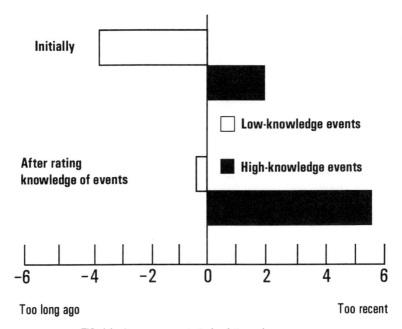

FIG. 4.4. Average error in judged time of occurrence.

off by a week, a month, or a year (Huttenlocher, Hedges, & Bradburn; Skow-ronski, Betz, Thompson, & Shannon, 1991).

3. As we have already seen, reports of elapsed time are subject to round-ing errors. Rounding occurs according to culturally shared algorithms, for example, 10 days, 2 weeks, 1 month (Huttenlocher, Hedges, & Bradburn, 1990).

4. Other things being equal, there is a general tendency to remember events as having happened more recently than they actually did. In the survey world, this is called telescoping and leads to overreporting of the frequency of events within a time period. Telescoping has been the object of research lately and appears to be the result of two aspects of memory for time discussed earlier—the increase in the variability of remembered dates as the event recedes into the past, and the tendency to round to canonical values that increase in distance the further back in time the event. The combined effect of rounding and bounding—that is, the specification of a cut-off date for the reference period—produces the net forward telescoping that is frequently observed (Huttenlocher, Hedges, & Bradburn, 1990; Neter & Waksberg, 1964; Rubin & Baddeley, 1989).

5. Events that are low-frequency or personally atypical are more often exactly dated (Brewer, 1988; Linton, 1979; Wagenaar, 1986; White, 1982). For example, Brewer (1988), in a study of randomly sampled autobiographical

events, found that subjects showed good recall for low-frequency events and for events occurring in low-frequency locations. This means, for example, that, if we attend NIH panel meetings often, the date of a panel meeting missed is more easily recalled than the ones to which we have gone.

6. Pleasant events are more often exactly dated than unpleasant events but the magnitude of dating errors is not associated with pleasantness (Banaji & Hardin, 1994; Skowronski et al., 1991; Wagenaar, 1986; White, 1982). Both the dates of atypical events and pleasant events may be better remembered because of their perceptual distinctness or may be rehearsed more. Although most people remember pleasant events better than unpleasant ones (Skowronski et al., 1991), this generalization is subject to considerable variance because some people seem to remember unpleasant events more vividly than pleasant events.

7. It should surprise no one that women are better at remembering dates than men (Skowronski & Thompson, 1990). That difference has caused many a tense moment in marriages.

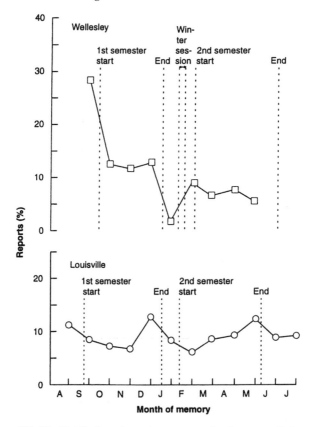

FIG. 4.5. Distribution of events over one school year recalled.

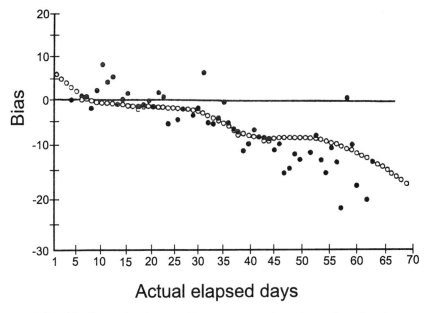

FIG. 4.6. Observed and modeled bias in reporting for each actual number of elapsed days.

8. Finally, there appears to be a not-well-understood tendency to remember more events that occur around boundaries of socially defined time periods, such as the beginning or ending of academic terms (Fig. 4.5). Given that events are remembered, however, there is a tendency to remember them as occurring further away from the boundaries than they actually did (Fig. 4.6; Huttenlocher, Hedges, & Prohaska, 1988; Pillemer, Rhinehart, & White, 1986; Robinson, 1987). This is a phenomenon that needs further research.

CONCLUSIONS

Chronological order is one of the most important aspects of our experience of events that make up what we call autobiographical memory, the memory system that is the basis for our self-reports. But calendar time is not a good cue to retrieve events and most events are not encoded with their calendar dates. Retrieval of event dates is largely a matter of the reconstruction of the dates through which we draw on other aspects of the autobiographical sequences within which events are encoded. Although we know that people are not very good at exact reconstructions and uncertain about exact dates, it appears that the temporal representation of events in memory is unbiased and that the observed errors in reporting come from as yet unknown processes that occur during the recall process. Such errors appear to be systematic across many groups and are subject to our understanding through further research. When the processes and the typical extent of these errors are fully understood, we will be in a position to use this information to evaluate the validity of self-reported dates and, perhaps, make adjustments to the data to increase the validity of event dating.

REFERENCES

Baddeley, A., Lewis, V., & Nimmo-Smith, I. (1978). "When did you last . . . ? In M. M. Gruneberg, P. E. Morris, & R. N. Sykes (Eds.), *Practical aspects of memory* (pp. 77–83). New York: Academic Press.

Banaji, M. R., & Hardin, C. (1994). Affect and memory in retrospective reports. In N. Schwarz & S. Sudman (Eds.), *Autobiographical memory and the validity of retrospective reports* (pp. 71–88). New York: Springer-Verlag.

Barsalou, L. W. (1988). The content and organization of autobiographical memory. In U. Neisser & E. Winograd (Eds.), *Remembering reconsidered: Ecological and traditional approaches to the study of memory* (pp. 193–243). Cambridge, England: Cambridge University Press.

Bradburn, N. M., Rips, L. J., & Shevell, S. K. (1987). Answering autobiographical questions: The impact of memory and inference on survey responses. *Science, 236,* 157–161.

Brewer, W. F. (1988). Memory for randomly sampled autobiographical events. In U. Neisser & E. Winograd (Eds.), *Remembering reconsidered: Ecological and traditional approaches to the study of memory* (pp. 21–90). Cambridge, England: Cambridge University Press.

Brown, N. R., Rips, L. J., & Shevell, S. K. (1985). The subjective dates of natural events in very long-term memory. *Cognitive Psychology, 17,* 139–177.

Brown, N. R., Shevell, S. K., & Rips, L. J. (1986). Public memories and their personal context. In D. C. Rubin (Ed.), *Autobiographical memory* (pp. 137–158). Cambridge, England: Cambridge University Press.

Burton, S., & Blair, E. A. (1991). Task conditions, response formulation processes, and response accuracy for behavioral frequency questions in surveys. *Public Opinion Quarterly, 55*(1), 50–79.

Ebbinghaus, H. (1964). *Memory: A contribution to experimental psychology.* New York: Dover. (Originally published in 1894).

Huttenlocher, J., Hedges, L. V., & Bradburn, N. M. (1990). Reports of elapsed time: Bounding and rounding processes in estimation. *Journal of Experimental Psychology: Learning, Memory and Cognition, 16,* 196–213.

Huttenlocher, J., Hedges, L. V., & Prohaska, V. (1988). Hierarchical organization in ordered domains: Estimating dates of events. *Psychological Review, 95,* 471–484.

Jobe, J. B., Tourangeau, R., & Smith, A. F. (1993). Contributions of Survey Research to the Understanding of Memory. *Applied Cognitive Psychology, 1*(7), 567–584.

Linton, M. (1978). Real-world memory after six years: An *in vivo* study of very long term memory. In M. M. Gruneberg, P. E. Morris, & R. N. Sykes (Eds.), *Practical aspects of memory* (pp. 69–76). London: Academic Press.

Miller, G. A. (1956). The magic number 7, plus or minus 2. *Psychological Review, 63,* 81–97.

Menon, G. (1994). Judgments of behavioral frequencies: Memory search and retrieval strategies. In N. Schwarz & S. Sudman (Eds.), *Autobiographical memory and the validity of retrospective reports* (pp. 161–172). New York: Springer-Verlag.

Neter, J., & Waksberg, J. (1964). A study of response errors in expenditures data from household interviews. *Journal of the American Statistical Association, 59*, 18–55.

Pillemer, D. B., Rhinehart, E. D., & White, S. H. (1986). Memories of life transitions: The first year of college. *Human Learning, 5*, 109–123.

Robinson, J. A. (1987). Autobiographical memory: A historical perspective. In D. C. Rubin (Ed.), *Autobiographical memory* (pp. 159–190). Cambridge, England: Cambridge University Press.

Rubin, D. C., & Baddeley, A. D. (1989). Telescoping is not time compression: A model of the dating of autobiographical events. *Memory and Cognition, 17*, 653–661.

Skowronski, J. J., Betz, A. L., Thompson, C. P., & Shannon, L. (1991). Social memory in everyday life: Recall of self-events and other events. *Journal of Personality and Social Psychology, 60*, 831–843.

Skowronski, J. J., & Thompson, C. P. (1990). Reconstructing the dates of personal events: Gender differences in accuracy. *Applied Cognitive Psychology, 4*, 371–381.

Sudman, S., Bradburn, N. M., & Schwarz, N. (1996). *Thinking about answers: The application of cognitive processes to survey methodology.* San Francisco: Jossey-Bass.

Thompson, C. P. (1982). Memory for unique personal events: The roommate study. *Memory & Cognition, 10*, 324–332.

Thompson, C. P., Skowronski, J. J., & Lee, D. J. (1988). Reconstructing the date of a personal event. In M. M. Gruneberg, P. E. Morris, & R. N. Sykes (Eds.), *Practical aspects of memory: Current research and issues: Vol. 1. Memory in everyday life* (pp. 241–246). New York: Wiley.

Wagenaar, W. A. (1986). My memory: A study of autobiographical memory over six years. *Cognitive Psychology, 18*, 225–252.

White, R. T. (1982). Memory for personal events. *Human Learning, 1*, 171–183.

5

The Use of Memory and Contextual Cues in the Formation of Behavioral Frequency Judgments

Geeta Menon
Eric A. Yorkston
New York University

Surveys often ask for the frequencies with which people engage in different behaviors. For example, a national consumer survey that attempts to capture the purchasing and lifestyle trends of consumers asks its respondents the frequency with which they go on weight-reducing diets. Further, the survey also elicits information such as the frequency of consumption of various products such as regular and diet soda, chocolate bars, yogurt, and artificial sweeteners. By coupling this information with respondents' opinions on various diet and nutrition statements, marketers may arrive at judgments of market-size and brand-share forecasts. Furthermore, they can uncover nutritional trends, design product tie-ins, and arrive at market segments based on usage occasion, psychographics, and, of course, demographics. Frequency judgments are a powerful tool for marketing managers and advertisers.

Government surveys also rely heavily on frequency questions. For example, the National Health Interview Survey on Epidemiology asks people how often they eat various kinds of foods such as broccoli, spinach, rice, beef, liver, and so forth, to determine people's level of health consciousness. The National Crime Survey asks people the frequency of exposure to various kinds of crimes such as robbery, physical abuse, and the frequency of someone taking something from a place where they were temporarily residing. From these responses, national health and crime rates are calculated. Therefore, ensuring the accuracy of these reports assumes the utmost importance.

Yet previous research indicates that individuals often cannot judge frequencies accurately (e.g., Burton & Blair, 1991; Menon, 1993). The extent of error associated with a frequency report may vary from 13% for a behavior that is reported most accurately to 130% for less accurately reported behaviors (Menon, 1993). The magnitude of these errors is enormous, and the consequence of these errors can be very expensive for a marketing manager who relies on these estimates for new product introductions, brand-share forecasts, or segmentation analysis. With corporations launching multimillion dollar campaigns and national public policy decisions relying on frequency reports, the need for eliciting accurate frequency reports is critical.

In order to elicit more accurate frequency reports in surveys, however, we need to first understand how respondents formulate behavioral frequency judgments. If we understand the process by which frequency judgments are generated, we are in a better position to facilitate the use of a response formulation strategy that enhances the accuracy of frequency reports.

In this chapter, we provide an integrative theory that predicts when and how respondents use different cognitive processes in order to report behavioral frequencies. We begin with a discussion of the two sources of information that respondents can tap into to arrive at frequency judgments: memory-based and context-based information. Although traditionally we would want to eliminate context effects and the bias that may result, we suggest that strategic use of contextual cues may enable more accurate memory-based processing. We then discuss the factors that moderate the manner in which these sources of information are combined to form a judgment. Of particular interest are the findings of several papers that indicate that the regularity (or periodicity) with which the behavior is engaged in by a person affects the way information is organized in memory. Finally, we prescribe questioning strategies that increase the accuracy of frequency judgments.

INPUTS FOR FREQUENCY JUDGMENTS

Ideally when respondents are asked to make a frequency judgment, they retrieve the information from memory (i.e., memory-based information). However, respondents do not always make memory-based judgments because constructing frequencies based on recall of the different episodes and events can be both effortful and cumbersome. The incentive to use the least-taxing cognitive strategy in a typical survey situation is fairly high. This prompts respondents to use judgment heuristics to reduce the task complexity and make the judgment process easier (March & Simon, 1958; Tversky & Kahneman, 1974). There are a variety of non-memory-based information sources, such as the judgment context (i.e., context-based information), that may require less processing and can be used as an alternate method to formulate judgments. We now review the role of these two sources of information as inputs for frequency judgments.

Memory-Based Information

How do consumers retrieve the necessary inputs from memory to form a frequency judgment? Previous work has assumed that respondents try to recall the occurrences of a behavior when asked to arrive at a frequency judgment. More recent evidence suggests that respondents rarely recall-and-count all the episodes of a frequent behavior (i.e., an episodic recall strategy). Instead, they rely on a heuristic and estimate the frequency from other, more available information. For example, a person may use 5 cups a day as the basis on which to arrive at 35 cups when asked how much coffee was consumed last week. The research that addresses what cognitive processes are involved while resorting to this heuristic and what conditions facilitate the usage of rates has been documented only within the last decade.

Blair and Burton (1987) established three factors that affect the use of an episodic recall versus an estimation strategy:

- the actual frequency of the event (more than six episodes triggers the use of an estimation strategy);
- the reference time frame (longer time frames enhance the use of an estimation strategy); and
- question wording ("how many" vs. "how many times," with the latter triggering an estimation strategy).

These findings provide a starting point for understanding the processes by which survey respondents generate frequency judgments. For instance, the findings indicate that both internal and external factors affect the frequency formulation process. Whereas the researcher has no control over internal factors, such as the actual frequency of the behavior, many of the external factors, including question wording and the reference time period, may be either manipulated or controlled by the researcher.

Menon (1993, 1994) demonstrated that, holding these three factors constant (i.e., frequency = behaviors engaged in once a day; reference time frame = one week; question wording = How many times), the use of episodic recall versus estimation strategies is a function of how information is organized in memory. These studies proposed a model of autobiographical memory for behaviors engaged in frequently and predicted under what circumstances each of the different frequency formulation strategies would be used. This model explicitly introduced the regularity (i.e., periodicity) of a behavior as a construct that determines whether or not a rate-of-occurrence is accessible in memory for use at a later point in time in computing a judgment. Because one of the fundamental principles that governs what information is used in constructing a judgment is the accessibility of the information memory (i.e., how easy it is to retrieve), the regularity of the behavior dictates the response formulation strategy that respondents use to construct a frequency report.

What is regularity? Suppose both Persons A and B consume 7 cans of soda a week. Whereas Person A may consume a can of soda a day, Person B may consume 2 cans on some days and no cans on others, averaging 7 cans a week. The time period between two consecutive episodes is less variable for Person A than Person B and, thus, more regular. Note that although these behaviors differ in their regularity, they both occur with the same frequency. Generally stated, a regular behavior has a fixed periodicity of occurrence, whereas an irregular behavior does not. This regularity of behaviors affects how people store information about their frequency in memory. Research on judgments of behavioral frequencies has suggested that a rate-of-occurrence may be stored in memory (Blair & Burton, 1987; Burton & Blair, 1991) because people have the ability to learn temporal and sequential patterns (Povel, 1981; Simon & Kotovsky, 1963). This, however, is more likely for regular behaviors (which contain simpler patterns) than for irregular behaviors (Menon, 1993).

Menon (1993) conducted three experiments employing different methodologies (verbal protocols, response latencies, and diaries) to demonstrate that:

- when an event is perceived to be a regular one, people have rates-of-occurrence encoded in memory that they retrieve to form a judgment and use an estimation strategy;
- in the case of irregular behaviors, such rates do not exist in memory and people are more likely to use an episodic recall strategy to arrive at a frequency judgment.

Most important, not only were regular behaviors easy to report about because of the easily accessible rate-of-occurrence in memory, respondents were also much more accurate about these judgments. This is presumably because such rates are developed over a period of one's lifetime and therefore tend to be very robust. In the case of irregular behaviors, respondents must rely on episodic recall. If the behavior is a frequently occurring one, then such episodes may not be easily accessible in memory. In the case of infrequent behaviors, however, episodic information may be easily accessible in memory and the subsequent frequency reports may be fairly accurate.

In sum, with all else being constant, whether or not a behavior is regular determines the cognitive process that respondents use, and for frequent behaviors also determines the accuracy of the associated frequency judgment.

Context-Based Information

Respondents can also use information provided by the response context, such as information appearing earlier in the questionnaire itself (e.g., Bickart, 1993; Bishop, Hippler, Schwarz, & Strack, 1988; Schwarz & Hippler, 1995), the ambiguity of the issue discussed (Strack, Schwarz, & Wänke, 1991), or even the moods previous questions have cued (Schwarz & Clore, 1988; Schwarz & Strack, 1991; for a detailed discussion or contextual effects in survey research see Schwarz & Sudman, 1991). One context-based heuristic that has recently received attention involves the use of information provided by the response alternatives (e.g., Menon, Raghubir, & Schwarz, 1995, 1997; Schwarz & Hippler, 1987; Schwarz, Hippler, Deutsch, & Strack, 1985; Schwarz & Scheuring, 1988). Specifically, respondents assume that the researcher constructed a meaningful set of response alternatives that reflects the frequency distribution of the behavior under study. Accordingly, they assume that the extreme alternatives correspond to the extremes of the distribution and that alternatives in the middle reflect the average or typical frequency of the behavior (Schwarz, 1990; Schwarz & Hippler, 1991). Based on this assumption, respondents use the range of the response alternatives provided to them as a frame of reference in estimating their own behavioral frequency. This results in reports of higher frequencies along response alternatives that present a high rather than a low range of frequencies. For example, Schwarz et al. (1985, Experiment 1) observed that 16.2% of a sample reported watching TV for more than 2½ hours per day when response alternatives ranged from "up to ½ hour" to "more than 2½ hours." The number of respondents that reported watching more than 2½ hours per day more than doubled to 37.5% when the response alternatives ranged from "up to 2½ hours" to "more than 4½ hours."

The Use of Memory-Based and Context-Based Information

Feldman and Lynch (1988) developed a framework that predicts that "an earlier response will be used as an input to a subsequent response if the former is accessible and if it is perceived to be more diagnostic than other accessible inputs" (p. 431). Whereas accessibility refers to ease of retrieving an input from memory, diagnosticity refers to the sufficiency of the retrieved input to arrive at a solution for the judgment task at hand. Therefore, the likelihood that the response to an earlier question will be used in a response to a later question is: (a) a positive function of the accessibility of the earlier question in memory; (b) a positive function of its diagnosticity for the later question; (c) a negative function of the accessibility of alternate inputs; and (d) a negative function of the diagnosticity of these accessible alternate inputs (Simmons, Bickart, & Lynch, 1993).

Using response alternatives to elicit frequency judgments, Menon, Raghubir, and Schwarz (1995, 1997) explored how information accessible in memory affects the use of contextual information used in arriving at judgments. Figure 5.1 captures the essence of their model. They theorized that the probability of using context-based information in forming a frequency judgment is inversely proportional to the diagnosticity (or sufficiency to arrive at a judgment) of the alternate inputs accessible in memory:

- when memory-based information is accessible and diagnostic, contextual information is not used unless the contextual information contributes to the overall diagnosticity of the available information;
- when memory-based information is accessible but not diagnostic, the use of contextual information depends on its perceived diagnosticity; and,

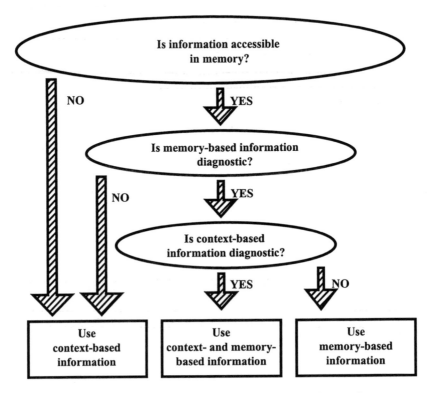

FIG. 5.1. The use of Memory and Contextual Information in Judgments. Source: Menon, Raghubir, and Schwarz (1997).

- when memory-based information is not accessible, contextual information is used even when its diagnosticity is questionable.

Response alternatives are readily accessible to respondents in the survey situation. They represent a source of relevant information that respondents could use to simplify a judgment task. As may be expected on theoretical grounds (Feldman & Lynch, 1988; Menon, Raghubir, & Schwarz, 1995, 1997), reliance on this source of information decreases when relevant behavioral information is easily accessible in memory. Specifically, Chassein, Strack, and Schwarz (1987) observed that subjects given an opportunity to refresh their episodic memory by browsing through last week's television schedule were able to eliminate the influence of the response scale. Similarly, Schwarz and Bienias (1990, Experiment 3) found that respondents who scored high on private self-consciousness, a trait associated with higher knowledge about oneself, were less affected by response alternatives than respondents who scored low on that trait. Finally, Schwarz and Bienias (1990, Experiments 1 and 2) also observed that because information regarding another's behaviors is less accessible than information about one's own behavior, proxy reports were more affected by response alternatives than self-reports. In addition, Bless, Bohner, Hild, and Schwarz (1992) observed that the impact of response alternatives decreased with decreasing complexity of the judgment task. All of these findings reflect the attenuating impact of alternative inputs on the influence of response alternatives.

Menon, Raghubir, and Schwarz (1995, 1997) found that the use of accessible and diagnostic information such as rates-of-occurrence (which exist for regular behaviors) lead to fewer influences by the context in which the question was asked. However, in the absence of such rate information in memory (as is the case for irregular behaviors), respondents attempted to infer the average frequency from the response alternatives provided to them and used this as the basis to compute their own frequency judgments.

Extending the theme of alternative inputs, Menon et al. (1995) also demonstrated that the impact of response alternatives on proxy reports depends on the proxy's similarity to the self and the accessibility of alternative information about one's own behavioral frequencies. Because respondents know more about their own than about another person's behavior (Schwarz & Bienias, 1990), Menon et al. ascertained that the information respondents infer from the context is used increasingly as they report about other people who they know less about. In other words, as specific information about the person the respondent is reporting about becomes less accessible or available in memory, contextual information becomes more and more diagnostic. Respondents rely less on memory-based information and more on the information provided by response alternatives. Of particular importance is the finding that the impact of response alternatives is strongly attenuated when the proxy is similar to the self and rate-based frequency information pertaining to the self is accessible, a contingency that had not been addressed in previous research (Schwarz & Bienias, 1990).

In short:

- the existence of a rate-of-occurrence in memory renders the information provided by the response alternatives less influential when respondents are asked about their own behavioral frequency;
- respondents rely on the information provided by response alternatives for irregular but not for regular behaviors.

Menon et al. (1995) demonstrated that there are two ways in which the response alternatives used to elicit self-reports may affect subsequent judgments about other people (see Fig. 5.2). The first way is indirect. Respondents may use information inferred from response alternatives to construct the earlier self-report and then use only their prior self-report as a basis for judging the other person. Paths 1 and 2 in Fig. 5.2 illustrate this indirect route. The second way is direct. Even if subjects did not incorporate information inferred from the response alternatives into their self-reports, the information from these alternatives from the prior self-report question is now accessible in memory. They can now use this accessible information to form judgments about the other person. Path 3 in Fig. 5.2 highlights this

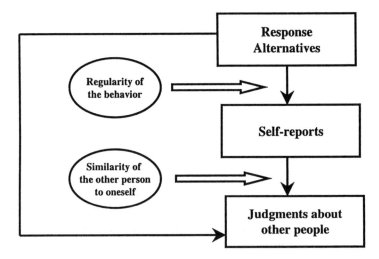

FIG. 5.2. Direct and indirect effects of response alternatives on frequency judgments. From "Behavioral frequency judgments: An accessibility-diagnosticity framework," by G. Menon, P. Raghubir, and N. Schwartz, 1995, *Journal of Consumer Research, 22*, pp. 212–228. Copyright © 1995 by The University of Chicago Press. Reprinted with permission.

direct influence. The direct versus the indirect use of response alternatives in formulating frequency judgments about other people varies as a function of: (a) the regularity of the behavior; and (b) the similarity of the other person to oneself. The results of mediational analyses (Baron & Kenny, 1986) provide support for these hypotheses of direct and indirect effects.

Theoretically, this model makes an important contribution by teasing apart the factors that make memory versus contextual cues diagnostic in judgment formation. Therefore, for regular behaviors, memory-based information should be accessible, leading to the lower use of context-based information. Although previous research demonstrated that the impact of response alternatives is less pronounced when memory-based information is accessible (Schwarz, 1990), this research has not addressed the moderating role of behavioral regularity. Rather, respondents in previous studies were given an opportunity to refresh their memory, for example, by browsing through a TV magazine prior to reporting their TV viewership during the last week. That such manipulations reduced the impact of response alternatives is consistent with the assumptions underlying the present studies. The Menon et al. studies extended the exploration of memory-based information by assessing the impact of a variable of considerable applied importance, namely the behavior's regularity.

TOWARD MORE ACCURATE DATA

Given what we know about the biases associated with judgments formed on the basis of memory-based and context-based information, the important question becomes what can we, as researchers, do to improve the accuracy of frequency judgments elicited. Traditionally, the approach to increasing accuracy has emphasized the elimination of contextual effects. For example, Schwarz and Hippler (N. Schwarz, personal communication, December 9, 1998) found that the impact of response alternatives is completely eliminated when the informational value of the response alternatives is called into question. Telling respondents that they were participating in a pretest designed to explore the adequacy of the scale erased the response alternative effect. Decreasing the diagnosticity of the scale was also accomplished by telling student respondents that the measurement scale had been borrowed from a disparate group, the elderly. Although it is important to decrease the inaccuracies of judgments that may result from contextual cues, it would also be beneficial if we could harness these context effects and enable respondents to increase the accuracy of their judgments elicited from memory.

One method that sheds insight into how this may be accomplished is by examining the process by which respondents form their behavioral judgments. Burton and Blair (1991) studied the effects of event frequency, question wording, and reference timeframe on the accuracy of frequency estimates. They hypothesized that respondents would tend to use more episodic recall strategies as the frequency of the event went up, with the use of open-ended (vs. closed-ended questions), and with a longer response time. They also hypothesized that the use of these strategies that were supposed to induce episodic recall would also enhance the accuracy of frequency estimates. However, they did not find strong support for their hypotheses. One of the reasons for this might be that episodic recall may not always be the best route for a respondent to take in a survey situation if more diagnostic, heuristic-type information is present in memory. For example, the presence of rates in memory for regular behaviors enhances the accuracy of frequency estimates of such behaviors.

When eliciting responses for irregular behaviors, an episodic recall strategy may provide a more accurate response. Still, inducing episodic recall does not guarantee greater accuracy. When respondents are asked how frequently they engage in a particular behavior in a survey, they search their memories trying to use some or all of the accessible information to form a judgment (Bradburn, Rips, & Shevell, 1987). Irregular behaviors are difficult to estimate precisely because information is not accessible. Therefore, besides eliciting episodic recall, we must also provide a method for making irregular behaviors more accessible.

Menon (1997) demonstrated that when information is not easily accessible in memory, providing contextual cues in the questionnaire increases the accuracy of the formulated judgment. The decompositional question, which involves providing cues, aims at making this process of recall easier. The decompositional question is hypothesized to counteract the effects of recency, vividness, or salience that make some episodes more easily accessible than others and lead to highly erroneous frequency judgments. This is because the cues provided draw the respondent's attention to various scenarios in which the behavior may have been engaged in, besides the ones that are salient in memory. However, the effectiveness of this cueing question form depends enormously on the quality of the cues developed and there may continue to remain instances that cannot be tapped through cues.

Breaking up a behavior into various subcategories eases the process by which the respondent generates frequencies by recalling specific instances. For example, suppose we want to measure the number of times a respondent has dined at a restaurant in the past month. Because this can be a frequent, yet irregular behavior, asking the respondent directly, "How many times have you eaten at a restaurant in the past month?" is likely to provide an inaccurate response. Greater accuracy could be achieved through a decompositional question. A decompositional question eliciting the frequency of eating at restaurants would provide a mutually exclusive, collectively exhaustive list of various occasions or situations under which a person would visit a restaurant (e.g., with friends, for lunch, for a date, and so on) and determine the number of times the person went to the restaurant for each of these occasions or situations. This process makes recall within each subcategory easier. For the cues provided through the decompositional question to be effective, they should coincide with the natural categories that are used by respondents to classify events (Barsalou, 1983; Hu, Toh, & Lee, 1996) because people are very sensitive to frequencies within such categories and are able to estimate such instances fairly accurately under diverse task instructions (Alba, Chromiak, Hasher, & Attig, 1980).

Providing cues through the use of a decompositional question serves to enhance the accuracy of the reports, contingent on the following conditions:

- the effectiveness of this question is moderated by the regularity of the target behavior such that the accuracy of frequency judgments pertaining to regular behaviors are not enhanced, but those pertaining to irregular behaviors are;
- the effectiveness of this question is mediated through the cognitive process used for the task, such that the use of the decompositional question enhances episodic recall. This works well for irregular behaviors (because episodes are not well represented in memory) and decreases the associated perceived cognitive effort, but not for regular behaviors (because memory-based information such as rates of occurrence are already highly accessible in memory and can be used in generating a frequency judgment), and increases the associated perceived cognitive effort.

Therefore, Menon (1997) proposed and found support for a mediated-moderation model of behavioral frequency judgments (cf. Baron & Kenny, 1986; see Fig. 5.3). She demonstrated that the use of the decompositional question enhances the use of episodic recall (Path 1). Decompositional questions also increased the perceived cognitive effort associated with generating a frequency judgment for regular behaviors and decreased it for irregular behaviors (Path 2). Similar effects manifested for the accuracy of the frequency judgment, where responses to questions about irregular behaviors were more accurate, but not for regular behaviors (Path 3). These effects on perceived cognitive effort and accuracy manifested because of the change in the cognitive process that the decompositional question triggers (i.e., Paths 1 & 4 and 1 & 5). Therefore, the effect of question wording on perceived cognitive effort and accuracy was mediated through the cognitive process.

In sum, Menon (1997) investigated the theoretical underpinnings of accuracy as a basis for demonstrating that contextual factors such as question

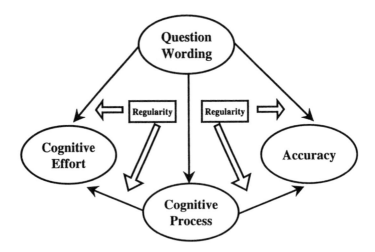

FIG. 5.3. A mediation–moderation model of frequency formulation. From "Are the parts better than the whole? The effects of decompositional questions on judgments of frequent behaviors," by G. Menon, 1997, *Journal of Marketing Research, 32*, pp. 212–228. Copyright © 1997 by the American Marketing Association. Reprinted with permission.

wording can be used to increase response accuracy by creating a better match between accessible information in memory and contextual cues. This work extends the work of Burton and Blair (1991) and demonstrates that the effects of question wording on perceived cognitive effort and accuracy are mediated by the cognitive process employed by respondents. It provides a specific method that marketing researchers can use to increase the accuracy of behavioral frequency judgments; that is, breaking up an overall frequency into parts decreases the cognitive load on respondents and increases the accuracy of frequency reports associated with irregular, but not regular, behaviors. These findings extend earlier work by showing that the accuracy of frequency reports is not only highly contingent on the regularity of the behavior but also the cognitive process used by the respondent. This is a particularly important finding given that regular behaviors are reported accurately in an open-ended question but for irregular behaviors, the use of cues enhances accuracy.

DISCUSSION

The focus of this chapter was to understand the cognitive mechanisms by which frequency judgments are generated in surveys, and to evaluate whether we can increase the accuracy of these frequency reports. Studies by Blair and Burton (1987) and Burton and Blair (1991) indicate that the cognitive processes that respondents use to arrive at a frequency depend on the relative frequency of the target event. Although it is easy to recall and count every instance of an infrequent behavior, it becomes more difficult to do so when a behavior occurs frequently. For frequent behaviors, respondents may use other strategies to provide an estimate (Blair & Burton, 1987; Burton & Blair, 1991; Menon, 1993; Ross, 1984; Schwarz, 1990; Strube, 1987). For example, one might use the rate-of-occurrence of twice a day in judging how many times one showered last week and arrive at the frequency judgment of 14 times. The use of such estimation procedures by survey respondents is consistent with current theory that people are cognitive misers who use heuristics to arrive at decisions and judgments efficiently (Newell & Simon, 1972; Taylor, 1981; Wyer & Srull, 1986, 1989). To the extent that behavioral frequencies are reported based on inferential heuristics, they are judgments and are subjective. This led Schwarz (1990) to conclude that the traditional distinction between opinion questions (presumably answered on the basis of somewhat unreliable judgmental processes) and factual questions (presumably answered on the basis of more reliable recall from memory) is misleading.

In this chapter, we have summarized the evidence that respondents in a survey situation tend to assess the accessibility of inputs in memory for the judgment task at hand. They evaluate the diagnosticity of this information, relative to the information that they infer from the context. They then combine the information to arrive at a judgment. What we then have are two sets of factors:

- information internal to the respondent (e.g., information they have in their memory) that researchers cannot control;
- information external to the respondent (e.g., contextual cues) that researchers have control over.

In the specific case of behavioral frequency judgments, we have reported the findings from various papers that indicate that such judgments are arrived at using different processing strategies, depending on the regularity of the behavior. The use of a rate-of-occurrence, as with a regular behavior, results in fairly accurate judgments. Therefore, it may be worthwhile eliciting rates-of-occurrence, whenever they exist, instead of frequency judgments. For irregular behaviors, however, a consumer researcher can either: (a) elicit rates-of-occurrence for regular subdomains, or (b) provide better episodic cues to enhance the accessibility of specific instances of the behavior and also provide a method by which respondents are better able to demarcate the reference period to minimize the overreporting that such cues may facilitate (e.g., Loftus & Marsburger, 1983).

From a practical standpoint, we can make the following recommendations for designing questions that elicit frequency judgments:

- Frequencies of regular behaviors can be elicited using open-ended questions with a fairly high level of accuracy. Further, the use of response alternatives does not bias the frequency judgments for these kinds of behaviors.
- Frequencies of irregular behaviors are more difficult to construct for respondents. Researchers should ensure that the cues provided by the context are ones that help respondents construct accurate judgments, and not ones that bias. We know from the literature on the effects of response alternatives that respondents are easily swayed by any information that they infer is being communicated to them.

In conclusion, understanding the organization of autobiographical memory in the interest of designing better questionnaires that elicit more accurate information is extremely important and is attracting more attention among researchers (see Sudman, Bradburn, & Schwarz, 1996, for a review). Although some research has focused solely on the effects of accessibility of alternate sources of information in memory on frequency judgments (e.g., Blair & Burton, 1987; Menon, 1993), others have examined the effects of contextual information on response accuracy (e.g., Burton & Blair, 1991; Menon et al., 1995). This chapter integrated these findings into a framework that examines the cognitive processes that underlie the estimates of frequency reports, with the objective of prescribing questioning tools that enhance their accuracy in surveys.

There are yet some unanswered questions that could be addressed in future research. For example, most of the empirical studies reported in this chapter have dealt with frequently occurring everyday behaviors. For infrequent behaviors, individual episodes are likely to be accessible for formulating frequency judgments. However, what if the infrequent behavior is also regular? One of the research questions of interest is whether the actual frequency of the behavior moderates the accuracy of rates-of-occurrence as a heuristic such that rates produce more accurate results for frequent behaviors, but not infrequently occurring ones. It is likely, therefore, that for low-frequency events, people will tend to use an episodic recall strategy that will lead to accurate results, just as rate-based estimation leads to more accurate results for high-frequency events.

As the literature suggests, regular behaviors are reported more accurately than irregular behaviors, presumably because people have access to robust rates-of-occurrence in memory that have been developed over one's lifetime and hence are very reliable. Therefore, accessibility of information in memory appears to be the key here. Another interesting area to pursue in the future is the role of individual characteristics (e.g., cognitive capacity), their effects on information accessibility, and on the subsequent use of different strategies (episodic recall vs. estimate) and how it moderates the effects on accuracy. For example, it is possible that inaccuracies result because of processes used at encoding versus retrieval. Specifically, the cognitive capacity that the person has at encoding may determine the accessibility of various inputs (e.g., episodes vs. rates-of-occurrence), and the cognitive capacity at retrieval will determine the kind of judgment strategy used (i.e., episodic recall vs. estimation). These questions still need to be addressed by future research.

REFERENCES

Alba, J. W., Chromiak, W., Hasher, L., & Attig, M. S. (1980). Automatic encoding of category size information. *Journal of Experimental Psychology: Human Learning and Memory, 6*(4), 370–378.

Baron, R. M., & Kenny, D. A. (1986). The moderator-mediator variable distinction in social psychological research: Conceptual, strategic, and statistical considerations. *Journal of Personality and Social Psychology, 51*(6), 1173–1182.

Barsalou, L. W. (1983). Ad hoc categories. *Memory and Cognition, 11*(3), 211–227.

Bickart, B. (1993, February). Carryover and backfire effects in marketing research. *Journal of Marketing Research, 30*, 52–62.

Bishop, G. F., Hippler, H. J., Schwarz, N., & Strack, F. (1988). A comparison of response effects in self-administered and telephone surveys. In R. M. Groves, P. Biemer, L. Lyberg, J. Massey, W. Nicholls, & J. Waksberg (Eds.), *Telephone survey methodology* (pp. 321–340). New York: Wiley.

Blair, E., & Burton, S. (1987, September). Cognitive processes used by survey respondents to answer behavioral frequency questions. *Journal of Consumer Research, 14*, 280–288.

Bless, H., Bohner, G., Hild, T., & Schwarz, N. (1992). Asking difficult questions: Task complexity increases the impact of response alternatives. *European Journal of Social Psychology, 22*, 309–312.

Bradburn, N. M., Rips, L. J., & Shevell, S. K. (1987). Answering autobiographical questions: The impact of memory and inference on surveys. *Science, 236*, 157–161.

Burton, S., & Blair, E. (1991). Task conditions, response formulation processes, and response accuracy for behavioral frequency questions in surveys. *Public Opinion Quarterly, 55*(1), 50–79.

Chassein, B., Strack, F., & Schwarz, N. (1987). *Erinnerungsstrategie und Häufigkeitsskala: Zum unterschiedlichen Einfluß von relationaler versus episodischer Erinnerung auf Häufigkeitsurteile* [Recall strategy and frequency scales: The differential impact of relational vs. episodic recall on frequency judgments]. 29th Tagung Experimentell Arbeitender Psychologen, Aachen, Germany.

Feldman, J. M., & Lynch, J. G. (1988). Self-generated validity and other effects of measurement on belief, attitude, intention, and behavior. *Journal of Applied Psychology, 73*, 421–435.

Hu, M. Y., Toh, R. S., & Lee, E. (1996). Impact of the level of aggregation on response accuracy in surveys of behavioral frequency. *Marketing Letters, 7*(4), 371–382.

Loftus, E. F., & Marsburger, W. (1983, March). Since the eruption of Mt. St. Helens, has anyone beaten you up? Improving the accuracy of retrospective reports with landmark events. *Memory and Cognition, 11*, 114–120.

March, J. G., & Simon, H. A. (1958). *Organizations*. New York: Wiley.

Menon, G. (1993, December). The effects of accessibility of information in memory on judgments of behavioral frequencies. *Journal of Consumer Research, 20,* 431–440.

Menon, G. (1994). Judgments of behavioral frequencies: Memory search and retrieval strategies. In N. Schwarz & S. Sudman (Eds.), *Autobiographical memory and the validity of retrospective reports* (pp. 161–172). New York: Springer-Verlag.

Menon, G. (1997, August). Are the parts better than the whole? The effects of decompositional questions on judgments of frequent behaviors. *Journal of Marketing Research, 32,* 335–346.

Menon, G., Raghubir, P., & Schwarz, N. (1995, September). Behavioral frequency judgments: An accessibility-diagnosticity framework. *Journal of Consumer Research, 22,* 212–228.

Menon, G., Raghubir, P., & Schwarz, N. (1997). How much will I spend? Factors affecting consumers' estimates of future expenses. *Journal of Consumer Psychology, 6*(2), 141–164.

Newell, A., & Simon, H. (1972). *Human problem solving.* Englewood Cliffs, NJ: Prentice Hall.

Povel, D. (1981, February). Internal representation of simple temporal patterns. *Journal of Experimental Psychology: Human Perception and Performance, 7,* 3–18.

Ross, L. (1984). Thoughts and research on estimates about past and future behaviour. In T. M. Jabine, M. Straf, J. M. Tanur, & R. Tourangeau (Eds.), *Cognitive aspects of survey methodology: Building a bridge between disciplines* (pp. 61–64). Washington, DC: National Academy Press.

Schwarz, N. (1990). Assessing frequency reports of mundane behavior: Contribution of cognitive psychology to questionnaire construction. In C. Hendrick & M. Clark (Eds.), *Research methods in personality and social psychology* (pp. 98–119). Newbury Park, CA: Sage.

Schwarz, N., & Bienias, J. (1990). What mediates the impact of response alternatives on frequency reports of mundane behaviors? *Applied Cognitive Psychology, 4,* 61–72.

Schwarz, N., & Clore, G. L. (1988). How do I feel about it? Informative functions of affective states. In K. Fiedler & J. Forgas (Eds.), *Affect, cognition, and social behavior* (pp. 544–620). Toronto: Hogrefe International.

Schwarz, N., & Hippler, H. J. (1987). What response scales may tell your respondents: Informative functions of response alternatives. In H. J. Hippler, N. Schwarz, & S. Sudman (Eds.), *Social information processing and survey methodology* (pp. 163–178). New York: Springer-Verlag.

Schwarz, N., & Hippler, H. J. (1991). Response alternatives: The impact of their choice and presentation order. In P. P. Biemer, R. M. Groves, L. E. Lyberg, N. A. Mathiowetz, & S. Sudman (Eds.), *Measurement errors in surveys* (pp. 41–56). New York: Wiley.

Schwarz, N., & Hippler, H. J. (1995). Subsequent questions may influence answers to preceding questions in mail surveys. *Public Opinion Quarterly, 59,* 93–97.

Schwarz, N., Hippler, H. J., Deutsch, B., & Strack, F. (1985). Response categories: Effects on behavioral reports and comparative judgments. *Public Opinion Quarterly, 49,* 388–395.

Schwarz, N., & Scheuring, B. (1988). Judgments of relationship satisfaction: Inter- and intraindividual comparisons as a function of questionnaire structure. *European Journal of Social Psychology, 18,* 485–496.

Schwarz, N., & Strack, F. (Eds.). (1991). Social cognition and communication: human judgment in its social context [Special Issue]. *Social Cognition, 9*(1), 1–125.

Schwarz, N., & Sudman, S. (Eds.). (1991). *Context effects in social and psychological research.* New York: Springer-Verlag.

Simmons, C. J., Bickart, B. A., & Lynch, J. G., Jr. (1993). Capturing and creating public opinion in survey research. *Journal of Consumer Research, 20*(2), 316–329.

Simon, H. A., & Kotovsky, K. (1963, November). Human acquisition of concepts for sequential patterns. *Psychological Review, 70,* 534–546.

Strack, F., Schwarz, N., & Wänke, M. (1991). Semantic and pragmatic aspects of context effects in social and psychological research. *Social Cognition, 9,* 111–125.

Strube, G. (1987). Answering survey questions: The role of memory. In H. J. Hippler, N. Schwarz, & S. Sudman (Eds.), *Social information processing and survey methodology* (pp. 86–101). New York: Springer-Verlag.

Sudman, S., Bradburn, N. M., & Schwarz, N. (1996). *Thinking about answers: The application of cognitive processes to survey methodology*. San Francisco: Jossey-Bass.

Taylor, S. E. (1981). The interface of cognitive and social psychology. In J. H. Harvey (Ed.), *Cognition, social behaviour and the environment* (pp. 189–211). Hillsdale, NJ: Lawrence Erlbaum Associates.

Tversky, A., & Kahneman, D. (1974). Judgment under uncertainty: Heuristics and biases. *Science, 185*, 1124–1131.

Wyer, R. S., & Srull, T. K. (1986). Human cognition in its social context. *Psychological Review, 93*(3), 322–359.

Wyer, R. S., & Srull, T. K. (1989). *Memory and cognition in its social context*. Hillsdale, NJ: Lawrence Erlbaum Associates.

6

Emotion and Memory: Implications for Self-Report

John F. Kihlstrom
University of California, Berkeley

Eric Eich
University of British Columbia

Deborah Sandbrand
University of California, Los Angeles

Betsy A. Tobias
University of Arizona

So much of social and behavioral science research on health and mental health depends on self-reports of current states, as when we collect information from patients about their presenting symptoms and complaints, or on self-reports of the past, as when we collect historical information about past episodes of illness and life experiences that may be risk factors for illness. The first is a problem of perception; the second is a problem of memory. Both perception and memory, especially as we encounter them in clinical research, are constructive and reconstructive activities in which judgment and inference play large roles. The study of perception, memory, and judgment is what cognitive psychology is all about, and indeed cognitive psychology has been quite successful in explaining how these basic mental functions operate. Over the past few years, however, psychologists have increasingly come to realize that cognitive processes are not isolated from the rest of mental life and in particular that our emotional and motivational states may affect what we perceive and remember as well as the judgments we make about the present and the past (for general reviews, see Blaney, 1986; Bower, 1981; Christianson, 1992b; Clark & Fiske, 1982; Eich, 1995a; Ekman

& Davidson, 1994; Ellis & Moore, in press; Fiedler & Forgas, 1988; Forgas, 1991; Johnson & Magaro, 1987; Kuiken, 1991; Niedenthal & Kitayama, 1994). Much of this literature has focused on memory.

AFFECTIVE VALENCE AND AFFECTIVE INTENSITY

Two emotional effects on memory have to do with the emotional valence, positive or negative, of the material to be remembered and the cues used for retrieval regardless of the mood state of the person doing the remembering. The more familiar of these is the affective valence effect: In general, information associated with positive affect is more easily remembered than that associated with negative affect (Fig. 6.1a). The tendency to remember that which is agreeable, and to forget that which is disagreeable, is some-

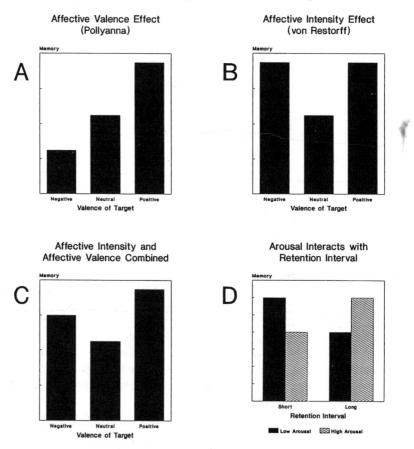

FIG. 6.1. Schematic depiction of affective arousal effects.

times taken as evidence for the psychoanalytic concept of repression (for reviews see Singer, 1990), but this is a mistake: As Rapaport (1942) noted, Freud's notion of repression covers material that is associated with primitive sexual and aggressive motives and the anxiety aroused by their conflict with social strictures, not the merely unpleasant. Nevertheless, the general tendency to favor positive over negative material is so intuitively appealing that it has acquired its own special label, the Pollyanna Principle (Boucher & Osgood, 1969; Matlin & Stang, 1978).

Matlin and Stang (1978) reviewed a wealth of literature indicating that, on average, subjects favor positive over negative material in attention, perception, language, word associations, learning, memory, thinking, judgment, and social cognition, and they concluded that, "This preference for the pleasant seemed to invade every area of experimental psychology that we examined, and the effects were usually remarkably robust" (pp. 2–3). They further proposed, following Erdelyi (1974), that human information processing is necessarily selective and that the seeking of pleasure and avoidance of displeasure are the most important principles on which this selectivity is based.

While focusing their attention on the Pollyanna Principle, Matlin and Stang (1978) also acknowledged the operation of another, secondary principle, the Intensity Principle: that intense or highly polarized items are processed more efficiently than neutral or less intense items (Dutta & Kanungo, 1975). We refer to this principle as the affective intensity effect: Memories associated with some affect, or emotional arousal, are better remembered than those that are affectively neutral, regardless of whether the emotional valence is positive or negative (Fig. 6.1b). In part, the affective intensity effect is a special case of the familiar salience effect on memory, also known as the von Restorff effect, after the researcher who first noted it: More salient events are more memorable than less salient ones (von Restorff, 1933; see also Fabiani & Donchin, 1995; Hunt, 1995; Tversky & Kahneman, 1973). Apparently, possessing some emotional valence is one of the things that can render a memory salient.

Matlin and Stang (1978) attempted to reconcile the effects of affective valence and affective intensity by proposing a J-shaped function relating emotional valence to memorability (Fig. 6.1c). Items associated with both negative and positive affective valence are more memorable than those with no valence but items with a positive valence are more memorable than those with a negative valence. Unfortunately, this compromise is threatened by a methodological flaw (Banaji & Hardin, 1994). Although studies of affective intensity have usually controlled for the conditions under which the memories in question were encoded, studies of affective valence generally have not done so. There is now reason to think that positive events are more arousing than negative ones, on average, and that when intensity is controlled, what looks like an affective valence effect may really resolve to an affective intensity effect (Banaji & Hardin, 1994). There may well be an affective valence effect on memory, independent of affective intensity, but further research will be necessary to demonstrate it convincingly.

An interesting aspect of the affective intensity effect is its interaction with time. More than 30 years ago, Kleinsmith and Kaplan (1963, 1964) performed an experiment in which they recorded physiological arousal during encoding and then tested memory at delays of 2 minutes to 7 days. At short intervals, items associated with relatively high arousal were poorly remembered; at long intervals, however, these same items were well remembered. The Kleinsmith and Kaplan effect has proved difficult to replicate but it shines through in a meta-analysis of replication attempts (Park & Banaji, 1997), and has been confirmed experimentally (Crowder et al., 1997).

The Kleinsmith and Kaplan (1963, 1994) effect is not an artifact of statistical regression but rather is a genuine crossover interaction: Memories associated with high levels of arousal are remembered poorly over the short term but well over the long term. The effect is of great interest in the context of the current controversy over recovered memories of childhood sexual abuse, although it should be noted that the retention intervals involved in these experiments, minutes and days, pale before the years and decades claimed in cases of recovered memory. In the final analysis, the important issue in the recovered memory debate remains that of providing independent corroboration for any incidents of abuse that a subject or patient might remember.

AROUSAL AND MOOD

The affective intensity and affective valence effects are sometimes construed as being generated by the affective properties of the memories themselves. But in the Kleinsmith and Kaplan (1963, 1964) experiment, the fate of the memories could not be predicted from the affective valence of the items in the abstract. The effect only emerged when the researchers considered the subject's actual affective response to each item. In other words, the subject's affective state is at least as important as the affective valence of what he or she is trying to remember—and, in fact, it may be that encoding or retrieving any affectively valenced material induces a corresponding emotional state in the subject.

Historically, perhaps the most familiar consequence of the subject's affective state is known as the Yerkes-Dodson Law (Yerkes & Dodson, 1908; for recent reviews, see Anderson, 1990; Neiss, 1988): Arousal is related to task performance by an inverted-U-shaped function (Fig. 6.2a). In the memory context, of course, arousal level may affect both encoding and retrieval

Yerkes-Dodson Effect

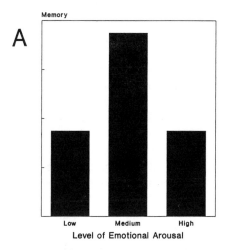

Resource Allocation Effects

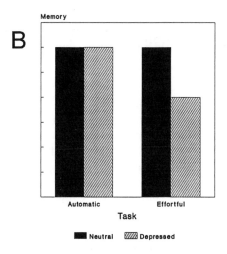

FIG. 6.2. Schematic depiction of arousal state effects.

operations. Although a number of competing explanations have been put forward for the effects of arousal on memory (for reviews, see Christianson, 1992a; Eysenck, 1976; Heuer & Reisberg, 1992; Mandler, 1992; Revelle & Loftus, 1992), in general terms we may hypothesize that low levels of arousal (e.g., during fatigue or drowsiness) are associated with low levels of attention, poor encodings of events as they occur, and poor memory for these events later. Increasing arousal also increases the deployment of attention, resulting in better memory, but very high levels of arousal may increase the information processing load and thus effectively reduce the amount of information being processed—the result, again, is poor encoding, and poor memory, especially of peripheral details.

Shifting from undifferentiated arousal to valenced mood, Fig. 6.2b shows that the effects on memory of low arousal levels are paralleled in the resource allocation effects of depression on ongoing information-processing tasks, including the encoding and retrieval of memories (Ellis & Ashbrook, 1988, 1989; see also Hertel, 1994). In particular, depressed mood appears to increase the person's information-processing load (Ellis & Ashbrook, 1988, 1989)—or, alternatively, his or her level of initiative (Hertel, 1994). In the former case, the added internal cognitive activity drains attentional resources that would otherwise be devoted to other tasks; in the latter case, available attentional resources simply are not devoted to the task in the first place. Either situation results in poor encoding of material presented during a depressed mood and performance deficits on subsequent retention tests—especially if these tasks themselves are cognitively demanding.

The resource allocation effects of negative moods are fairly well documented at this point, but we have little information about comparable effects of positive mood states. Comparing the effects of positive and negative moods is of considerable theoretical importance in determining underlying mechanisms (Kihlstrom, 1989). For example, if resource allocation effects are mediated by the distracting effect of the person's mood-relevant thoughts, as Ellis and Ashbrook (1988, 1989) suggested, we should expect happy and sad moods to have the same effects on information processing. On the other hand, it might be that depressed moods have a more specific effect on attentional allocation policy—for example, by reducing people's interest in their surroundings and consequently their motivation to pay attention to them, as suggested by Hertel (1994). In this case, happiness and sadness should have opposite effects: The sad person's disinterest should impair cognitive processing, whereas the happy person's peppiness should facilitate it.

MOOD-DEPENDENT MEMORY

Perhaps the most dramatic and controversial effects of the person's mood state are seen in mood-dependent memory, which occurs when retrieval of material is enhanced by reinstating the mood that the individual was in when the material was initially encoded (Bower, 1981). The notion of mood-dependent memory, illustrated in Fig. 6.3a, is based on an analogy with the state-dependent memory produced by pharmacological substances that act

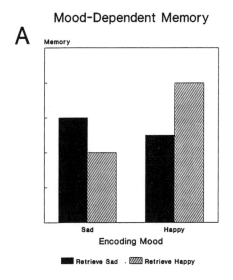

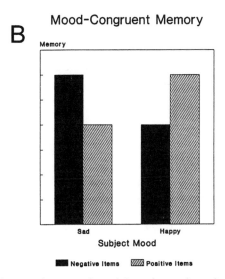

FIG. 6.3.   Schematic depiction of mood-dependent and mood-congruent memory effects.

directly on the central nervous system (Overton, 1984; for reviews see Eich, 1980, 1989); conceptually similar environment-dependent memory effects have been observed in experiments where the encoding and retrieval phases take place in different physical environments (e.g., Godden & Baddeley, 1975; Smith, Glenberg, & Bjork, 1978), at different times of day (e.g., Holloway, 1978), or while listening to different kinds of music (e.g., Balch & Lewis, 1996).

In all these cases, the memorability of an event is a function of the congruence between the context in which the memory is encoded and that in which retrieval is attempted. These context effects, in turn, exemplify a more general encoding specificity principle in memory, which states that memory is best when the processing operations performed at the time of retrieval match those that were performed at the time of encoding (Tulving & Thomson, 1973; see also Kihlstrom & Barnhardt, 1993).

Some early support for mood-dependent memory came from studies of patients with bipolar affective disorder (Weingartner, Miller, & Murphy, 1977) and normal subjects threatened with electric shock (Macht, Spear, & Levis, 1977). Following those early studies, however, mood dependence assumed a "now you see it, now you don't" quality. Mood-dependent memory has rarely been observed in straightforward designs in which subjects study a single word list in one mood and are tested for memory in the same or a different mood (e.g., Bower, Monteiro, & Gilligan, 1978). Bower et al. (1978) were able to produce the effect using an interference design employing two word lists but subsequent conceptual replications have yielded mixed results (e.g., Bower, Gilligan, & Monteiro, 1981); interestingly, environment-dependent effects on memory also appeared to be unreliable (Fernandez & Glenberg, 1985). In the face of these failures to replicate, Bower and Mayer (1989) concluded that mood dependence was evanescent rather than robust and that most of the earlier positive results, including Bower's own, may well have been spurious outcomes—a point of view apparently shared by some other reviewers of this literature (Blaney, 1986; Leventhal & Tomarken, 1986).

In the most recent turn of events, Eich and his colleagues developed a paradigm in which mood dependence can be reliably produced in the laboratory (Eich, 1995b). For example, Eich and Metcalfe (1989) employed a musical mood-induction procedure and asked subjects to study a list of words; later, they went through the musical mood-induction procedure again and attempted to remember the items they had studied previously. Testing revealed strong evidence of mood dependence: Items studied while subjects were sad were remembered better when the subjects were also sad during the memory test and items studied while they were happy were remembered better when they were happy. The same experiment also illustrated the resource allocation effects of sad mood on encoding and retrieval: Compared to the condition where subjects were happy during both encoding and retrieval, memory was relatively poor when subjects were sad while encoding, regardless of whether the retrieval state was happy or sad, and when subjects were sad while retrieving, regardless of whether the encoding state was happy or sad. Other experiments in Eich's laboratory have yielded similar effects for the retrieval of autobiographical memories as opposed to word lists (Eich, Macaulay, & Ryan, 1994). Eich, Macaulay, and Lam (1997) reported good evidence for mood-dependent memory in bipolar affective disorder (manic-depressive illness).[1]

Mood dependence can affect memory processes even if subjects are not engaged in tasks that would ordinarily be considered to involve memory. At issue here is the distinction between explicit memory, or conscious recollection, and implicit memory, or the influence of memory on task performance, independent of conscious recollection (Schacter, 1987). Almost all studies of emotion and memory involve explicit memory tasks such as free recall, cued recall, and recognition. Implicit memory tasks have been studied in the literature on resource allocation effects, where it has been found that depression impairs performance on explicit memory tasks, which typically make considerable demands on attentional resources but not on implicit memory tasks, which are less dependent on attention (e.g., Ellis & Ashbrook, 1988, 1989). Macaulay, Ryan, and Eich (1993) found evidence of mood dependence in performance on a category-generation test of implicit memory.

From one point of view, it might be thought that mood dependence would have little or no effect on implicit memory. After all, as a general rule, implicit memory transfers when explicit memory does not (Roediger & McDermott, 1993). As an example, performance on at least some implicit memory tasks is spared in cases of multiple personality disorder (also known as dissociative identity disorder), even when the interpersonality amnesia profoundly impairs performance on explicit memory tasks (e.g., Eich, Macaulay, Loewenstein, & Dihle, 1997; Nissen, Ross, Willingham, MacKenzie, & Schacter, 1988; for a review, see Kihlstrom & Schacter, 1995). On the other hand, Tobias (1992; Tobias, Kihlstrom, & Schacter, 1992) suggested that mood dependence might be greater in implicit, compared to explicit, memory. It is known that drug-state dependency effects on explicit memory are cue dependent: The effect is found when the memory task employs relatively impoverished retrieval cues, such as free recall, but not with relatively rich cues, such as cued recall or recognition (Eich, 1980, 1989). According to Tobias (1992), implicit memory tasks involve the most impoverished retrieval cues of all—after all, they do not even specify that the subject should retrieve a memory. Her first study, which compared stem-cued recall to stem completion, found no evidence of mood dependence on either explicit or implicit memory. However, her second study, which compared free recall to a novel test of free association, found a small but significant mood-dependent effect on implicit, but not explicit, memory. Although further studies along these

---

[1]Interestingly, Eich (1995a; Eich & Birnbaum, 1988) argued that drug state- and environment-dependent memory is, in turn, mediated by emotional states; Balch and Lewis (1996) made the same claim for music-dependent memory, and given what we know about circadian effects on arousal levels, it may well be that emotional state accounts for time-dependent memory as well.

lines need to be performed, the important point is that mood-dependent memory may affect performance even on tasks that do not seem to involve conscious recollection of the past.

Mood-dependent memory is not merely a curiosity of mental life but may have broad practical and theoretical implications. For example, mood-dependent memory may be implicated in the perseveration of clinical episodes of depression in affective disorder patients. That is to say, negative mood may make negative memories more available, thus reinforcing the negative mood, which makes negative memories even more available, and so on in a vicious cycle. More important, in the present context, it means that it may be hard for people who are currently depressed to remember times when they were happy, and vice versa, making cognitive-behavioral therapy more difficult and distorting their memories of childhood and other possibly critical events.

MOOD-CONGRUENT MEMORY

Concern about memory distortion is strengthened by another set of mood-memory effects, which go by the label of mood-congruent memory: Mood state facilitates the processing of material with a similar emotional valence and impairs the processing of material with the opposite valence (for reviews, see Blaney, 1986; Bower & Forgas, in press; Johnson & Magaro, 1987; Leventhal & Tomarken, 1986). The effect is illustrated in Fig. 6.3b. Conceptually, mood-congruent memory effects can be separated into those that operate at the encoding stage (mood-congruent encoding) and those that operate at the retrieval stage (mood-congruent retrieval) but the outcome of these processes is the same: better memory for information whose affective valence matches the valence of the person's mood at the time information processing occurs.

Mood-congruent encoding appears to be mediated by attentional processes: Happy subjects pay more attention to positive items, whereas sad subjects pay more attention to negative ones. Among patients, mood-dependent encoding is more likely to occur in cases of depression than of anxiety disorder, perhaps because anxious individuals are hypervigilant and deploy attention away from threat cues (Mathews & MacLeod, 1994; Mineka, 1992). In the present context, however, mood-congruent retrieval is the more important effect because it raises the possibility that the subject's mood state at the time of inquiry may bias his or her self-reports of past experiences—happy subjects more likely to retrieve happy memories, and sad subjects more likely to retrieve sad ones. In fact, *prima facie* evidence for mood-congruent retrieval comes from studies of autobiographical memory where both clinical and nonclinical subjects have been found to access personal memories that are affectively congruent with mood state at time of retrieval more readily than incongruent ones (e.g., Lloyd & Lishman, 1975; Teasdale & Fogarty, 1979; Teasdale & Russell, 1983).

Demonstrations of mood-congruent memory have sometimes been interpreted as instances of mood dependence on the assumption that unpleasant events induce unpleasant mood states in those who experience them and pleasant events induce pleasant mood states. This is an interesting theoretical controversy—unfortunately, one with little empirical evidence on either side. As a practical matter, however, whether taken together or separately, mood dependence and mood congruence raise the question of whether subjects' self-reports of past experience might be distorted by the mood state they are in at the time they make the report. Thus, for example, depressed or anxious individuals might exaggerate the frequency or severity of trauma, loss, abuse, or other negative events from childhood because such memories are more accessible to them at the time of retrieval. This is an extremely important empirical question, but it is also a fiendishly difficult one to answer. One reason for the difficulty, of course, is that the best way to evaluate memory bias is to compare the subject's memories to an objective record of what happened in his or her life and this sort of information is generally not available except in longitudinal databases. As an alternative, one could test memory when people were in a negative mood state and then again in neutral and positive mood states, but this is also difficult to manage.[2]

PUTTING RESEARCH INTO PRACTICE

In principle, mood-dependent retrieval is a big problem for investigators who rely on self-reports. But is it a problem in actual practice? A recent study by Brewin and his colleagues (Brewin, Andrews, & Gotlib, 1993) concluded that it is not. Brewin et al. covered three common criticisms of retrospective reports of early experiences: (a) that memories of childhood are imperfect and unreliable; (b) that syndromes such as anxiety and depression generally impair memory function; and (c) that depression biases retrieval away from positive material and toward negative material. They

---

[2]Complicating the picture somewhat, Parrott and Sabini (1990) also obtained evidence for mood-incongruent memory: Subjects in positive moods recalled more negative autobiographical memories than did subjects in negative moods, and vice versa. Although the conditions under which mood incongruence occurs are not well understood, Parrott and Sabini suggested that mood congruence occurs when subjects perceive the memory task as related to their current mood, and mood incongruence when they perceive it to be unrelated. Mood incongruence, in their view, occurs by virtue of a self-regulatory process in which subjects recall mood-incongruent memories in an attempt to produce a balanced self-concept and autobiographical record.

find the evidence for the first two criticisms wanting. They concluded that, in general, our recollection of the past is "reasonably free of error" (Baddeley, 1990, p. 310), and that anxiety and depression confer no special impairment on memory functioning. Most important, Brewin et al. found inconsistent and unconvincing evidence that negative mood biases memory toward negative events and they concluded that although mood may distort memory for relatively recent events, it has little impact on memory for childhood. This led them to conclude that retrospective reports of childhood experiences can be taken at face value, although they did propose some strategies for enhancing accurate recall and minimizing bias and error.

Our view is that Brewin et al. (1993) were premature in their conclusions about the accuracy of childhood memory and its invulnerability to emotional distortion. Remembering is inherently a reconstructive process (Bartlett, 1932; Ross, 1989) with lots of opportunity for bias and error (Roediger, 1996) and one's emotional state must cast a light—or a shadow—over that process. Moreover, anxiety and depression very likely put a considerable drain on cognitive resources—even if, like sleep-deprived subjects, the anxious and the depressed can pull themselves together for a short while and perform adequately on standard laboratory tests.

Most important, the evidence on which Brewin et al. (1993) based their sanguine conclusions about mood-congruent memory seems inadequate. Very few experimental studies involve clinically significant alterations in mood, or, for that matter, clinically significant memories; very few have independent confirmation of the quality that is really necessary to evaluate memories for distortion and bias. Moreover, surprisingly little of the evidence pertaining to childhood memory comes from the recall and interpretations of discrete events. In fact, a great deal of it involves test–retest correlations on scales rating such things as parental discord or care; another large segment involves factual knowledge, such as where the subject lived or who took care of the subject during the birth of a sibling. This is not within the definition of episodic memory.

In this context, a strong cautionary note is offered by a recent study of memory in soldiers who participated in the Persian Gulf War (Southwick, Morgan, Nicolaou, & Charney, 1997). One month after their return from the theater of operations, the soldiers completed a questionnaire concerned with combat-related traumatic events (e.g., an extreme threat to personal safety, observing bizarre disfigurement from wounds, seeing others killed or wounded). Two years later, they completed the questionnaire again, and this time they reported significantly more traumatic experiences than they had initially. Moreover, scores on a scale of combat-related post-traumatic stress disorder (PTSD) were significantly correlated with these changes in the follow-up reports. One interpretation of these findings is that individuals who show symptoms of PTSD exaggerate their histories of traumatic events, possibly as part of an attempt to explain their current problems. The same danger exists in other studies of memory in individuals with anxiety, depression, and PTSD.

One area in which we agree with Brewin et al. (1993) is in their call for more research in this area. Beginning with classical psychoanalysis, a variety of theories implicate childhood experiences as the cause of adult psychopathology—a viewpoint that has been revived in recent speculations about the role of incest and child sexual abuse in eating disorders and other mental illnesses. It is a fact that many mental patients frequently report a high level of childhood trauma, abuse, and neglect, but what we need to know is whether these reports are reliable and whether there is any causal relation between the trauma and the illness. We do not know this for sure. Everything we know about mood and memory justifies our suspicion that memory-based self-reports may not be reliable, but this knowledge is also limited. Therefore, clinical practitioners and researchers should treat retrospective reports of childhood and adult experiences as just that—reports to be verified, not historical truth. If we want to know the truth about such things as the association between childhood experience and adult depression, the approach is not through memory, with all its vagaries, but through history: not through retrospective self-reports, but through prospective studies of objective data.

ADDENDUM: WHY RETROSPECTIVE ANALYSES CAN GIVE FALSE IMPRESSIONS OF CAUSAL RELATIONS

Certainly the commonest approach to questions such as the relation between childhood experience and adult psychopathology is retrospective: Subjects who have been classified as depressed or nondepressed, for example, are then asked to report on their childhood experiences; or, in some cases, objective data is available concerning these experiences. Such analyses frequently provide evidence for an association between antecedent and consequent—giving the impression, for example, that certain kinds of childhood experiences are actually associated with depression in adults. It cannot be said too often that such retrospective methods tend to overestimate the strength of the relation between antecedent and consequent (Dawes, 1993, 1994).

To give an example (which in turn we owe to Dawes), consider the relation between smoking and lung cancer. We know from solid epidemiological research that smoking is a huge risk factor for lung cancer: About 1 in 10 smokers contract lung cancer, compared to about 1 in 200 nonsmokers, an increased risk of about 2,000%. Consider now a study in which an investigator compares smoking history in 400 individuals with lung cancer, compared to 400 cancer-free controls. The resulting table, conditioning on the consequent lung cancer, would look something like Fig. 6.4a: The vast majority of cancer victims would be found to be smokers, and smoking would be very rare in controls. The diagonal formed by the two critical cells, smoker-with-cancer and nonsmoker-without-cancer, accounts for 82% of the sample and the resulting correlation is a very high *phi* = .64.

But this turns out to be a gross overestimate of the actual relation between smoking and lung cancer. The reason is that there are relatively few smokers in the population and a study that conditions on the consequent oversamples this group and inflates the correlation between antecedent and consequent. Assume, for the purposes of illustration, that the base rate of smoking in the population is 25%. If we drew a random sample of the population for study, the actual relation between smoking and lung cancer proves to be quite a bit weaker: As illustrated in Fig. 6.4b, the diagonal still accounts for 77% of the cases, but taking the base rates into account, the correlation coefficient drops to *phi* = .25. The correlation remains significant (statistically and clinically), but it is greatly diminished in strength.

Conditioning on
the Consequence

	Cancer	No Cancer
Smoker	348	93
Nonsmoker	52	307

A

Diagonal = 82%   phi = .64

Compound Probabilities

	Cancer	No Cancer
Smoker	20	180
Nonsmoker	3	597

B

Diagonal = 77%   phi = .25

Conditioning on
the Antecedent

	Cancer	No Cancer
Smoker	40	360
Nonsmoker	2	398

C

Diagonal = 55%   phi = .22

FIG. 6.4. Varieties of antecedent-consequent relations (after Dawes, 1993).

Now what happens if we condition on the antecedent, that is, if we follow 400 smokers and 400 nonsmokers to determine how many contract lung cancer? When we do this, applying the probabilities known from a study with proper sampling, we find (see Fig. 6.4c) that the diagonal is reduced still more, to 55%, but that correlation is not distorted, *phi* = .25.

The distorting effects of conditioning on the consequent, which is the typical method in these kinds of studies, is inevitable—as Dawes (1993, 1994) showed, the source of the distortion is in the algebra by which probabilities are calculated. This distortion is inevitable so long as the base rate of the antecedent is substantially different from 50%, and it increases the further the base rate departs from this value. The proper way to determine the strength of relation between antecedent and consequent is to study a random (or stratified, or otherwise unbiased) sample of the population; failing that, it is far better to condition on the antecedent than to condition on the consequent. Longitudinal follow-up studies, then, have two virtues: They obviate many of the problems involved in collecting self-reports of potentially important antecedent variables, and they introduce relatively little distortion into the relations between the variables of interest.

ACKNOWLEDGMENTS

This chapter was presented at a conference, "The Science of Self-Report: Implications for Research and Practice," sponsored by the Office of Behavioral and Social Sciences Research, National Institutes of Health, Bethesda, Maryland, November 1996. An earlier version of this chapter was presented at a workshop on Mood and Memory: Effects on Decision-Making and Risk-Taking Behaviors sponsored by the Office of AIDS Research, National Institute of Mental Health, Washington, D.C., November 1990. The point of view represented here is based on research supported in part by Grants MH-44739 and MH-48502 from the National Institute of Mental Health. We thank Mahzarin Banaji, Robert Crowder, Lucy Canter Kihlstrom, Regina Miranda, and Jason Mitchell for their comments.

REFERENCES

Anderson, K. J. (1990). Arousal and the inverted-U hypothesis: A critique of Neiss's "Reconceptualizing arousal." *Psychological Bulletin, 107*, 96–100.

Baddeley, A. D. (1990). *Human memory: Theory and practice*. Hove, UK: Lawrence Erlbaum Associates.

Balch, W. R., & Lewis, B. S. (1996). Music-dependent memory: The roles of tempo change and mood mediation. *Journal of Experimental Psychology: Learning, Memory, & Cognition, 22*, 1354–1363.

Banaji, M. R., & Hardin, C. (1994). Affect and memory in retrospective reports. In N. Schwarz & S. Sudman (Eds.), *Autobiographical memory and the validity of retrospective reports* (pp. 71–86). New York: Springer-Verlag.

Bartlett, F. C. (1932). *Remembering: A study in experimental and social psychology.* Cambridge, England: Cambridge University Press.

Blaney, P. H. (1986). Affect and memory: A review. *Psychological Bulletin, 99,* 229–246.

Boucher, J., & Osgood, C. E. (1969). The Pollyanna hypothesis. *Journal of Verbal Learning & Verbal Behavior, 8,* 1–8.

Bower, G. H. (1981). Mood and memory. *American Psychologist, 36,* 129–148.

Bower, G. H., & Forgas, J. P. (in press). Affect, memory, and social cognition. In E. Eich, J. F. Kihlstrom, G. H. Bower, J. P. Forgas, & P. M. Niedenthal (Eds.), *Counterpoints: Cognition and emotion.* New York: Oxford University Press.

Bower, G. H., Gilligan, S. G., & Monteiro, K. P. (1981). Selectivity of learning caused by affective states. *Journal of Experimental Psychology: General, 110,* 451–473.

Bower, G. H., & Mayer, J. D. (1989). In search of mood-dependent retrieval. *Journal of Social Behavioral & Personality, 4,* 133–168.

Bower, G. H., Monteiro, K. P., & Gilligan, S. G. (1978). Emotional mood as a context for learning and recall. *Journal of Verbal Learning and Verbal Behavior, 17,* 573–585.

Brewin, C. R., Andrews, B., & Gotlib, I. H. (1993). Psychopathology and early experience: A reappraisal of retrospective reports. *Psychological Bulletin, 113,* 82–98.

Christianson, S.-A. (1992a). Emotional stress and eyewitness memory: A critical review. *Psychological Bulletin, 112,* 284–309.

Christianson, S.-A. (Ed.). (1992b). *Handbook of emotion and memory.* Hillsdale, NJ: Lawrence Erlbaum Associates.

Clark, M. S., & Fiske, S. T. (Eds.). (1982). *Affect and cognition.* Hillsdale, NJ: Lawrence Erlbaum Associates.

Crowder, R. G., Banaji, M. R., Wenk, H. E., Hardin, C., Phelps, E. A., & Ziv, O. (1997). *It's true: A replication of the classic Kleinsmith & Kaplan (1963) arousal and memory study.* Unpublished manuscript, Yale University.

Dawes, R. (Ed.). (1994). On the necessity of examining all four cells in a 2×2 table. *Making Better Decisions, 1*(2).

Dawes, R. M. (1993). Prediction of the future versus an understanding of the past: A basic asymmetry. *American Journal of Psychology, 106,* 1–24.

Dutta, S., & Kanungo, R. N. (1975). *Affect and memory: A reformulation.* London: Pergamon.

Eich, J. E. (1980). The cue-dependent nature of state-dependent retrieval. *Memory & Cognition, 8,* 157–173.

Eich, E. (1989). Theoretical issues in state-dependent memory. In H. L. Roediger & F. I. M. Craik (Eds.), *Varieties of memory and consciousness: Papers in honor of Endel Tulving* (pp. 331–352). Hillsdale, NJ: Lawrence Erlbaum Associates.

Eich, E. (1995a). Mood as a mediator of place dependent memory. *Journal of Experimental Psychology: General, 124,* 293–308.

Eich, E. (1995b). Searching for mood-dependent memory. *Psychological Science, 6,* 67–75.

Eich, E., & Birnbaum, I. M. (1988). On the relationship between the dissociative and affective properties of drugs. In G. M. Davies & D. M. Thomson (Eds.), *Memory in context: Context in memory* (pp. 81–93). Sussex, England: Wiley.

Eich, E., Macaulay, D., & Lam, R. W. (1997). Mania, depression, and mood dependent memory. *Cognition & Emotion, 11,* 607–618.

Eich, E., Macaulay, D., Loewenstein, R. J., & Dihle, P. H. (1997). Memory, amnesia, and dissociative identity disorder. *Psychological Science, 8,* 417–423.

Eich, E., Macaulay, D., & Ryan, L. (1994). Mood dependent memory for events of the personal past. *Journal of Experimental Psychology: General, 123,* 201–215.

Eich, E., & Metcalfe, J. (1989). Mood dependent memory for internal versus external events. *Journal of Experimental Psychology: Learning, Memory, and Cognition, 15*, 443–445.

Ekman, P., & Davidson, R. J. (Eds.). (1994). *The nature of emotion: Fundamental questions*. New York: Oxford University Press.

Ellis, H. C., & Ashbrook, P. W. (1988). Resource allocation model of the effects of depressed mood states on memory. In K. Fiedler & J. Forgas (Eds.), *Affect, cognition, and social behavior* (pp. 25–43). Toronto: Hogrefe.

Ellis, H. C., Ashbrook, P. W. (1989). The "state" of mood and memory research: A selective review. *Journal of Social Behavior and Personality, 4*, 1–21.

Ellis, H. C., & Moore, B. A. (in press). Mood and memory. In T. Dalgleish & M. Power (Eds.), *Handbook of cognition and emotion*. Chichester, England: Wiley.

Erdelyi, M. H. (1974). A new look at the New Look: Perceptual defense and vigilance. *Psychological Review, 81*, 1–25.

Eysenck, M. H. (1976). Arousal, learning, and memory. *Psychological Bulletin, 83*, 389–404.

Fabiani, M., & Donchin, E. (1995). Encoding processes and memory organization: A model of the von Restorff effect. *Journal of Experimental Psychology: Learning, Memory, & Cognition, 21*, 224–240.

Fernandez, A., & Glenberg, A. M. (1985). Changing environmental context does not reliably affect memory. *Memory and Cognition, 13*, 333–345.

Fiedler, K., & Forgas, J. (Eds.). (1988). *Affect, cognition, and social behavior*. Toronto: Hogrefe.

Forgas, J. (Ed.). (1991). *Emotion and social judgments*. Oxford, England: Pergamon.

Godden, D. R., & Baddeley, A. D. (1975). Context-dependent memory in two natural environments: On land and underwater. *British Journal of Psychology, 66*, 325–331.

Hertel, P. T. (1994). Depression and memory: Are impairments remediable through attentional control? *Current Directions in Psychological Science, 3*, 190–193.

Heuer, F., & Reisberg, D. (1992). Emotion, arousal, and memory for detail. In S.-A. Christianson (Ed.), *Handbook of emotion and memory* (pp. 151–180). Hillsdale, NJ: Lawrence Erlbaum Associates.

Holloway, F. A. (1978). State dependent retrieval based on time of day. In B. Ho, D. W. Richards, & D. L. Chute (Eds.), *Drug discrimination and state dependent learning* (pp. 319–343). New York: Academic Press.

Hunt, R. R. (1995). The subtlety of distinctiveness: What von Restorff really did. *Psychonomc Bulletin & Review, 2*, 105–112.

Johnson, M. H., & Magaro, P. A. (1987). Effects of mood and severity on memory processes in depression and mania. *Psychological Bulletin, 101*, 28–40.

Kihlstrom, J. F. (1989). On what does mood-dependent memory depend? *Journal of Social Behavior and Personality, 4*, 23–32.

Kihlstrom, J. F., & Barnhardt, T. M. (1993). The self-regulation of memory, for better and for worse, with and without hypnosis. In D. M. Wegner & J. W. Pennebaker (Eds.), *Handbook of mental control* (pp. 88–125). Englewood Cliffs, NJ: Prentice-Hall.

Kihlstrom, J. F., & Schacter, D. L. (1995). Functional disorders of autobiographical memory. In A. Baddeley, B. A. Wilson, & F. Watts (Eds.), *Handbook of memory disorders* (pp. 337–364). London: Wiley.

Kleinsmith, L. J., & Kaplan, S. (1963). Paired-associate learning as a function of arousal and interpolated interval. *Journal of Experimental Psychology, 65*, 190–193.

Kleinsmith, L. J., & Kaplan, S. (1964). Interaction of arousal and recall interval in nonsense syllable paired-associate learning. *Journal of Experimental Psychology, 67*, 124–126.

Kuiken, D. (1991). Mood and memory: Theory, research, and applications. Newbury Park, CA: Sage.

Leventhal, H., & Tomarken, A. J. (1986). Emotion: Today's problems. *Annual Review of Psychology, 37*, 565–610.

Lloyd, G. G., & Lishman, W. A. (1975). Effect of depression on the speed of recall of pleasant and unpleasant experiences. *Psychological Medicine, 5*, 173–180.

Macaulay, D., Ryan, L., & Eich, E. (1993). Mood dependence in implicit and explicit memory. In P. Graf & M. E. J. Masson (Eds.), *Implicit memory: New directions in cognition, development, and neuropsychology*, (pp. 75–94). Hillsdale, NJ: Lawrence Erlbaum Associates.

Macht, M. L., Spear, N. E., & Levis, D. J. (1977). State-dependent retention in humans induced by alterations in affective state. *Bulletin of the Psychonomic Society, 10*, 415–418.

Mandler, G. (1992). Memory, arousal, and mood: A theoretical integration. In S.-A. Christianson (Ed.), *Handbook of emotion and memory* (pp. 93–110). Hillsdale, NJ: Lawrence Erlbaum Associates.

Mathews, A. M., & MacLeod, C. (1994). Cognitive approaches to emotion and emotional disorders. *Annual Review of Psychology, 45*, 25–50.

Matlin, M., & Stang, D. (1978). *The Pollyanna principle: Selectivity in language, memory, and thought.* Cambridge, MA: Schenkman.

Mineka, S. (1992). Evolutionary memories, emotional processing, and the emotional disorders. In D. L. Medin (Ed.), *The psychology of learning and motivation* (Vol. 28, pp. 161–206). New York: Academic Press.

Neiss, R. (1988). Reconceptualizing arousal: Psychobiological states in motor performance. *Psychological Bulletin, 103*, 345–366.

Niedenthal, P. M., & Kitayama, S. (1994). *The heart's eye: Emotional influences in perception and attention.* San Diego, CA: Academic Press.

Nissen, M. J., Ross, J. L., Willingham, D. B., MacKenzie, T. B., & Schacter, D. L. (1988). Memory and awareness in a patient with multiple personality disorder. *Brain & Cognition, 8*, 21–38.

Overton, D. A. (1984). State-dependent learning and drug discriminations. In L. L. Iverson, S. D. Iverson, & S. H. Snyder (Eds.), *Handbook of psychopharmacology* (Vol. 18, pp. 59–127). New York: Plenum.

Park, J., & Banaji, M. R. (1997). *Arousal and memory: A meta-analytic confirmation.* Unpublished manuscript.

Parrott, W. G., & Sabini, J. (1990). Mood and memory under natural conditions: Evidence for mood-incongruent recall. *Journal of Personality & Social Psychology, 59*, 321–336.

Rapaport, D. (1942). *Emotions and memory.* Baltimore: Williams & Wilkins.

Revelle, W., & Loftus, D. A. (1992). The implications of arousal effects for the study of affect and memory. In S.-A. Christianson (Ed.), *Handbook of emotion and memory* (pp. 113–149). Hillsdale, NJ: Lawrence Erlbaum Associates.

Roediger, H. L. (1996). Memory illusions. *Journal of Memory & Language, 35*, 76–100.

Roediger, H. L., & McDermott, K. B. (1993). Implicit memory in normal human subjects. In F. Boller & J. Grafmann (Eds.), *Handbook of neuropsychology* (Vol. 8, pp. 63–131). Amsterdam: Elsevier.

Ross, M. (1989). Relation of implicit theories to the construction of personal histories. *Psychological Review, 96*, 341–357.

Schacter, D. L. (1987). Implicit memory: History and current status. *Journal of Experimental Psychology: Learning, Memory, and Cognition, 13*, 501–518.

Singer, J. L. (Ed.). (1990). *Repression and dissociation: Implications for personality theory, psychopathology, and health.* Chicago: University of Chicago Press.

Smith, S. M., Glenberg, A. M., & Bjork, R. A. (1978). Environmental context and human memory. *Memory & Cognition, 6*, 342–353.

Southwick, S. M., Morgan, C. A., Nicolaou, A. L., & Charney, D. S. (1997). Consistency of memory for combat-related traumatic events in veterans of Operation Desert Storm. *American Journal of Psychiatry, 154*, 173–177.

Teasdale, J. D., & Fogarty, S. J. (1979). Differential effects of induced mood on retrieval of pleasant and unpleasant events from episodic memory. *Journal of Abnormal Psychology, 88*, 248–257.

Teasdale, J. D., & Russell, M. L. (1983). Differential effects of induced mood on the recall of positive, negative and neutral words. *British Journal of Clinical Psychology, 22,* 163–171.

Tobias, B. A. (1992). *Mood effects on explicit and implicit memory.* Unpublished doctoral dissertation, University of Arizona.

Tobias, B. A., Kihlstrom, J. F., & Schacter, D. L. (1992). Emotion and implicit memory. In S.-A. Christianson (Ed.), *Handbook of emotion and memory* (pp. 67–92). Hillsdale, NJ: Lawrence Erlbaum Associates.

Tulving, E., & Thomson, D. M. (1973). Encoding specificity and retrieval process in episodic memory. *Psychological Review, 80,* 352–373.

Tversky, A., & Kahneman, D. (1973). Availability: A heuristic for judging frequency and probability. *Cognitive Psychology, 5,* 207–232.

von Restorff, H. (1933). Uber die Wirkung von Bereichsbildungen im Spurenfeld. *Psychologie Forschung, 18,* 299–342.

Weingartner, H., Miller, H., & Murphy, D. L. (1977). Mood-state-dependent retrieval of verbal associations. *Journal of Abnormal Psychology, 86,* 276–284.

Yerkes, R. M., & Dodson, J. D. (1908). The relation of strength of stimulus to rapidity of habit-formation. *Journal of Comparative and Neurological Psychology, 18,* 459–482.

III

SELF-REPORTING SENSITIVE EVENTS AND CHARACTERISTICS

Christine A. Bachrach
National Institute of Child Health and Human Development

Beginning in the late 1940s, survey experts and behavioral scientists began to notice systematic biases in the self-reports of certain kinds of behaviors and characteristics. People reported voting and having a library card when they did not and failed to report bankruptcy and arrests for drunken driving even when these events had occurred (Parry & Crossley, 1950). Given the heavy reliance on self-report as a measurement tool in the social and behavioral sciences, these findings carried serious implications. Although measurement error is a natural and expected phenomenon in all fields of science, serious and systematic bias in measurements can lead to erroneous inferences and undermine the validity of otherwise sound scientific research.

The two chapters that follow provide insight into our evolving understanding of the sources of self-report bias in sensitive domains—domains that encompass behaviors, events, and characteristics that are disapproved of, embarrassing, or illegal. The chapters also furnish evidence that these sources of bias can be addressed by manipulating the ways in which self-report data is elicited and recorded and describe methodological advances that hold great promise for strengthening scientific studies on sensitive topics.

In the first chapter, Nora Cate Schaeffer presents an overview of theory and evidence relating to bias in self-reports. A central concept motivating work on this topic is *social desirability*—that is, the tendency of informants to present information about themselves in a way that enhances their worth in the eyes of an interviewer. To the extent that attributes, attitudes, or behaviors are socially valued, they are emphasized or exaggerated; to the extent they are socially disapproved, they are minimized or underreported (DeMaio, 1985). Many of the approaches that have been used to address the problem of self-report bias flow from social desirability theory, and an increasing body of evidence (described in the chapters that follow) shows that they work. For example, self-administered questionnaires have been employed to reduce the motivation for socially desirable reporting by permitting subjects to provide information without communicating it to an interviewer. The introduction of computer interviewing has greatly expanded techniques for enhancing privacy (see also chapter 8, this volume).

Other approaches stemming from social desirability theory involve manipulating the context or presentation of questions so as to create a more permissive frame of reference for responses. These techniques are also proving effective (e.g., Tourangeau, Rasinski, Jobe, Smith, & Pratt, 1997; Tourangeau & Smith, 1996) although much research remains to be done to inform their use. Yet other approaches seek to offset the costs to subjects of providing socially undesirable answers—by providing financial incentives or by attempting to enhance the perceived legitimacy and value of the research (Mosher & Duffer, 1994; Tourangeau et al., 1997; Tourangeau & Smith, 1996).

In her chapter, Schaeffer offers suggestions for the extension of theory on the sources of self-report bias. Her ideas draw on the concepts of information processing but extend them to suggest that "errors of memory and processing may be biased toward a conventional, socially nonthreatening answer" (chapter 7, p. 116). She suggests that responses to threatening questions may derive from routine habits of self-presentation that draw on public biographies that people construct about themselves and furnish more or less automatically unless competing values and beliefs are made conscious. These ideas are distinct from other prevailing theories in that they do not require that respondents consciously weigh the costs of admitting censured behaviors to another person; rather, they suggest that nondisclosure is rooted in the very schema and processes that structure the memory and retrieval of information. They suggest that new approaches that circumvent the tendency of cognitive structures and processes to produce biased reports could lead to further improvement of self-report data.

In the final chapter in this section, Heather Miller and her associates provide an excellent case study of why it is important to advance theoretical and experimental work on self-report bias. After presenting a careful review of mode effects in self-reports on sensitive topics, Miller describes a case-control study that linked risk of breast cancer to a self-reported history of abortion. Miller explores the possibility that these findings could have resulted from underreporting of abortion, a well-documented bias in interview studies of reproductive health. In doing so, she emphasizes a point made also by Nora Schaeffer: that the sources and extent of self-report bias are likely to vary depending on the personal experience of each respondent. Miller points out that differential accuracy in reporting by cases and controls can lead to misleading conclusions about the sources of health risk.

The chapters in this section touch on topics of research that are central to public health and public policy. Illicit drug use and risky sexual behavior are but a few of the private behaviors of individuals that—because they have important consequences for health and well-being of individuals and communities—are important foci of health research. Strategies to prevent or reduce the risk associated with these behaviors must depend on sound scientific research on their antecedents and consequences. Self-report data are a necessary and valuable element in research on these topics. As these chapters make clear, much progress has been made in identifying and addressing sources of bias in self-reports of sensitive topics, and many promising avenues of further inquiry remain to be explored.

REFERENCES

DeMaio, T. J. (1985). Social desirability and survey measurement: A review. In C. F. Turner & E. Martin (Eds.), *Surveying subjective phenomena* (Volume 2, pp. 257–282). New York: Russell Sage Foundation.

Mosher, W. D., & Duffer, A. P., Jr. (1994, May). *Experiments in survey data collection: The National Survey of Family Growth Pretest.* Paper presented at the Annual Meeting of the Population Association of America.

Parry, H., & Crossley, H. (1950). Validity of responses to survey questions. *Public Opinion Quarterly, 14*, 61–80.

Tourangeau, R., Rasinski, K., Jobe, J. B., Smith, T. W., & Pratt, W. F. (1997). Sources of error in a survey on sexual behavior. *Journal of Official Statistics, 13*, 341–352.

Tourangeau, R., & Smith, T. W. (1996). Asking sensitive questions: The impact of data collection mode, question format, and question context. *Public Opinion Quarterly, 60*, 275–304.

7

Asking Questions About Threatening Topics: A Selective Overview

Nora Cate Schaeffer
University of Wisconsin—Madison

This view [that not all intentionally false statements ought to count as lies] found powerful expression in Grotius. He argued that a falsehood is a lie in the strict sense of the word only if it conflicts with a right of the person to whom it is addressed.

—Bok (1978, p. 37)

In their 1950 study that included a comparison between survey responses and records, Parry and Crossley (1950) showed that respondents overreported voting, having a library card, and several other socially desirable characteristics as compared to information about the respondents in external records. In a 1976 record-check study, Locander, Sudman, and Bradburn reported similar findings and also showed that respondents underreport bankruptcy and being charged with drunken driving. These classic studies addressed a key concern of those who rely on survey data—the accuracy of responses to questions that respondents might perceive as threatening.

All self-reports are subject to response error. But validation studies, which incorporate a comparison between self-reports and records, suggest that some respondents sometimes perceive some topics as threatening, so that reports about threatening topics are subject to more than the usual errors caused by omissions, telescoping, and the like. Results like those just mentioned suggest that asking a threatening question seems to elicit from some respondents a tendency to present themselves in a socially desirable way. This tendency may lead to overreports of socially desirable behaviors or to underreports of threatening behaviors.

Instead of beginning with a discussion of what makes a question sensitive in a way that is socially or interactionally threatening, I first present excerpts from research on three topics that could be considered threatening. The topics, which have all been the subject of recent studies, are the number of sex partners a person has had, whether a woman has ever had an abortion, and the use of marijuana. The discussion will illustrate why we think we know the direction of errors in self-reports on these topics and the range of techniques that have been used in an attempt to reduce the component of response error caused by the threatening nature of the topics. The techniques that have been used include varying the mode of asking and answering questions, varying the context of the questions within the interview, and varying the structure or wording of the questions. After presenting illustrative results, I will then consider what theoretical developments have attempted to integrate these findings, what makes a question threatening, and what other avenues might be investigated to improve the accuracy of self-reports on such topics.

REPORTING OF THE NUMBER OF SEX PARTNERS

Consider first reporting about the number of sex partners by heterosexuals. In a series of comparisons, Smith (1992) found that, on average, men report many more sex partners than do women. Table 7.1 illustrates his findings. The first row presents the unadjusted estimate from the 1989 General Social Survey; the second row presents the results with some reasonable adjustments made to include nonrespondents; and the third row adds an adjustment that reduces the impact of extreme values, which are more likely to be reported by men, on estimates of the means. The table shows that the difference is substantial and that it persists despite attempts to correct for

TABLE 7.1
Mean Number of Adult Lifetime Sex Partners
Reported by Heterosexual Men and Women

	Males	Females	Males:Females
Unadjusted	13.00	3.24	4.06:1
Adjusted for nonresponse*	12.05	3.03	3.98:1
Adjusted for extreme values**	9.36	3.02	3.10:1

Note. Male and female means different at < .01 in all rows.

Source: 1989 General Social Survey. From Table 7 in Smith (1992). Copyright © 1992 by Statistics Sweden. Reprinted by permission of the author and Statistics Sweden.

*Values of 1.0 given to males and females with missing data.

**Values of 50 and greater recoded to 50.

possible sources of the discrepancy other than response error. Smith reported finding the difference in other surveys, and the difference is large enough that adjustments for obvious possible sources of the discrepancy, such as differences between the men and the women who participate in surveys or in the way men and women use extreme values when answering, do not make men's and women's reports the same. This comparison involves a relatively closed population; thus, reports from men and from women should yield similar estimates of population means. The fact that they do not, even when attempts are made to adjust the data, suggests that the number of sex partners is being misreported. Smith (1992) argued that, "most probably there is a combination of male overreporting and female underreporting" (p. 320). Thus, methods that decrease the number of partners that men report or increase the number reported by women might be interpreted as improving reports.

A series of experiments tested several methods for improving reporting of sex partners. These experiments varied the mode of response, the structure of the question, and question context. The results presented here from the Women's Health Study are based on a sample of women selected by area probability methods in Chicago and women selected from two Chicago health clinics. A comparison of self-administered questions with interviewer-administered questions (Table 7.2), found that, overall, the mean number of sex partners reported by women was significantly higher when self-administered methods of answering questions were used, and the effect was significant for three reference periods: the past year, the past 5 years, and over the respondent's lifetime.

A later experiment (referred to by the investigators as the ACASI experiment) compared audio-enhanced, computer-assisted self-interviewing (ACASI),

TABLE 7.2
Mean Number of Sex Partners Reported by Women, by Mode of Interview

Mode of Interview (Experimental Group)	Mean Reported Sex Partners		
	Past Year	Past 5 Years	Lifetime
Self-administered questions (self-administered or CASI)	1.72	3.88	6.54
Interviewer-administered questions (paper or CAPI)	1.44	2.82	5.43

Note. Self-administration elicits significantly more partners for all three time periods. Cell size is approximately 500. Significance tests were computed on logged data.

Source: Women's Health Study. From Table 22.2 (p. 440) in Tourangeau, R., & Smith, T. W. (1998). Collecting sensitive information with different modes of data collection. In M. Couper, R. Baker, J. Bethlehem, C. Clark, J. Martin, W. Nicholls, & J. O'Reilly (Eds.), *Computer-assisted survey information collection* (pp. 431–454). Copyright © 1998 by John Wiley & Sons, Inc. Reprinted by permission of authors and John Wiley & Sons, Inc.

computer-assisted self-interviewing (CASI), and computer-assisted personal interviewing (CAPI) to collect reports of the number of sex partners among an area probability sample in Cook County, Illinois. The results of this study are complex, involving three-way interactions, and the investigators present tabulated means only for the main effects. Table 7.3 shows the mean number of sex partners reported in each of three modes for each of three reference periods. The table combines responses of men and women because the mode-by-sex interaction was not significant, even though the expected pattern of men reporting fewer partners and women reporting more partners with self-administration was found (Tourangeau & Smith, 1996, p. 293). In this study, the mean number of partners reported was higher when ACASI was used, but not when CASI was used, and the effect was significant only for reports of the number of partners in the past 5 years and over the respondent's lifetime.

The ACASI experiment also manipulated question format and context to attempt to improve reports about threatening behaviors. In the question format manipulation, one version of the closed question about the number of sex partners presented high-frequency response categories and another version of the closed question presented low-frequency response categories. Each of these was followed by an open question that asked for an exact number of partners. This second response was compared with answers obtained to an open question administered as a third treatment. The main effects from this experiment are summarized in Table 7.4. The question format had a significant effect on the reports of the number of sex partners in the last year and last 5 years. The mean number of partners reported was highest with the high-frequency categories, lowest with the low-frequency categories, and intermediate with the open question. For the 5-year

TABLE 7.3
Mean Reported Sex Partners by Mode of Interview

Mode	Past Year	Past 5 Years	Lifetime
ACASI	2.26	4.52	7.05
CASI	1.87	2.99	5.75
CAPI	2.14	3.44	5.51

Note. The interview modes are audio-enhanced computer-assisted self-interviewing (ACASI), computer-assisted self-interviewing (CASI), and computer-assisted personal interviewing (CAPI). The effect of mode is significant for lifetime reports and marginally significant for 5-year reports. ACASI yields higher reports than CASI for lifetime and 5-year reports. There are higher order interactions involving mode of data collection. Cell sizes range from 86 to 104. Significance tests are based on logged data.

Source: ACASI Experiment. From Table 3 (p. 292) in Tourangeau and Smith (1996). Copyright © 1996 by the American Association for Public Opinion Research. Reprinted by permission of the University of Chicago Press and the author.

TABLE 7.4
Mean Reported Sex Partners by Question Format

Question Format	Past Year	Past 5 Years	Lifetime
Open	1.65	3.12	7.20
Closed-low	1.43	2.62	4.73
Closed-high	3.38	5.33	6.28

Note. The closed-low question format presented categories that implied a low frequency range; the closed-high question format presented categories that implied a high frequency range. The effect of question format is significant for the past year and past 5 years, and there is a significant interaction involving question format and mode of data collection. Significance tests are based on logged data.

Source: ACASI Experiment. From Table 3 (p. 292) in Tourangeau and Smith (1996). Copyright © 1996 by the American Association for Public Opinion Research. Reprinted by permission of the University of Chicago Press and the author.

and lifetime reports, there was an interaction between question format and mode that suggests that the effect of item format is reduced in the CAPI mode.

A third manipulation in the ACASI experiment placed questions that expressed either restrictive or permissive attitudes about sexual attitudes before the questions about the number of sex partners. The main effects reported in Table 7.5 suggest that the number of partners reported is higher in the restrictive context, but the difference is significant only for reports about partners in the last 5 years. There is a three-way interaction involving sex of the respondent, mode of asking the question, and context, such that the average number of sex partners reported by men and women is similar when a restrictive context and self-administration are used. Although such a complex three-way interaction requires replication, the results of these studies indicate that these methods can affect reporting of sex partners.

In all of these experiments about the reporting of sex partners, no external criterion is available, but a criterion of internal consistency in a closed

TABLE 7.5
Mean Reported Sex Partners by Question Context

Context	Past Year	Past 5 Years	Lifetime
Permissive	1.88	2.95	5.77
Restrictive	2.28	4.24	6.34

Note. The permissive context preceded the question about sex partners with attitude items expressing permissive attitudes toward sexual behavior; the restrictive context presented items expressing restrictive attitudes. The effect of question context is significant for the past 5 years but is qualified by higher order interactions. Significance tests are based on logged data.

Source: ACASI Experiment. From Table 3 (p. 292) in Tourangeau and Smith (1996). Copyright © 1996 by the American Association for Public Opinion Research. Reprinted by permission of the University of Chicago Press and the author.

population is used to diagnose the presence of response error. Evidence about men's and women's attitudes toward sexual behavior provide a basis for speculations about the different probable direction of reporting error for men and women (e.g., Smith, 1992, p. 320). But because there is no criterion, we cannot say which experimental manipulations produce more accurate reports in any absolute sense, although we can identify which manipulations produce reports that seem to be consistent with accurate reports. That is, we tend to interpret manipulations that reduce the number of partners reported by men or increase the number of partners reported by women as increasing the accuracy of self-reports.

REPORTING OF ABORTION

The second example to be considered here is the reporting of abortion. A comparison between responses to the National Survey of Family Growth (NSFG) and data compiled from abortion providers by the Alan Guttmacher Institute (AGI) illustrates the use of aggregate comparisons to diagnose the existence of a problem with self-reports and the direction of overall error. Jones and Forrest (1992) used the detailed retrospective fertility histories in the NSFG that cover the 3 or 4 years preceding the interview to estimate the number of abortions performed in the United States based on the NSFG. They compute these estimates for 11 years covered by the fertility histories in the 1976, 1982, and 1988 NSFG surveys. They then compare the survey-based estimates to the estimates of the number of abortions performed in each year that the AGI compiles from abortion providers. Their analysis suggests that, for example, 45% of the abortions actually performed in the 3 years covered by the 1976 NSFG were reported in the survey. (See Table 7.6, which shows the proportion of the abortions estimated from AGI data that are reported for the period covered by each of the three NSFG surveys.) In each of the 11 years for which Jones and Forrest used the NSFG fertility histories to make this comparison, the NSFG yields a substantially lower estimate of the number of abortions performed in that year than the AGI

TABLE 7.6
Percentage of Abortions Estimated as Actually Having Occurred in the
United States as Reported in the 1976, 1982, and 1988 Cycles of the NSFG

	Percentage Reported
Cycle II, 1976 (1973–1975)	45
Cycle III, 1982 (1979–1982)	48
Cycle IV, 1988 (1984–1987)	35

Note. Source: National Survey of Family Growth. From Table 1 in Jones, E. F., & Forrest, J. D. (1992). Underreporting of abortion in surveys of U.S. women: 1976 to 1988. *Demography, 29,* 113–126. Reprinted by permission of the Population Association of America and the authors.

data. In reviewing these data, Jones and Forrest concluded that "... neither the incidence nor the trend in the number of abortions [using the AGI data as the criterion] can be inferred from the NSFG data" (p. 117), and they found similar deficiencies with the National Surveys of Young Women and the National Longitudinal Surveys of Work Experience of Youth (NLSY). (They also note that confidential questions in the 1988 NSFG and NLSY show promise for increasing the number of abortions reported.)

A portion of the sample for the Women's Health Study was selected from two Chicago clinics so that reports about abortion experiences could be validated by comparison with clinic records. This study illustrates the reverse record-check methodology, in which a sample is drawn from a source that can provide records to use in validating responses. The study attempted to improve the reporting of abortion by varying several factors: whether questions were self-administered or interviewer-administered, whether the medium for recording answers was paper or computer, whether the interview took place in the woman's home or at a neutral site, whether nurses or regular field staff conducted the interview, and whether questions about abortion were initially asked as part of a series of questions about medical procedures or in a series of questions about pregnancies and their outcomes. None of these experimental variables affected reports of having had at least one abortion. About 74% of the women in the clinic sample reported having ever had an abortion, and only 52% reported an abortion at roughly the time recorded in the clinic records (Tourangeau, Rasinski, Jobe, Smith, & Pratt, 1997, p. 359).

An experimental pretest for Cycle V of the NSFG that was conducted in 1993 tested methods that might improve the reporting of abortion (Lessler, Weeks, & O'Reilly, 1994). The pretest used a sample of women in three pairs of matched sites who had participated in the 1991 National Health Interview Survey. Results from the NSFG pretest, shown in Table 7.7, unlike those just reported for the Women's Health Study, which used a different sampling strategy, show some increases in the level of reporting. The study manipulated features of the interview and incentives. Women were assigned to one

TABLE 7.7
Percentage of Women Reporting They Ever Had an
Abortion by Site, Incentive, and Mode

	In-Home (No Money)	In-Home ($20)	Neutral Site ($40)
No ACASI	14	22	29
ACASI	25	30	Not applicable

Note. ACASI administration followed interviewer administration. Both the neutral site-$40 incentive and ACASI increase the number of women reporting they ever had an abortion.

Source: NSFG Cycle V Pretest. From Exhibit C in Lessler, Weeks, and O'Reilly (1994). Reprinted by permission of the authors.

of three interview treatments: CAPI interview in the home, CAPI in the home with a short ACASI supplement, or CAPI interview at a neutral site. For the incentive manipulation, $20 was offered to all in-home respondents in three of the sites and no incentive was provided to their in-home counterparts in the matched sites; all respondents interviewed in a neutral site were paid $40 and reimbursed some expenses. The results of the experiment suggest that interviewing in a neutral site (with a $40 incentive) and using ACASI both similarly increase the proportion of women who report that they ever had an abortion.

REPORTING OF MARIJUANA USE

The final example concerns reporting of marijuana use. Unlike the previous two behaviors, for marijuana use there are neither records from providers or a closed population comparison to use in evaluating estimates or identifying, even experimentally, the direction of reporting error. Instead, reasoning by analogy with other behaviors for which records or other criteria are available and knowing that marijuana use is illegal, researchers make the assumption that marijuana use is underreported and that methods that increase reporting improve reporting.

The 1990 National Household Survey of Drug Abuse (NHSDA) Field Test drew on extensive preliminary investigations to test methods that might improve the reporting of drug use. The study used a multistage probability sample of households in 33 metropolitan areas. The experimental treatments included the 1990 NHSDA questionnaire and a new instrument crossed with two modes of administration, self-administered questionnaire (SAQ) and interviewer-administered paper-and-pencil interview (PAPI). The new instrument revised the 1990 NHSDA questions in an attempt to make them more internally consistent and to remove ambiguities. Results from these experiments are illustrated by the result in Table 7.8. These results show that the proportion of the sample reporting marijuana use is higher when questions are self-administered than when they are administered by an interviewer. The new question wording did not have a significant effect.

These examples illustrate that reports about very different types of threatening behaviors can be affected—and possibly improved—by manipulating the mode of interview and other features of the interview. Although the use of a self-administered instrument does not affect reporting in the direction we think of as improving reporting in every experiment in which it has been used, it has been evaluated frequently, and it often seems to improve reporting of threatening behaviors. Moreover, the effect is often greatest for reports about recent behavior, which are arguably more threatening. (See Tourangeau & Smith, 1998, for a summary).

TABLE 7.8

Estimates of Prevalence of Reported Marijuana Use (Percentage)
by Questionnaire Wording and Mode of Administration

	By Question Wording		By Mode	
	Current	New (Clarified)	SAQ	PAPI
Lifetime	35.47	36.18	36.71	34.96
Past year	7.72	7.53	8.64	6.63
Past 30 days	3.94	4.16	5.02	3.11

Note. Effect of mode is significant for past 30 days and past year. Effect of question wording is not significant. Effect is clearest for most recent use.

Source: 1990 National Household Survey of Drug Abuse Field Test. From Table 7-1 in Turner, Lessler, and Devore (1992). Reprinted by permission of the author.

Two important questions raised by these experiments are (a) the extent to which the experimental treatments actually address sources of error associated with the sensitivity of the topics as opposed to other sources of reporting error, and (b) whether there are other sources of error due to the sensitivity of the topic that remain to be addressed. I consider next some issues suggested by these questions.

A MODEL OF MODE EFFECTS

Tourangeau and Smith (1996) have developed a model of mode effects that summarizes how self-administration and the use of computer-assisted data collection might affect the accuracy of self-reports. The model suggests that self-administration is effective because it increases the privacy of reporting, and the use of computer-assisted modes is effective because it enhances the perceived legitimacy of the data collection effort.

Their interpretation of the effect of privacy is supported by experiments that apply utility theory to studying threatening questions. When used to study answers to threatening questions, utility theory is concerned with how a respondent's risk-taking behavior (reporting disapproved facts about oneself) is affected by their perception of what is to be lost or gained by reporting (see Nathan, Sirken, Willis, & Esposito, 1990). In these experiments, subjects were presented with hypothetical scenarios describing a respondent in an interview. The subject rated the likelihood that the respondent would answer truthfully about a specific threatening topic in the situation described in the scenario. As the results in Table 7.9 indicate, the rated likelihood of a truthful response is greater in the more private situation; that is, when the respondent's family is not at home, at least when the interviewer is in her 50s. Moreover, other ratings by subjects (not shown in

TABLE 7.9
Effects of Interviewer Age and Privacy on Likelihood of Truthful Response

| | Interviewer Age | | |
	20s	50s	Overall
Privacy			
Family not home	6.19	7.81	7.00
Family home	6.50	5.40	5.96

Note. Higher number means a greater likelihood of a truthful response. Main effect of privacy and privacy by interviewer age interaction are significant.

Source: Rasinski, K. A., Baldwin, A. K., Willis, G. B., & Jobe, J. B. (1994). Risk and loss perceptions associated with survey reporting of sensitive behaviors. In *Proceedings of the Section on Survey Research Methods of the American Statistical Association* (pp. 497–502). Washington, DC: The American Statistical Association. Reprinted by permission of the author.

Table 7.9) indicated that the perceived risk of disclosure to one's spouse and of embarrassment in front of the interviewer affected how likely the subjects thought it was that the respondent would tell the truth for a more threatening and a less threatening survey topic, respectively.

These vignette studies, and the results from the experiments reviewed earlier suggest that respondents are more comfortable revealing socially threatening things about themselves when they can do so privately. Thus, the process of reporting about sensitive topics is affected by situational variables. It is tempting to conclude that the response processes that are affected by manipulating the mode of the interview are conscious processes, but even the vignette studies, which simulate conscious decision making, do not demonstrate that the actual behavior of respondents during an interview is guided by conscious calculation. And it is quite possible that it is not.

WHAT MAKES A QUESTION THREATENING

With these examples as background, I would like to consider what directions the research just reviewed suggests for future research about reports of threatening behaviors. To do this, I first consider where errors in self-reports about threatening topics might originate and then what makes a question threatening.

Current views of errors in reports of threatening questions suggest four origins for reporting errors. Three of these—cognitive processing, the social organization of the behavior being reported about, and task requirements—affect all reports of behaviors. But the pattern of overreporting of desirable behaviors and underreporting of undesirable behaviors that is often

found when there is a criterion available to determine the direction of
reporting error suggest that there are also sources of error specific to
threatening topics.

The application of information-processing models to the question–answering process suggests that errors may originate at the stages of comprehension and interpretation of the question, retrieval, evaluation of the candidate answer, and reporting. Similarly, the way events are organized in respondents' lives may make them more or less difficult to report about accurately, particularly given the estimation methods and heuristics that respondents use to construct self-reports. Behaviors are organized in socially patterned ways in respondents' lives, and this affects how important the behavior is to the respondent, how frequently and regularly the behavior is engaged in, how similar each instance of the behavior is to other instances, how much social reinforcement the behavior receives, and how distinct it is from other, similar, behaviors. Because these features of a behavior interact with the estimation methods respondents use to affect how easy it is to report accurately about the behavior, accuracy and inaccuracy in reporting are also socially patterned. Thus, information about a class of events that is salient to the respondent and simple in its structure may be easier to report about accurately than other classes of events or behaviors.

Table 7.10 speculates that the three threatening topics I have reviewed probably differ in how they are organized in the experience of respondents (see Schaeffer, 1994). For example, sex partners are probably not acquired nor abortions undergone at regular intervals, but the use of marijuana may be regularly patterned for some respondents. The speculations in Table 7.10 are a reminder that the patterning and organization of threatening behaviors varies across respondents (and across groups of respondents) who engage

TABLE 7.10
Speculation on Social Organization of Three Threatening Behaviors

	Sex Partners	Abortion	Drug Use
Importance of category to respondent	variable	probably often high	variable, probably increases with frequency
Frequency	low for most, high for a few	.low for most, high for a few	low for most, high for a few
Regularity	low	low	variable
Similarity	probably increases with number	low for most	increases with frequency and regularity
Social reinforcement	low to moderate	low	may be high among social group
Clarity (distinct from similar events)	generally high	generally high	may be reduced if multiple drugs used

in such behaviors. Reports of such behaviors are subject to the same memory errors (such as omissions) as are reports of more mundane activities. But in the case of threatening behaviors, even errors of memory and processing may be biased toward a conventional, socially nonthreatening answer. That is, the nonthreatening answer to a threatening question—and an important source of response bias—may be incorporated in the heuristics that respondents use to construct their answers during an interview.

Consider sources of response error that are associated with the level of threat presented by the survey question. To be comprehensive, a theory of question threat would have to encompass topics as diverse as income, voting, intravenous drug use, and masturbation, and I have not found such a fully developed theory in the literature. But to begin, we can distinguish, as others have, between threatening questions and threatening answers. Threatening questions pose what Lee and Renzetti (1990) called an intrusive threat. Their discussion suggests that respondents may perceive a question as an intrusive threat if they consider the topic private or personal, if the question concerns deviant acts, if the topic is of interest to those in power, or if it is sacred to the respondent. Thus, respondents may consider a question threatening regardless of their answer. For example, they may consider their income to be "nobody's business" in general, no matter what their income, even if they might discuss it frankly under certain circumstances.

Most studies have been concerned with response situations in which a respondent perceives a question as threatening because of the respondent's (true) answer. A respondent who has never used intravenous drugs may recognize the question as intrusive, but answer "no" to the question without objecting. If the threat of a question varies depending on the answer, then the risks associated with admitting threatening behaviors depend on the respondent's behavior in that specific behavioral domain. A comprehensive list of the risks involved in giving a threatening answer, such as that begun in Table 7.11, would include the risks associated with having the respondent's answer disclosed to others outside the interview situation. These risks include the risk that others would be in a position to do any of the following: have information that would help them obtain access to the respondent, know that the respondent has something that the others want, know that the respondent has engaged in illegal behaviors, know that the respondent has engaged in behaviors counter to values that the others (or some third party) might hold, make other negative inferences about the respondent, or learn that the respondent has kept the information secret. Even if respondents were not concerned about the risks of disclosure, their answers might reflect the pressures of answering to an interviewer in a social situation. Thus, respondents might take into account (although not necessarily consciously) that an answer might reveal that they engaged in behaviors that are counter to values that the interviewer might hold, or that

TABLE 7.11
Risks and Losses in Answering Truthfully

Risk	Loss
Disclosure to Outsiders	
Improved access to R	Further intrusions
R has something others want	Further solicitations
Illegal behavior	Embarrassment, punishment
Counter (others') values	Embarrassment
Negative inferences	Embarrassment
Reveal past secrecy	Embarrassment, violation of openness
Disclosure to Interviewer	
Counter interviewer's (possible) values	Disagreement, embarrassment
Negative inferences by interviewer	Embarrassment
Painful feelings	Remember painful feelings
Counter (own) values	Threat to self

the interviewer might make negative inferences about them based on an answer. Finally, giving a threatening answer might raise painful or stressful feelings or require that respondents admit to having done things that they wish they had not.

Each of these risks has threatened losses associated with it. These losses include further intrusions or solicitations, embarrassment, painful memories, and threat to the respondent's self-concept. Experimental manipulations that increase the legitimacy of the survey or reduce interaction with the interviewer presumably reduce these perceived risks of disclosure and embarrassment and also any lack of frankness that might result from these sources. In contrast, threats to the respondent's self-concept have not been addressed by the experimental manipulations described earlier. A possible exception is the restrictive–permissive context manipulation in the reporting of sex partners, which may work, in part, by making specific personal values salient to the respondent when they construct their answers.

It is not obvious exactly how the mode of interview or other such manipulations might affect cognitive processing. Manipulations such as the use of a self-administered response mode or computerized instruments certainly could affect respondents' conscious calculations of risks and their likelihood and thereby influence a respondent's decision to report. This possibility is compatible with the view that overreporting of desirable behaviors and underreporting of undesirable behaviors is intentional or deliberate. Using the terms of the information-processing model described earlier, this might suggest that when a respondent retrieves a sensitive answer, he or she then decides whether or not to modify it before reporting. Manipulations such as the use of self-administered or computerized instruments may reduce such errors due to the sensitivity of a topic that occur in the final stages of processing.

But whereas such conscious calculations may be responsible for some reporting errors due to the sensitivity of the topic, and for part of the effect of interview mode described earlier, other processes may be relevant for some respondents or some behaviors. I have already suggested that nonthreatening answers may be incorporated into the heuristics and estimation methods that respondents use to construct survey answers. For example, a nonthreatening value may be retrieved and used as an anchor in an anchor-and-adjust response strategy.

And there are other related possibilities. For example, as my epigraph indicates, ethicists have argued about whether a falsehood told to someone who has no right to the requested information is a lie. Regardless of the moral status of such falsehoods, they have a routine social function in smoothing casual interactions and deflecting rude inquiries of all kinds: If someone asks a question that is none of their business, the recipient of that question may prefer a routine denial to the dispreferred (and possibly implicating) act of refusing to answer. Furthermore (and partly because of their conventional nature), nonthreatening answers may be embedded in the public biographies—personal histories available for public consumption—that people construct about themselves. For some people, parts of these public biographies may, over time, become incorporated into a public self-concept or may replace actual history in memory. Thus, a denial that one has used marijuana may be produced almost automatically because it is the conventional answer to a question that is nobody's business or because it is part of a public self. As such, the denial requires no extensive retrieval or active judgment about the risks of reporting in an interview—it is a fast and safe solution to the task of answering a threatening question. And with repetition, the public, socially acceptable answer may replace other historical answers entirely.

We can find some insight into automatic processing and the role of cognitive structures in such processing in research on racial stereotypes, a kind of cognitive structure (Devine, 1989). This research suggests that relevant cues from the environment may automatically evoke stereotypes that are used in cognitive processing. Processing and decision making will draw on these automatic structures unless competing values and beliefs are made conscious. When competing values and beliefs are made conscious, they may then guide actual behavior.

In the survey interview, automatic processing could be activated by cues that a question presents and could affect the reporting of answers to threatening questions in at least two ways. First, a question may activate what Dykema (1996) called a personal-event schema. This cognitive structure incorporates the individual's definition of the behavior, information about its frequency, as well as links to affect and the self-concept. We might also think of this schema as having several layers that distinguish information about the individual's behavior in a public biography, which can be readily reported, from information that is to be kept more private. Second, a question about a threatening topic might evoke interactional conventions for dealing with intrusive questions. These conventions could also affect answers to a self-administered form, as Schwarz (1990) argued. I would speculate that recipients of intrusive questions routinely use denial as an automatic, socially routine, defensive strategy. Such conventional denials could be offered simply because an intrusive question was asked and without any calculation of risks. In other words, respondents may deny engaging in threatening behaviors partly because they routinely do so.

Automatic processing of this type could affect several stages of cognitive processing—for example, how the question or the cognitive task is understood, retrieval, or evaluation of a candidate answer (see Table 7.12). Respondents might interpret threatening questions in a way that makes the behavior being asked about different from the behaviors they themselves engage in and thereby distance themselves from the behavior. Respondents may also treat the cognitive task posed by the question as one of classifying themselves as more like someone who engages in the behavior or more like someone who does not. For example, the pragmatic meaning of a question about abortion that a respondent constructs may be to determine whether the respondent is more like someone who has an abortion or more like someone who does not. If some respondents treat threatening questions in this way, there is an opportunity for other cognitive structures (e.g., a stereotype of what someone who has an abortion is "like") to play a role in the response process. In either of these two cases, the respondent's cogni-

TABLE 7.12
Examples of Possible Automatic Processing in
Reports of Sensitive (Threatening) Behaviors

Stage	Example—Threat to Self
Comprehension of question	(Ambiguous) terms interpreted in ways that distance R from threatening events or behaviors
Interpretation of cognitive task	Question is asking R to classify self as more like someone who engages in behavior or more like someone who does not
	Question is "nobody's business," further processing is not required, standard social answer may be given
Retrieval	Full search not undertaken because question "does not apply" to R
Judgment	Standard socially acceptable answer is adequate

tive processing may be superficial because once the question has been redefined, it no longer requires a threatening answer.

CONCLUSION

Improving the accuracy of answers to questions on threatening topics has proved particularly challenging and somewhat daunting. As the review with which I began this chapter suggests, recent research appears to have made some progress in reducing errors due to the sensitivity of a topic, principally by increasing the privacy of responding. However, as this more speculative discussion suggests, further improvements are likely to require more specific theorizing about the stages of processing at which errors arise and about the role of automatic processing and conscious decision making in that processing. In addition, we must probably consider that such response errors may have different origins for different respondents and different topics and thus require multiple solutions.

REFERENCES

Bok, S. (1978). *Lying: Moral choice in public and private life*. New York: Pantheon.

Devine, P. G. (1989). Stereotypes and prejudice: Their automatic and controlled components. *Journal of Personal and Social Psychology, 56*, 5–18.

Dykema, J. (1996). *Events, instruments, and reporting errors: Combining knowledge from multiple perspectives*. Unpublished Master's Thesis, University of Wisconsin–Madison.

Jones, E. F., & Forrest, J. D. (1992). Underreporting of abortion in surveys of U.S. women: 1976 to 1988. *Demography, 29*, 113–126.

Lee, R. M., & Renzetti, C. M. (1990). The problems of researching sensitive topics. *American Behavioral Scientist, 33*, 510–528.

Lessler, J. T., Weeks, M. F., & O'Reilly, J. M. (1994). Results from the National Survey of Family Growth Cycle V Pretest. In *Proceedings of the American Statistical Association, the Section on Survey Research Methods* (pp. 64–70). Washington, DC: American Statistical Association.

Locander, W. B., Sudman, S., & Bradburn, N. (1976). An investigation of interview method, threat and response distortion. *Journal of the American Statistical Association, 71*, 269–275.

Nathan, G., Sirken, M., Willis, G., & Esposito, J. (1990, November). *Laboratory experiments on the cognitive aspects of sensitive questions*. Paper presented at the International Conference on Measurement Errors in Surveys, Tuscon, Arizona.

Parry, H. J., & Crossley, H. M. (1950). Validity of responses to survey questions. *Public Opinion Quarterly, 14*, 61–80.

Rasinski, K. A., Baldwin, A. K., Willis, G. B., & Jobe, J. B. (1994). Risk and loss perceptions associated with survey reporting of sensitive behaviors. In *Proceedings of the Section on Survey Research Methods of the American Statistical Association* (pp. 497–502). Washington, DC: The American Statistical Association.

Schaeffer, N. C. (1994). Errors of experience: Response errors in reports about child support and their implications for questionnaire design. In N. Schwarz & S. Sudman (Eds.), *Autobio-*

graphical memory and the validity of retrospective reports (pp. 141–170). New York: Springer-Verlag.

Schwarz, N. (1990). Assessing frequency reports of mundane behaviors: Contributions of cognitive psychology to questionnaire construction. In C. Hendrick & M. S. Clark (Eds.), *Research methods in personality and sociology* (pp. 98–119). Newbury Park, England: Sage.

Smith, T. W. (1992). A methodological analysis of the sexual behavior questions on the General Social Surveys. *Journal of Official Statistics, 8*(3), 309–325.

Tourangeau, R., Rasinski, K., Jobe, J., Smith, T. W., & Pratt, W. F. (1997). Sources of error in a survey on sexual behavior. *Journal of Official Statistics, 13*, 341–365.

Tourangeau, R., & Smith, T. W. (1996). Asking sensitive questions: The impact of data collection mode, question format, and question context. *Public Opinion Quarterly, 60*, 275–304.

Tourangeau, R., & Smith, T. W. (1998). Collecting sensitive information with different modes of data collection. In M. Couper, R. Baker, J. Bethlehem, C. Clark, J. Martin, W. Nicholls, & J. O'Reilly (Eds.), *Computer-assisted survey information collection* (pp. 431–454). New York: Wiley.

Turner, C. F., Lessler, J. T., & Devore, J. (1992). Effects of Mode of Administration and Wording on Reporting of Drug Use. In C. F. Turner, J. T. Lessler, & J. C. Gfroerer (Eds.), *Survey measurement of drug use* (pp. 177–220). Rockville, MD: National Institute on Drug Abuse, U.S. Department of Health and Human Services.

8

The Association Between Self-Reports of Abortion and Breast Cancer Risk: Fact or Artifact

Heather G. Miller
James N. Gribble
Leah C. Mazade
Susan M. Rogers
Charles F. Turner
Research Triangle Institute, Washington, DC

All measurements, whether generated in the laboratory or in the field, are vulnerable to error. Yet all too often, public health policymaking and practice base decisions on such empirical data without taking their methodological limitations fully into account. For example, findings from studies that use small samples of convenience are often given the same weight as the results from larger, population-based samples. And the reporting bias that may afflict self-disclosure of information is not always explored and assessed. Of concern to scientists attending the 1996 National Institutes of Health (NIH) conference and contributing to this volume is the quality of self-reported measurements found in many health studies that address such factors as symptoms, exposures, compliance with treatment, and utilization of health care services.

As researchers have long recognized, several kinds of bias can afflict self-reports. Thus, some understanding of the validity and reliability of measurements is vital to drawing reasonable inferences from them, for methodological artifacts can not only mask important associations between self-reported measures and health outcomes of interest but produce spurious linkages as well. For example, one recent study found no association between self-reported measures of the use of condoms and incident sexually transmitted diseases, or STDs (Turner & Miller, 1997; Zenilman et al., 1995); respondents who reported always using condoms were just as likely to have an incident STD as people who reported that they never used them. The findings raised troubling questions: Is consistent, correct condom use, a behavior widely considered to prevent transmission of infection, inadequate to protect a person from acquiring an STD? Or is social desirability bias obscuring the protective effect of condoms?

The problem of bias is well documented in the scientific literature but has proved difficult to study. To highlight the importance of exploring bias in self-reports and the challenges involved in such research, this chapter reviews several recent case-control studies that have noted a weak but persistent association between induced abortion and breast cancer. Unfortunately, the findings of two recent studies are being used without qualification in campaigns to discourage women from seeking an abortion. They have appeared in widely disseminated, fear-arousing messages that ignore the uncertainty and inconsistencies in the data. Those problems are carefully referenced in the scientific literature, but advertisements on public transportation in several East Coast cities merely warn that "women who choose abortion suffer more and deadlier breast cancer" (Estrich, 1996). That message delivers misinformation about the severity of the disease in that group of women, and the confusion it may generate among women who are at greatest risk for breast cancer may make them discredit prevention messages about effective strategies, such as mammographic screening.

Sound guidelines for prevention require solid empirical data. Thus, it is crucial to know whether the relationship between induced abortion and breast cancer is real or spurious—that is, an artifact resulting from bias in self-reports of abortion. In this chapter, we examine several potential sources of bias and the quality of existing self-reported data from case-control studies of abortion and breast cancer. Such studies play an important role in the development of public health policies that can affect the lives of millions of women. The scale of that impact argues strongly for improving not only our understanding of bias in key measures but ultimately the quality of those measures.

INTERVIEW CONDITIONS AND BIAS IN
SELF-REPORTS OF SENSITIVE BEHAVIORS

Measurements of sensitive behaviors contain many potential sources of bias.[1] Chapter 7, this volume, notes several, including complexities and

---

[1]Other biases may exist in case-control studies linking abortion and breast cancer besides those discussed in this section. Bias in ascertaining cases, which may result from differential surveillance, diagnosis, or referral, is a well-recognized problem in case-control studies. Case-control research is also vulnerable to biases associated with nonparticipation. Women who have already been identified as cases may be more willing than controls to participate in research studies—with the result that recruitment rates can differ across the two groups.

problems associated with cognitive processing, the social organization of the behavior of interest, task requirements to provide the data, and management of the threat associated with some questions on sensitive or illegal behaviors. Certainly, those sources of bias could be found in measures of abortion as well. Recall bias or difficulties with cognitive processing can be particularly problematic when respondents are asked to report on a lengthy retrospective period. And generally, a diagnosis of breast cancer occurs later in life; it may thus be quite distant from hypothesized causal factors, including abortion. In addition, the task of providing specific information on the timing and outcomes of all conceptions can be enormously complex, especially for women who have suffered multiple miscarriages.

A further consideration is that the social organization of abortion has changed dramatically during the lifetimes of women who are currently diagnosed with breast cancer. What was once an illegal medical procedure no longer carries legal sanctions—yet it remains controversial. A number of psychological and social factors come into play when a woman is asked about a behavior that was once illegal and continues to carry significant stigma.

In recent years, evidence has been building to confirm that the way questionnaires are administered during a survey can affect the quality of self-reported measures of sensitive behaviors. In this chapter, we explore whether the increased privacy afforded by self-administered questionnaires (SAQs) decreases the threat associated with questions about abortion. We also consider whether there are ways to manage the costs associated with SAQs; that is, the task requirements and cognitive complexities inherent in filling out a questionnaire without the assistance of an interviewer.

Paper-and-Pencil Self-Administered Questionnaires

Interviewer-administered questionnaires (IAQs) that contain items on sensitive or illegal behaviors may present problems for both the interviewer and the interviewee. Asking or answering questions, for example, about a respondent's recent history of STDs or date rape could conceivably generate anxiety for both individuals in the interview—for the interviewer, who might worry about losing the case, and for the interviewee, who may fear a "loss of face." Historically, surveys have attempted to deal with the potential for such discomfort by using paper-and-pencil self-administered questionnaires (PAPI SAQs) to increase privacy for both parties.

Data from surveys of several sensitive behaviors, including drug use, sexual behavior, and induced abortion (see the later discussion), support the notion that increased privacy during the interview results in increased reporting of those behaviors. A 1990 field test of the National Household Survey on Drug Abuse (NHSDA) included a methodological experiment that randomized subjects to either PAPI SAQs or IAQs for sensitive portions of the questionnaire. Overall, PAPI SAQs yielded higher estimates of illicit drug use than did IAQs (Turner, Lessler, & Devore, 1992). However, the relative advantage of PAPI SAQs appeared to be a direct function of the sensitivity of the behavior being reported. Thus, the prevalence of recent cocaine use among NHSDA participants assigned to the PAPI SAQ mode was 2.4 times higher than the prevalence among participants in the IAQ mode. The interview mode effect was less pronounced for reports of marijuana use and was almost nonexistent for reports of alcohol use by adults.[2] The National Longitudinal Survey of Labor Market Experience, Youth Cohort (NLS–Y), also found that PAPI SAQs yielded more frequent reports of illicit drug use than did IAQs (Shober, Fe Caces, Pergamit, & Branden, 1992), as have other such surveys (see, for example, Aquilino, 1994; Gfroerer & Hughes, 1992).

Although few studies have investigated the effect of the mode of interview in surveys of self-reported sexual behavior (Catania, McDermott, & Pollack, 1986), those that have report a mode effect for some but not all sexual behaviors. For example, Millstein and Irwin (1983) found that girls completing IAQs reported significantly lower levels of masturbation and vaginal intercourse (25% and 63%, respectively) compared with girls assigned to either one of the SAQ formats (38% and 74%, respectively).

The increased reports of sensitive behavior associated with more privacy during the interviewing process seem to be a stable finding, but do such reports actually constitute a decrease in reporting bias? In general, survey methodologists believe that biases in the reporting of illicit or stigmatized behavior in general population surveys result in a net negative bias in estimates of the prevalence of those behaviors in the population. The direction of the bias is negative because the number of survey respondents who deny engaging in stigmatized or sensitive behavior in which they have, in fact, engaged is expected to be larger than the number who falsely report behavior in which they have not engaged (Bradburn et al., 1979; Catania, Gibson, Chitwood, & Coates, 1990; Miller, Turner, & Moses, 1990; Turner, Lessler, & Gfroerer, 1992). Thus, researchers believe that higher levels of such reports reflect a reduction in reporting bias and thereby an increase in the accuracy of the measurements.

Concerns about the quality of data gathered in a survey would argue for using PAPI SAQs, which are relatively easy and inexpensive to produce. Nevertheless, their limitations should not be overlooked. Extensive use of contingent questioning—that is, branching or skip patterns—may not be possible in a PAPI SAQ because some respondents have trouble following the complex instructions required to make their way through a self-admin-

---

[2] A mode effect was found for 12- to 17-year-olds—a group for whom the use of alcohol is illicit. For that group, estimates of the prevalence of recent alcohol use were 1.4 times greater when PAPI SAQs were used.

istered form (Lessler & Holt, 1987). Moreover, according to the National Center for Education Statistics (1993), the reading skills of a sizable segment of the U.S. population are limited, which means that some proportion of survey respondents will not be able to complete these forms by themselves. Because literacy is correlated with education and other indicators of socio-economic status, the resulting measurements from surveys that cannot hold privacy constant across all subjects may be afflicted with other biases as well. For example, surveys that use PAPI SAQs for sensitive portions of the questionnaire run the risk of producing differences in response distributions if participants of limited literacy cannot be randomized to that mode. More-over, some investigators have noted higher rates of item nonresponse with PAPI SAQs in comparison to IAQs (Cox, Witt, Traccarella, & Perez-Michael, 1992; Fay, Turner, Klassen, & Gagnon, 1989; Rogers & Turner, 1991; Turner, Miller, & Moses, 1989). And among participants who do respond to all items, the number who provide logically inconsistent answers on PAPI SAQs can be substantial (see, for example, Cox et al., 1992, and Smith, 1992).

Audio Computer-Assisted Self-Interviewing

Until recently, the problems just noted were for the most part unavoidable but advances in interviewing technology now offer some hope of overcoming them. Specifically, the use of audio computer-assisted self-interviewing (audio-CASI) appears to reduce some of the measurement biases that have been problematic in prior surveys of sensitive behavior (Cooley, Turner, O'Reilly, Allen, & Paddock, 1996; Johnston, 1992; O'Reilly & Turner, 1992; O'Reilly, Hubbard, Lessler, Biemer, & Turner, 1994).

With audio-CASI, respondents use portable laptop computers and listen to questions through headphones; they enter their answers by pressing labeled keys. The system does not rely on synthesized voices, and the recorded audio component is equivalent to a high-quality tape recording. In addition, there are no significant delays in playing back the audio-deliv-ered questions. Unlike some earlier efforts (e.g., Camburn, Cynamon, & Harel, 1991), audio-CASI is capable of executing skip patterns, checking for out-of-range responses and inconsistencies across similar questions, and generating data files. Every respondent hears the questions asked in the same neutral manner, regardless of the question's substance or the re-sponse it elicits from a participant. The technology can be used with any respondent who can hear and speak and does not require literacy in any language (see, for example, Hendershot, Rogers, Thornberry, Miller, & Turner, 1996; Turner, Rogers, Hendershot, Miller, & Thornberry, 1996).

Early studies hypothesized that the use of audio-CASI would reduce re-porting bias by increasing privacy during the interview for all respondents, even those of limited literacy. The results of several large studies (Duffer,

Lessler, Weeks, & Mosher, 1996; Turner, Ku, Sonenstein, & Pleck, 1996; Turner, Lessler, & Devore, 1992; Turner, Miller, & Rogers, 1997) that contained an audio-CASI component, including studies on drug use and AIDS-related sexual behaviors, indicate just such a reduction.

Mail and Telephone Interviews

Because studies that collect interview data from large population-based samples can be very expensive, many researchers have used mailed questionnaires and telephone interviews when logistic and economic constraints precluded face-to-face interviews. (See, for example, two recent telephone surveys: the National AIDS Behavioral Survey, Catania et al., 1992, and a French survey of AIDS-related sexual behavior, ACSF Investigators, 1992.) Yet each mode of data collection has its own set of limitations. Surveys that are conducted by mail afford participants privacy but often have poor response rates. Telephone surveys generally have better response rates but are not similarly private because they require participants to report information to another human being, albeit over the phone rather than face to face. The problem of privacy in telephone interviewing and the apparent success of audio-CASI in reducing bias in self-reports led scientists at Research Triangle Institute to explore the potential of audio-CASI for use in telephone interviewing.

A New Telephone Interviewing Technology

Telephone audio-CASI, or T-ACASI, is built on the audio-CASI platform but uses a touchtone telephone instead of a laptop computer. It thus offers the same advantages as audio-CASI in terms of survey administration, although operationally it replicates many of the procedures of standard telephone interviewing.[3]

Results from two T-ACASI pilot studies (Miller et al., 1997; Turner, Miller, Smith, Cooley, & Rogers, 1996) indicate that the system is stable and easy to use and respondents prefer it to a live interviewer when sensitive questions are being asked. Moreover, a study that compared data from standard telephone interviewing with data collected by T-ACASI found that T-ACASI interviews produced higher rates of prevalence of several sensitive behaviors, including anal intercourse, and lower rates of normative behaviors, such as condom use (Turner, Miller et al., 1996). Furthermore, T-ACASI

---

[3]In a T-ACASI interview, a human telephone interviewer calls and recruits an eligible respondent. After eliciting consent and collecting data on nonsensitive items, the interviewer transfers the call to the T-ACASI system, which administers the sensitive part of the questionnaire.

participants were two times more likely than respondents assigned to the live interviewer to report never using a condom.

The potential value of T-ACASI in reducing bias in self-reports has yet to be fully explored, although several studies are under way. Its application to measures of abortion, a major topic of interest here, may offer a way to investigate whether a link indeed exists between induced abortion and breast cancer—or whether the association observed in other case-control studies reflects differential reporting of cases versus controls. The next section reviews the evidence from case-control studies on the role that reporting bias may play in that research.

EVIDENCE OF A LINK BETWEEN ABORTION AND BREAST CANCER

Two recent case-control studies (Daling, Malone, Voigt, White, & Weiss, 1994; Newcomb et al., 1996) reported a modest but statistically significant association between breast cancer and induced abortion. Because of the intensity of the abortion debate in this country, the finding was quickly seized on and widely publicized. Left behind was a carefully balanced review of existing data provided by the Daling team, the caveats included by Newcomb and her colleagues, and statements issued by researchers from the National Cancer Institute and other scientific authorities advising caution. All of those qualifying comments went virtually unheeded in the lay press, written off, perhaps, as academic methodological hair-splitting. The National Cancer Institute (1994), in its presentation and review of the findings of Daling and coworkers, summarized some of the methodological concerns that make it difficult to draw inferences from the studies, noting that small relative risks, such as those reported by Daling and by Newcomb, are "usually difficult to interpret. Such increases may be due to chance, statistical bias, or effects of confounding factors that are sometimes not evident" (p. 2).

We reviewed the epidemiological literature for other studies of the relationship between breast cancer and abortion (see Table 8.1) and found no definitive answers. Abundant and solid empirical evidence supports the premise that full-term pregnancy reduces the risk of breast cancer (e.g., Kelsey, Gammon, & John, 1993; MacMahon et al., 1970). But the picture offered by studies of the relationship between pregnancies that do not go to full term and the risk of breast cancer is much less clear. Some investigators report no significant increase in the risk of breast cancer with either spontaneous or induced abortion (Adami, Bergstrom, Lund, & Meirik, 1990; Brinton, Hoover, & Fraumeni, 1983; La Vecchia et al., 1987; Lipworth, Katsouyanni, Ekbom, Michels, & Trichopoulos, 1995; Parazzini, La Vecchia, & Negri, 1991; Rosenberg et al., 1988). Others have found increased risk asso-

TABLE 8.1
Selected Major Case-Control Studies of Breast Cancer and Abortion

Citation	N	Response Rate	Mode	Population	RR Induced Abortion (95% CI)	RR Spontaneous Abortion (95% CI)
Newcomb et al., 1996	Cases: 6,888 Controls: 9,529	Case: 81% Control: 84%	IAQ (phone)	U.S. women < 75 years old	1.23 (1.00–1.51)	1.11 (1.02–1.20)
Lipworth et al., 1995	Cases: 820 Controls: 1,548	Case: 94% Control: 94%	IAQ	Greek women (nulliparous)	0.98 (0.56–1.73)	1.17 (0.64–2.13)
				Greek women (parous)	0.99 (0.56–1.74)	0.61 (0.33–1.14)
Daling et al., 1994	Cases: 845 Controls: 961	Case: 84% Control: 74%	IAQ	U.S. White females < 46 years old	1.5 (1.2–1.9)	0.9 (0.7–1.2)
Parazzini et al., 1991	Cases: 2,394 Controls: 2,218	Case: 97% Control: 98%	IAQ	Italian females < 75 years old	0.9 (0.7–1.1)	0.8 (0.7–1.1)
Adami et al., 1990	Cases: 422 Controls: 527	Case: 89% Control: 81%	IAQ	Scandinavian women < 45 years old	1.3* (0.6–3.0)	1.3* (0.7–2.6)
Ewertz and Duffy, 1988	Cases: 1,486 Controls: 1,336	Case: 88% Control: 79%	SAQ (mail)	Danish women < 70 years old (no full-term pregnancy)	3.85 (1.08–13.6)	2.63 (0.83–8.32)
				Danish women < 70 years old (full-term pregnancy)	N.S.**	N.S.**

Study	Cases/Controls	Response	Method	Population	RR (95% CI)	RR (95% CI)
Rosenberg et al., 1988	Cases: 3,200 / Controls: 4,844	***	IAQ	U.S. women < 70 years old (nulliparous)	1.3 (0.9–2.2)	0.9 (0.5–1.5)
				U.S. women < 70 years old (parous)	1.2 (0.9–1.6)	0.9 (0.8–1.0)
La Vecchia et al., 1987	Cases: 1,108 / Controls: 1,281	Case: 98% Control: 98%	IAQ	Italian women < 75 years old	0.7 (0.5–1.1)	0.9 (0.7–1.3)
Hirohata et al., 1985	Cases: 212 / Controls: 424	Case: 99% Controls: 87%	IAQ	Japanese women	1.19 (0.7–1.9)	1.53 (1.01–2.3)
Brinton et al., 1983	Cases: 1,362 / Controls: 1,250	Case: 86% Control: 74%	IAQ	U.S. White females (before live birth)	1.34 (0.3–5.6)	1.09 (0.8–1.5)
				U.S. White females (after live birth)	0.89 (0.4–2.0)	1.2 (0.9–1.6)

Note. IAQ = interviewer-administered questionnaire; SAQ = self-administered questionnaire.
*Adjusted risk ratio (RR) for women reporting 2 or more abortions (spontaneous or induced).
**N.S. (no significant association).
***The authors do not provide response rates for cases and controls. They do state that 5% of patients (which would include both cases and controls) declined participation.

ciated with both types of abortion (Howe, Senie, Bzduch, & Herzfeld, 1989; Newcomb et al., 1996). Some studies report increased risk associated with induced but not spontaneous abortion (Daling et al., 1994; Ewertz & Duffy, 1988), and at least one has found increased risk only with spontaneous abortion (Hirohata et al., 1985). Several large cohort studies have also looked at the association between breast cancer and abortion, but again, their data do not allow definitive statements about any such link (see Calle et al., 1995; Hadjimichael, Boyle, & Meigs, 1986; Kvale, Heuch, & Eide, 1987; Lindefors-Harris, Eklund, Meirik, Rutqvist, & Wiklund, 1989).

The variation in findings across case-control studies may reflect small samples, differences in the populations being sampled, or differences in design and analysis, including controlling for different covariates. Case-control studies—like all experimental designs—have strengths and weaknesses that are known to affect the quality of the data they produce (see, for example, Breslow & Day, 1980; Sackett, 1979; Schlesselman, 1982). When such studies produce small risk ratios or findings at tenuous levels of significance, bias as an alternative explanation of those findings becomes more plausible. Because the size of the effect in much of the research is small, several investigators have wondered whether the abortion–breast cancer association might be an artifact of reporting bias (Daling et al., 1994; Gammon, Bertin, & Terry, 1996; Henshaw, 1996; Lindefors-Harris et al., 1989; Lindefors-Harris, Eklund, Adami, & Meirik, 1991; Lipworth et al., 1995; Michels, Hsieh, Trichopoulos, & Willett, 1995; Newcomb et al., 1996). Evidence from other large-scale studies of women that included items on abortion supports the notion that measurements of this sensitive topic are vulnerable to reporting bias.

Reporting of Abortions

There are two sources of data on induced abortions in the United States: clinicians who perform abortions and the women who undergo them. Surveillance data from clinicians are collected by the Centers for Disease Control and Prevention (CDC); self-reported data come from health surveys conducted among women of childbearing age.[4] Comparing surveillance data with self-reported data provides estimates of some of the bias in the self-reported measures.

According to CDC data, 1,429,577 abortions were performed in 1990 (Koonin, Smith, & Ramick, 1993). Overall, the majority of women who underwent abortion in 1990 were young, and almost half did not report a previous live birth. In an independent survey of abortion providers, Henshaw, Koonin,

---

[4]That is, the National Survey of Family Growth (NSFG), the National Surveys of Young Women (NSYW), and the National Longitudinal Survey of Labor Market Experience, Youth Cohort.

and Smith (1991) found few induced abortions among women older than 40 but substantial differences by race: The abortion rate among non-White females was 2.7 times the rate among White females.

Self-reported data confirm some of the patterns seen in surveillance data but show major dissimilarities in other areas. Like the surveillance data, self-reports show that younger women were more likely than older women to report an abortion and that abortions were most frequently reported by women who reported no previous live births (Jones & Forrest, 1992; Miller et al., 1997). The completeness of the self-reporting, however, differs substantially from the CDC data. Overall, the abortions reported by women taking part in health surveys accounted for only 35% to 40% of the abortions enumerated in surveillance data (Jones & Forrest, 1992). Moreover, completeness of reporting appears to vary by race: A slightly greater proportion of Black females versus White females reported a lifetime history of abortion. But the actual racial difference appears to be even greater. Comparing data from the 1988 wave of the NSFG with abortion surveillance data, Jones and Forrest found that White females reported 38% of the abortions noted in surveillance records, whereas non-White females reported 27% of such abortions.[5]

Reporting bias may also vary by the conditions under which data are collected. Under standard interview conditions in the NSFG, interviewers asked respondents about their abortion history during a face-to-face interview using IAQs. But in an experiment embedded in the 1988 wave of the NSFG, respondents were also given a PAPI SAQ to offer them a second, private opportunity to report past abortions. Use of the PAPI SAQs increased women's reporting of abortions from 39% to 71% of the level reported by abortion providers (Jones & Forrest, 1992). The impact of the interview mode may also vary by race. Data from the experiment showed that the level of completeness of abortion reporting among White females increased from 46% in the IAQ mode to 74% in the PAPI SAQ mode (Jones & Forrest, 1992). However, the increase among Black women was greater, rising from 26% in the IAQ mode to 67% in the PAPI SAQ mode.

In 1994, RTI conducted a pilot test for the 1995 wave of the NSFG that included a mode experiment. In the pilot study, interviewers asked women about their sexual history, including any abortions they might have had. At the end of the IAQ portion of the interview, women were reinterviewed using audio-CASI.[6] The proportion of women who reported abortions in the private

---

[5]Comparing data from the NLS-Y with surveillance data indicated approximately the same rate of underreporting, with White females reporting 45% of abortions, Black females 27%, and Hispanic females 19%.

[6]The audio-CASI interview included some items that the interviewer had asked before as well as a second section of new questions about such sensitive behaviors as injecting drugs, needle sharing, and same-gender sex.

audio-CASI condition (23.6%) was 1.4 times greater than the proportion who reported them in the less-private IAQ mode (17.3%; Duffer et al., 1996). Black women were more than twice as likely as White women (31% versus 14%) to report more abortions or sexual partners in the past 12 months in the audio-CASI mode (Kinsey, Thornberry, Carson, & Duffer, 1995).

The now completed 1995 wave of the NSFG replicated the pilot study's mode experiment for sensitive items, including abortion. All of the women who completed the NSFG's face-to-face IAQ (10,847 respondents) were asked to complete a smaller, self-administered reinterview using RTI's audio-CASI system. Preliminary analyses of the data from the 1995 wave (Miller et al., 1997) appear to confirm the findings of the mode experiment from the 1988 wave (see Table 8.2). That is, among sexually active women, the number who reported a history of abortion in the more private audio-CASI mode was greater than in the interviewer-administered mode. Of the women who did not report an abortion in the original IAQ mode, 4.5% reported one or more abortions in the audio-CASI mode.[7] Among women reporting one abortion in the IAQ mode, 5.8% reported two or more abortions in the audio-CASI mode.[8] Most of the discrepancies in reports of abortion across modes occurred in only one direction. Thus, among women reporting two or more abortions in the IAQ mode, only 0.4% reported no abortions in the audio-CASI mode. As the earlier wave found, the mode effect was greater among Black women than among Whites: 7.3% of Black females who reported no abortions in the IAQ mode reported one or more abortions when using audio-CASI; the comparable percentage for White participants was 4.2%. In addition, 10.3% of Black females reporting one abortion in the IAQ mode reported two or more abortions in the audio-CASI mode, compared with 5.0% of White women. Overall, the odds of reporting an abortion were approximately 1.3 times greater when information was collected using the audio-CASI technology compared with the IAQ.

At least two arguments support the hypothesis that data from the NSFG experiment provide a lower-bound estimate of the effect of the interview mode on measures of abortion. First, the design of the NSFG experiment required that all women complete the IAQ before the audio-CASI reinterview. A woman who wanted to answer the question about abortion more honestly

---

[7]Of 9,674 sexually active respondents who were interviewed in the IAQ mode, 2,121 reported no history of pregnancy, and consequently interviewers did not administer the questions concerning abortion. In this analysis, those women are considered as reporting no abortions. All women, regardless of pregnancy history, received questions on abortion in the audio-CASI mode.

[8]All percentages are weighted to account for variation in the probability of selection and nonresponse. (Weighting allows for comparison of these estimates with 1995 census projections.)

TABLE 8.2
Comparison of Abortion Reporting by Interview Mode
Among Sexually Active Women: 1995 NSFG

ORIGINAL IAQ REPORT	SUBSEQUENT REPORT IN A-CASI			Unweighted N
	No Abortions %	1 Abortion %	2+ Abortion %	
All Women				
No Abortions*	95.4	3.5	1.0	7,827
1 Abortion	1.8	92.5	5.8	1,265
2+ Abortions	0.4	2.2	97.4	582
White Women				
No Abortions	95.8	3.3	0.9	5,675
1 Abortion	1.1	93.9	5.0	850
2+ Abortions	0.6	2.5	96.9	343
Black Women				
No Abortions	92.8	5.3	2.0	1,742
1 Abortion	4.4	85.3	10.3	355
2+ Abortions	0.0	1.8	98.2	217

Note. The analyses exclude 230 cases with missing data.
*In the 1995 IAQ, women were asked to report pregnancy histories for up to 15 pregnancies, and abortion was listed as one of the possible pregnancy outcomes. Therefore, women who reported never being pregnant were not questioned about abortion. Included in these estimates are 54 women (16 Black, 37 White, 1 other race) who reported in the IAQ mode that they had never been pregnant but who reported at least one abortion in the audio-CASI mode.

(i.e., differently) in the audio-CASI mode may have found herself in a quandary. Answering more honestly in the audio-CASI mode would reveal her dishonesty on the IAQ. To prevent that, some women may have chosen to be consistent rather than honest. Second, the NSFG sample included only women between 15 and 44 years of age. The older cohort of women who could report an illegal abortion (i.e., one that occurred prior to 1971) was not represented in the sample.

Despite clear evidence of bias in self-reported measures of abortion, researchers have few alternatives to self-disclosure for gathering retrospective data on a controversial procedure. Improving our understanding of reporting bias in measures of abortion becomes critical when abortion is being considered as a potential risk factor for a serious medical condition or disease such as breast cancer. The next section reviews the evidence available from case-control studies of abortion and breast cancer risk and how reporting bias may affect inferences drawn from those results.

Potential Sources of Bias in Case-Control Studies
of Abortion and Breast Cancer

Recall bias, or the differential ability to remember a specific piece of information, is not unique to case-control studies, but in case-control studies, it
may have an additional dimension. Compared with controls, cases may have
a differential capacity to remember their medical history. During diagnosis
and treatment of their disease, women who have recently been diagnosed
with breast cancer have been asked questions about many possible risk
factors. They may thus be cognitively primed to remember historical events
of interest to researchers. That argument, however, does not seem very
compelling for abortion. Given the psychological and physical trauma surrounding induced abortion, it is difficult to believe that women who have
ever had an abortion will forget it. What is more plausible is that cases may
be more motivated to provide a complete medical history because they may
feel that they have much to gain from cooperating with people who are
trying to understand their disease. Prospective studies, which are less vulnerable to recall bias, have generally not found an increase in the risk of
breast cancer among women who report abortions (Calle et al., 1995; Kvale
et al., 1987; Lindefors-Harris et al., 1989; Sellers et al., 1993).

Several investigators have hypothesized that differential reporting of
abortion by cases and controls may play a role in findings of a link between
abortion and breast cancer. They speculate that women without the disease
may have less compelling reasons for participating in research and thus
may be less inclined to report prior abortions. A study conducted in Sweden
lends some support to that hypothesis (Lindefors-Harris et al., 1991); in
comparing registry reports of induced abortions with interview data, the
investigators found greater underreporting of induced abortion among
healthy controls than among women with newly diagnosed breast cancer.
The study compared interview data with registry data that covered legally
induced abortions in Sweden for the 1966 to 1974 period. Interviews were
conducted with 317 women with a history of breast cancer and 512 female
controls; the study used IAQs to collect retrospective data on induced and
spontaneous abortions. Cases and controls were identified by their national
registration number, which allowed researchers to link data from study
participants with data from national health registries, including the abortion
registry, and assess their concordance. Among cases, 26 women admitted
to abortion, but the registry only identified 24 cases. Among controls, 44
women admitted to abortion, but the registry identified 59 controls.

Finally, there are questions about social desirability bias, which can result
when subjects feel constrained to report the socially acceptable response.
In trying to probe differential bias in cases versus controls, Newcomb et al.
(1996) looked at reports of induced abortion by legal status (that is, before

1973, when abortions were illegal, compared with after 1973, when they were legal). They found that the risk ratio was greater for reports of illegal induced abortion than for reports of legal abortion, which suggests that cases were more likely than controls to report those events when they occurred under conditions of greater social and legal constraint.

CONCLUSION

The scientific literature leaves little doubt that self-reported measures of sensitive behaviors, including abortion, are vulnerable to bias. Moreover, findings from case-control studies indicate that the magnitude of that bias may not be constant across all subjects. The question that remains is what to do about the problem of bias and flawed estimates of critical variables. The availability of new automated interview technology holds promise for further methodologic research to improve our understanding of bias in sensitive data gathered in future case-control studies.

Although methodologic research is often viewed as esoteric, myopic, or worse, the pursuit of methodological research on the quality of self-reported data on abortion holds promise of some very concrete benefits. For example, improved measures of abortion could improve our capability to evaluate new contraceptive technologies and to interpret abortion surveillance data. Moreover, efforts to bring improved data to address the reported link between breast cancer and abortion potentially could affect a broader range of individuals, all of whom are currently operating in a politically charged atmosphere. Individual women, policy makers, service providers, and professionals crafting prevention messages all need to know whether the relationship between abortion and breast cancer is real or a methodologic artifact. To be able to speak with more confidence about the association between breast cancer and abortion would certainly be a step forward.

ACKNOWLEDGMENTS

This chapter draws on a presentation (Turner and Miller) at the 1996 Conference on the Science of Self-Reports, sponsored by the National Institutes of Health, and a related research proposal (Miller, Turner, Helzlsouer, Zenilman, & Newcomb, 1997). Coinvestigators Polly Newcomb, Kathy Helzlsouer, and Jonathan Zenilman contributed to the latter effort, but they are not responsible for any errors that may appear in this chapter. Its preparation was supported by grant RO1-HD/AG31067-03 from the National Institute of Child Health and Human Development and the National Institute on Aging, and grant R01-MH56318-01 from the National Institute of Mental Health.

REFERENCES

ACSF Investigators. (1992). Analysis of sexual behavior in France: A comparison between two modes of investigation: Telephone survey and face-to-face survey. *AIDS, 6*, 315–323.

Adami, H. O., Bergstrom, R., Lund, E., & Meirik, O. (1990). Absence of association between reproductive variables and the risk of breast cancer in young women in Sweden and Norway. *British Journal of Cancer, 62*, 122–126.

Aquilino, W. S. (1994). Interview mode effects in surveys of drug and alcohol use. *Public Opinion Quarterly, 58*, 210–240.

Bradburn, N. M., Sudman, S., Blair, S., Locander, W., Miles, C., Singer, E., & Stocking, C. (1979). *Improving interview method and questionnaire design.* San Francisco: Jossey Bass.

Breslow, N. E., & Day, N. E. (1980). *Statistical methods in cancer research. Vol. 1: The analysis of case-control studies.* Lyon, France: International Agency for Research on Cancer.

Brinton, L. A., Hoover, R., & Fraumeni, J. F. (1983). Reproductive factors in the aetiology of breast cancer. *British Journal of Cancer, 47*, 757–782.

Calle, E. E., Merris, C. A., Wingo, P. A., Thun, M. J., Rodriguez, C., & Heath, C. W., Jr. (1995). Spontaneous abortion and risk of fatal breast cancer in a prospective cohort of United States women. *Cancer Causes and Control, 6*, 460–468.

Camburn, D., Cynamon, D., & Harel, Y. (1991, May). *The use of audio tapes and written questionnaires to ask sensitive questions during household interviews.* Presentation to the National Field Technologies Conference, San Diego, CA.

Catania, J. A., Coates, T. J., Stall, R., Turner, H., Peterson, J., Hearst, N., Dolcini, M. M., Hudes, E., Gagnon, J., Wiley, & Groves, R. (1992). Prevalence of AIDS-related risk factors and condom use in the United States. *Science, 258*, 1101–1106.

Catania, J. A., Gibson, D. R., Chitwood, D. D., & Coates, T. J. (1990). Methodological problems in AIDS behavioral research: Influences on measurement error and participation bias in studies of sexual behavior. *Psychology Bulletin, 108*, 339–362.

Catania, J., McDermott, L., & Pollack, L. (1986). Questionnaire response bias and face-to-face interview sample bias in sexuality research. *Journal of Sex Research, 22*, 52–72.

Cooley, P. C., Turner, C. F., O'Reilly, J. M., Allen, D. R., & Paddock, R. E. (1996). Audio-CASI: Hardware and software considerations in adding sound to a computer-assisted interviewing system. *Social Science Computer Review, 14*, 197–204.

Cox, B., Witt, M., Traccarella, M., & Perez-Michael, A. (1992). Inconsistent reporting of drug use in 1988. In C. F. Turner, J. T. Lessler, & J. D. Gfroerer (Eds.), *Survey measurement of drug use* (pp. 109–153). DHHS Publication No. 92-1929. Washington, DC: Government Printing Office.

Daling, J. R., Malone, K. E., Voigt, L. F., White, E., & Weiss, N. S. (1994). Risk of breast cancer among young women: Relationship to induced abortion. *Journal of the National Cancer Institute, 86*, 1584–1592.

Duffer, A. P., Lessler, J. T., Weeks, M. F., & Mosher, W. D. (1996). Impact of incentives and interviewing modes: Results from the National Survey of Family Growth Cycle V pretest. In R. Warnecke (Ed.), *Health survey research methods: Conference proceedings* (pp. 147–151). DHHS Pub No. (PHS) 96-1013. Hyattsville, MD: National Center for Health Statistics.

Estrich, S. (1996, February 1). Right plays politics with breast cancer. *USA Today*, p. A9.

Ewertz, M., & Duffy, S. W. (1988). Risk of breast cancer in relation to reproductive factors in Denmark. *British Journal of Cancer, 58*, 99–104.

Fay, R., Turner, C. F., Klassen, A., & Gagnon, J. (1989). Prevalence and patterns of same-gender sexual contact among men. *Science, 243*, 338–348.

Gammon, M. D., Bertin, J. E., & Terry, M. B. (1996). Abortion and the risk of breast cancer: Is there a believable association? *Journal of the American Medical Association, 275*, 321–322.

Gfroerer, J. C., & Hughes, A. L. (1992). Collecting data on illicit drug use by phone. In C. F. Turner, J. T. Lessler, & J. D. Gfroerer (Eds.), *Survey measurement of drug use* (pp. 277–295). DHHS Publication No. 92-1929. Washington, DC: Government Printing Office.

Hadjimichael, O. C., Boyle, C. A., & Meigs, J. W. (1986). Abortion before first live birth and risk of breast cancer. *British Journal of Cancer, 53*, 281–284.

Hendershot, T. P., Rogers, S. M., Thornberry, J. T., Miller, H. G., & Turner, C. F. (1996). Multilingual audio-CASI: Using English-speaking field interviewers to survey elderly Korean households. In R. B. Warnecke (Ed.), *Health survey research methods: Conference proceedings* (pp. 165–169). DHHS Pub. No. (PHS) 96-1013. Hyattsville, MD: National Center for Health Statistics.

Henshaw, S. K. (1996). Pregnancy termination and risk of breast cancer. *Journal of the American Medical Association, 276*, 31.

Henshaw, S. K., Koonin, L. M., & Smith, J. C. (1991). Characteristics of U.S. women having abortions, 1987. *Family Planning Perspectives, 23*, 75–81.

Hirohata, T., Shigematsu, T., Nomura, A. M. Y., Nomura, Y., Horie, A., & Hirohata, I. (1985). Occurrence of breast cancer in relation to diet and reproductive history: A case-control study in Fukuoka, Japan. *National Cancer Institute Monograph, 69*, 187–191.

Howe, H. L., Senie, R. T., Bzduch, H., & Herzfeld, P. (1989). Early abortion and breast cancer risk among women under 40. *International Journal of Epidemiology, 18*, 300–304.

Johnston, G. (1992, January). *Demonstration of computer-administered audio survey technology.* Seminar presented at the National Center for Health Statistics, Hyattsville, MD.

Jones, E. F., & Forrest, J. D. (1992). Underreporting of abortion in surveys of U.S. women: 1976 to 1988. *Demography, 29*, 113–126.

Kelsey, J. L., Gammon, M. D., & John, E. M. (1993). Reproductive factors and breast cancer. *Epidemiology Review, 15*, 36–47.

Kinsey, S., Thornberry, J., Carson, C., & Duffer, A. (1995). Respondent preferences toward audio-CASI and how that affects data quality. In *Proceedings of the joint ASA/AAPOR meeting, 1995.* Washington, DC: American Statistical Society.

Koonin, L. M., Smith, J. C., & Ramick, M. (1993). Abortion surveillance: United States, 1990. *Morbidity and Mortality Weekly Review, 42(SS-6)*, 29–57.

Kvale, G., Heuch, I., & Eide, G. E. (1987). A prospective study of reproductive factors and breast cancer. *American Journal of Epidemiology, 126*, 831–841.

La Vecchia, C., Decarli, A., Parazzini, F., Gentile, A., Negri, E., Cecchetti, G., & Franceschi, S. (1987). General epidemiology of breast cancer in Northern Italy. *International Journal of Epidemiology, 16*, 347–355.

Lessler, J. T., & Holt, M. (1987). Using response protocols to identify problems in the U.S. Census long form. In *Proceedings of the Section on Survey Methods Research, American Statistical Association*, pp. 262–265.

Lindefors-Harris, B. M., Eklund, G., Adami, H. O., & Meirik, O. (1991). Response bias in a case-control study: Analysis utilizing comparative data concerning legal abortions from two independent Swedish studies. *American Journal of Epidemiology, 134*, 1003–1008.

Lindefors-Harris, B. M., Eklund, G., Meirik, O., Rutqvist, L. E., & Wiklund, K. (1989). Risk of cancer of the breast after legal abortion during first trimester: A Swedish registry study. *British Medical Journal, 299*, 1430–1432.

Lipworth, L., Katsouyanni, K., Ekbom, A., Michels, K. B., & Trichopoulos, D. (1995). Abortion and the risk of breast cancer: A case-control study in Greece. *International Journal of Cancer, 61*, 181–184.

MacMahon, B., Cole, P., Lin, T. M., Lowe, C. R., Mirra, A. P., Ravnihar, B., Salber, E. J., Valaoras, V. G., & Yuasa, S. (1970). Age at first birth and breast cancer risk. *Bulletin of the World Health Organization, 43*, 209–221.

Michels, K. B., Hsieh, C. C., Trichopoulos, D., & Willett, W. C. (1995). Abortion and breast cancer risk in seven countries. *Cancer Causes and Control, 6*, 75–82.

Miller, H. G., Turner, C. F., & Moses, L. E. (Eds.). (1990). *AIDS: The second decade.* Washington DC: National Academy Press.

Miller, H. M., Turner, C. F., Helzlsouer, K. J., Zenilman, J. M., & Newcomb, P. A. (1997). Abortion, breast cancer, and reporting bias. Unpublished proposal submitted to the National Institute of Child Health and Human Development and the National Cancer Institute. Research Triangle Park, NC: Research Triangle Institute.

Millstein, S., & Irwin, C. (1983). Acceptability of computer-acquired sexual histories in adolescent girls. *Journal of Pediatrics, 103,* 815–819.

National Cancer Institute. (1994, December). Abortion and possible risk for breast cancer: Analysis and inconsistencies. In *Cancer Facts.* Bethesda, MD: Author.

National Center for Education Statistics. (1993). *Adult literacy in America: A first look at the results of the National Adult Literacy Survey.* Washington, DC: U.S. Department of Education.

Newcomb, P. A., Storer, B. E., Longnecker, M. P., Mittendorf, R., Greenbert, E. R., & Willett, W. C. (1996). Pregnancy termination in relation to risk of breast cancer. *Journal of the American Medical Association, 275,* 283–287.

O'Reilly, J., Hubbard, M., Lessler, J., Biemer, P., & Turner, C. F. (1994). Audio computer-assisted self-interviewing: New technology for data collection on sensitive issues and special populations. *Journal of Official Statistics, 10,* 197–214.

O'Reilly, J., & Turner, C. F. (1992, March). *Survey interviewing using audio format, computer-assisted technologies.* Presentation to the Washington Statistical Society.

Parazzini, F., La Vecchia, C., & Negri, E. (1991). Spontaneous and induced abortions and risk of breast cancer. *International Journal of Cancer, 48,* 816–820.

Rogers, S. M., & Turner, C. F. (1991). Patterns of same-gender sexual contact among men in the U.S.A., 1970–1990. *Journal of Sex Research, 28,* 491–519.

Rosenberg, L., Palmer, J. R., Kaufman, D. W., Strom, B. L., Schottenfeld, D., & Shapiro, S. (1988). Breast cancer in relation to the occurrence and time of induced and spontaneous abortion. *American Journal of Epidemiology, 127,* 981–989.

Sackett, D. L. (1979). Bias in analytic research. *Journal of Chronic Diseases, 32,* 51–68.

Schlesselman, J. J. (1982). *Case control studies: Design, conduct, analysis.* New York: Oxford University Press.

Sellers, T. A., Potter, J. D., Severson, R. K., Bostick, R. M., Nelson, C. L., Kushi, L. H., & Folsom, A. R. (1993). Difficulty becoming pregnant and family history as interactive risk factors for post-menopausal breast cancer: The Iowa Women's Health Study. *Cancer Causes and Control, 4,* 21–28.

Shober, S. E., Fe Caces, M., Pergamit, M. R., & Branden, L. (1992). Effect of mode of administration on reporting in the National Longitudinal Survey. In C. F. Turner, J. T. Lessler, & J. D. Gfroerer (Eds.), *Survey measurement of drug use* (pp. 267–276). DHHS Publication No. 92-1929. Washington, DC: Government Printing Office.

Smith, T. (1992). A methodological analysis of the sexual behavior questions on the General Social surveys. *Journal of Official Statistics, 8,* 309–325.

Turner, C. F., Ku, L., Sonenstein, F. L., & Pleck, J. H. (1996). Impact of Audio-CASI on bias in reporting of male-male sexual contacts. In R. B. Warnecke (Ed.), *Health survey research methods: Conference proceedings* (pp. 171–176). DHHS Pub. No. (PHS) 96-1013. Hyattsville, MD: National Center for Health Statistics.

Turner, C. F., Lessler, J., & Devore, J. (1992). Effects of mode of administration and wording on reporting of drug use. In C. F. Turner, J. T. Lessler, & J. D. Gfroerer (Eds.), *Survey measurement of drug use: Methodological issues* (pp. 177–219). DHHS Pub. No. 92-1929, Washington, DC: Government Printing Office.

Turner, C. F., Lessler, J., & Gfroerer, J. (1992). Future directions for research and practice. In C. F. Turner, J. T. Lessler, & J. D. Gfroerer (Eds.), *Survey measurement of drug use: Methodological issues* (pp. 299–306). DHHS Pub. No. 92-1929, Washington, DC: Government Printing Office.

Turner, C. F., & Miller, H. G. (1997). Zenilman's anomaly reconsidered: Fallible reports, *ceteris paribus,* fragile condoms, and other hypotheses. *Sexually Transmitted Diseases, 24,* 522–527.

Turner, C. F., Miller, H. G., & Moses, L. E. (Eds.). (1989). *AIDS, sexual behavior, and intravenous drug use.* Washington, DC: National Academy Press.

Turner, C. F., Miller, H. G., & Rogers, S. M. (1997). Survey measurement of sexual behaviors: Problems and progress. In J. Bancroft (Ed.), *Researching sexual behavior* (pp. 37–60). Bloomington: Indiana University Press.

Turner, C. F., Miller, H. G., Smith, T. K., Cooley, P. C., & Rogers, S. M. (1996). Telephone audio computer-assisted self-interviewing (T-ACASI) and survey measurements of sensitive behaviors: Preliminary results. In R. Banks, J. Fairgrieve, L. Gerrard, T. Orchard, C. Payne, & A. Westlake (Eds.), *Survey and statistical computing 1996* (pp. 121–130). Chesham, Bucks, UK: Association for Survey Computing.

Turner, C. F., Rogers, S. M., Hendershot, T., Miller, H., & Thornberry, J. (1996). Improving representation of linguistic minorities in health surveys: A preliminary test of multilingual audio-CASI. *Public Health Reports, 111*, 276–279.

Zenilman, J. M., Weisman, C. S., Rompalo, A. M., Ellish, N., Upchurch, D. M., Hook, E. W., & Celentano, D. (1995). Condom use to prevent STDs: The validity of self-reported condom use. *Sexually Transmitted Diseases, 22*, 15–21.

PART

IV

SPECIAL ISSUES ON SELF-REPORT

Virginia S. Cain
Office of Behavioral and Social Sciences Research,
National Institutes of Health

The chapters in this section address issues that arise in gathering information from populations presenting unique challenges in data collection, in particular, immigrants, children, and drug abusers. In the case of immigrants to the United States from Mexico, many of the standard data collection approaches have been deficient. The dynamic, and sometimes clandestine, nature of migration may lead to undercounts and data of questionable quality. Even a large general-purpose data set may be too small to contain a sample of migrants sufficiently large for analytic purposes or may only have data on legal migrants, thereby missing approximately 30% of the migrants from Mexico to the United States. Dr. Douglas Massey has developed an alternative approach to collecting data, an ethnosurvey, which uses both ethnographic and survey methods to create a large, reliable, and valid data set covering a wide range of life events. In this chapter, he describes the rationale and process for conducting an ethnosurvey.

Although collecting data from children can be challenging, some information can only be obtained through interviews with the children themselves. A researcher working with children is faced with a wide range of developmental levels across ages and the inherent power differential when an adult is interviewing a child. In his chapter, Johnny Blair describes and compares a number of techniques for obtaining dietary information from children. He further explores the children's knowledge of surveys and of their roles as survey respondents.

Self-reported data are crucial for understanding drug dependence. Dr. James Anthony and his colleagues provide a thorough description of the role of self-report methodologies in this field, including some of the newer techniques for collecting self-report data systematically via computers and with momentary assessment methods. Other methods for determining drug exposure are also discussed and are contrasted with self-report methods. This chapter provides an excellent example of a field that has addressed self-report issues seriously and with creativity.

9

When Surveys Fail:
An Alternative for Data Collection

Douglas S. Massey
University of Pennsylvania

Immigration to the United States has grown steadily since the 1960s and is now one of the most important demographic factors affecting U.S. society. Between 1980 and 1990, immigration accounted for more than one third of net U.S. population growth, and over the next 50 years, two thirds of net growth will stem from the arrival of immigrants or the birth of their children. By far, the most important source country is Mexico. During the 1980s, 3 million Mexicans entered the United States legally and another 800,000 arrived without documents; and in the first half of the 1990s, 2.2 million Mexicans entered legally and 900,000 arrived illegally (Passel, 1995; U.S. Immigration and Naturalization Service, 1992).

As with any complicated and controversial social issue, access to reliable, high-quality data is crucial to understanding the causes and consequences of international migration, but the fact that so much of it is temporary and undocumented has hampered data collection efforts. Punitive laws enacted by Congress have driven the immigrant population further underground, making measurement even more challenging.

To date, the transitory, clandestine, and circular nature of Mexico–U.S. migration has defeated standard approaches to data collection and diminished the utility of conventional data sets for studying the issue. Although the U.S. Census contains a large sample of persons born in Mexico, it provides no information on their legal status and undercounts them irrespective of legal status. Moreover, even though the census contains a question on time of arrival, permitting investigators to construct synthetic cohorts of immigrants entering the United States at the same time, the data are still cross-sectional (gathered at a single point in time) and thus subject to methodological shortcomings stemming from selective processes of migration and return (Lindstrom & Massey, 1994). In addition, the census provides little information on immigrants before they enter the United States, and, as it occurs just once a decade, it is perpetually out of date. Although the Current Population Survey offers more timely data, it suffers from the same methodological problems as the census and has the additional liability of a small sample size.

The Immigration and Naturalization Service (INS) offers another potential source of data on Mexican immigration. Each year the agency tabulates data from applications for permanent residence and publishes them in both printed and machine-readable forms, allowing researchers to construct an annual profile of immigrants. Available indicators include age, sex, country of birth, country of last residence, occupation, place of intended residence, and class of admission (U.S. Immigration and Naturalization Service, 1992). Obviously, many important variables (notably education) are missing from this list, and the data shed little light on what happens to immigrants after they enter the country or the characteristics of those who later depart.

Another serious problem is that the INS only collects information on immigrants as they become legal residents, not when they actually enter the country. In 1994, 39% of all new immigrants were already living in the United States (as students, visitors, temporary workers, employees, asylees, or refugees). In addition, an unknown but presumably large number were already present as undocumented migrants (U.S. Immigration and Naturalization Service, 1995). When Portes (1979) surveyed arriving legal Mexican immigrants in 1972 and 1973, for example, he found that 62% had prior experience living in the country without documents.

The INS also tabulates and publishes data from a form known as the Report of Deportable Alien, filed by Border Patrol agents whenever they arrest someone entering the country without inspection. When summed, these records yield a count of apprehensions that investigators have used to measure undocumented migration (U.S. Immigration and Naturalization Service, 1995). Apprehensions statistics are flawed in several ways, however: They reflect enforcement efforts as well as attempted entries; they yield little information on the characteristics of the undocumented migrants; and they provide no data on what happens to undocumented migrants after they enter the United States.

Some of the most important advances in social science in recent years have come from longitudinal data sets such as the National Longitudinal Survey (Borus & Wolpin, 1984); but such nationally representative samples generally do not contain enough immigrants to support reliable study. Although the Panel Study of Income Dynamics recently added a subsample of

Hispanic respondents, the number of Mexican immigrants within it is still quite small, around 382 according to Padilla (1996) and as with the census and Current Population Survey, it does not identify undocumented migrants, who are probably underenumerated in any event.

To circumvent the deficiencies encountered in standard data sets, social scientists have turned to alternative means of securing data on Mexico–U.S. migration. One such method is the ethnosurvey, a multimethod data-gathering technique that simultaneously applies ethnographic and survey methods within a single study. Developed initially by Massey, Alarcón, Durand, and González (1987) to study emigration from four Mexican communities, ethnosurveys have since been applied in a variety of locations throughout Mexico to create a large, reliable, and valid public use data set on immigration to the United States.

Unlike other sources of information on Mexican immigration, ethnosurveys yield data that allow investigators to: (a) compare the characteristics and behavior of documented and undocumented migrants; (b) measure trends in the characteristics of both groups over time; (c) undertake longitudinal studies of the migration process; (d) discern the background and characteristics of migrants before and after they enter the United States; (e) undertake detailed cross-tabulations of Mexican based on large samples; (f) study transitions between different legal statuses and model selective movements back and forth across the border; and (g) provide an ongoing source of longitudinal data capable of monitoring the effect of shifting U.S. and Mexican policies.

THE ELEMENTS OF AN ETHNOSURVEY

Basic Philosophy

The underlying philosophy of the ethnosurvey is that qualitative and quantitative procedures complement one another and that when properly combined, one's weaknesses become the other's strength, yielding a body of data with greater reliability and more internal validity than would be possible to achieve using either method alone. Whereas survey methods produce reliable quantitative data for statistical analysis, generalization, and replication, in guaranteeing quantitative rigor, they lose historical depth, richness of context, and the intuitive appeal of real life. Ethnographic studies, in contrast, capture the richness of the phenomenon under study: Oral histories supplemented with archival work provide historical depth and firsthand experiences in the field give insight into the real life of a community. The lack of quantitative data, however, makes it difficult to demonstrate the validity of conclusions to other scientists, and subjective elements of interpretation are more difficult to detect and control. Qualitative field studies are also difficult to replicate.

The ethnosurvey was developed to capitalize on the strengths of both methods while minimizing their respective weaknesses. It shifts back and forth between quantitative and qualitative modes during all phases of design, data collection, and analysis. Consequently, ethnographic and survey methods inform one another throughout the study. Once a site is selected for study, the ethnosurvey begins with a phase of conventional ethnographic fieldwork, including participant observation, unstructured in-depth interviewing, and archival work. Early materials from this fieldwork are then made available for use in designing the survey instrument. After the instrument has been designed, it is applied to a probability sample of respondents selected according to a carefully designed sampling plan. During the implementation of the survey, qualitative fieldwork continues, or resumes after the survey's completion. The flow of analysis is organized so that preliminary quantitative data from the survey are made available to ethnographic investigators before they leave the field so that patterns emerging from quantitative analysis shape qualitative fieldwork, just as insights from early ethnographies guide later statistical studies.

Quantitative Components: The Interview Schedule

Semistructured Interviews. In an ethnosurvey, quantitative data are gathered using a semistructured interview schedule that in design is midway between the highly structured instrument of the survey researcher and the guided conversation of the ethnographer. When interviewing respondents about sensitive subjects or clandestine behavior such as undocumented migration, rigidly structured instruments and closed-form questions are inappropriate, impractical, and excessively obtrusive, yet some standardization is essential in order to collect comparable information across subjects. The ethnosurvey questionnaire is a compromise instrument that balances the goal of unobtrusive measurement with the need for standardization and quantification. It yields an interview that is informal, nonthreatening, and natural, but one that allows the interviewer some discretion about how and when to ask sensitive questions. Ultimately, it produces a standard set of reliable information that carries greater validity than that obtained using normal survey methods.

The ethnosurvey interview schedule is laid out in a series of tables with variables arranged in columns across the top and the rows referring variously to persons, events, years, or other meaningful categories. The interviewer holds a naturalistic conversation with the subject and fills in the cells of the table by soliciting required information in ways that the situation seems to demand, using his or her judgment as to the timing and wording of specific questions or probes.

Each table is organized around a particular topic, giving coherence and order to the conversation, and certain specialized probes may be included to elaborate particular themes of interest. The usual place to begin is with a simple roster that describes the household's demographic and social composition, where each household member is listed in rows down the side and columns give each person's sex, relationship to household head, year of birth, place of birth, marital status, schooling, current labor force status and occupation, and present income. Special probes are included to make sure that household members temporarily absent from the home are not overlooked.

Because the interview schedule is semistructured and does not employ fixed-question wording, it is crucial that each fieldworker has the same understanding of what information is being sought and why. Thus, interviewer training assumes great importance in an ethnosurvey. Rather than being trained by rote to ask specific questions exactly as written, interviewers are educated to be conversant with the goals, background, and nature of the study. Rather than following a scripted interaction, they tailor the interview to the respondent in ways the situation seems to demand.

Life Histories. A fundamental feature of any ethnosurvey is the collection of life histories. Within the quantitative survey, the semistructured questionnaire is readily adapted to compile event histories on specific aspects of life, such as employment, migration, marriage, childbearing, and property ownership. Different facets of a respondent's life are covered by different tables in the event history questionnaire. Rows refer to specific years or periods in the respondent's life, and columns correspond to variables relating to the facet of life under investigation. These tables provide structure to the gathering of life histories by guiding the flow of conversation between interviewer and respondent.

For each table, the interviewer begins at an appropriate starting point in the respondent's life and moves chronologically forward in time, asking about the timing of events and changes in status. When one aspect of life has been exhausted by reaching the present, the next facet of life is considered in parallel fashion. To compile a labor history, for example, each row of the table would list a specific job, spell of unemployment, or period of nonlabor-force activity. Moving from age 15 to the present, the columns would give the year when the job or spell of nonwork began, the respondent's age at the time, the duration of the job or spell, the place where the job or spell transpired, the respondent's occupational category, his or her industrial category, and, when relevant, the wages or salary earned. When all information on the first job or spell has been collected, the interviewer asks about the next job or spell and compiles the same information about it, proceeding systematically up to the present. When the labor history is done, the investigator might direct the conversation to other issues, compiling the respondent's marital history, for example, by asking about his or her first marriage or cohabitation and moving forward to more recent relationships. When the marital history is done, the interviewer may turn to a fertility history, then onto a residence history, and so on.

Event histories gathered from randomly selected respondents yield a representative sample of life histories. When properly compiled and coded, the various event histories (employment, marriage, fertility, etc.) can be combined with the aid of a computer to construct a comprehensive life history for each respondent, summarizing key events for each person-year of life from birth (or some other relevant starting point) to the survey date. The construction of such retrospective life histories takes the ethnosurvey design considerably beyond the cross-sectional approach usually applied to census or survey data and permits the estimation of dynamic, developmental models using sophisticated methods of longitudinal data analysis.

Multilevel Data Collection. Although individuals may be the ultimate units of analysis, their decisions are typically made within larger social and economic contexts. These contexts structure and constrain individual decisions so that analyses conducted only at the micro level are perforce incomplete. The ethnosurvey design is therefore explicitly multilevel, compiling data simultaneously for individuals, households, communities, and even the nations in which they reside.

In the case of migration, although individuals ultimately make the decision to go or stay, it is typically reached within some larger family or household unit. Likewise, households exist within larger communities that influence family decision making. Examples of community-level variables likely to influence the migration decision include local employment opportunities, wage levels, land tenure arrangements, inheritance systems, transportation and communication linkages, access to community facilities, economic and political power structures, climatic factors, governmental policies, and kinship networks.

The ethnosurvey is explicitly designed to collect such data for multilevel statistical analysis. Information is solicited from all household members, which enables the estimation of household contextual variables like dependency, family income, life-cycle stage, and kinship connections to other migrants. At the same time, other modules gather information on variables that pertain directly to households themselves, such as property ownership, dwelling construction, home furnishings, length of residence, and tenure in the home.

If communities themselves are sampling units and quantitative information is gathered on multiple communities as part of a cluster sampling design, then fieldworkers also complete community inventories that later enable researchers to construct aggregate-level data files. Individual, household, and community-level data may be organized into separate data sets or combined into a single multilevel file. Either way, variables defined at various levels are available for analysis. This file structure enables the systematic statistical evaluation of community on household outcomes and household context on individual decision making.

Quantitative Components: Sampling

Representative Multisite Sampling. A distinguishing feature of the ethnosurvey is the careful selection of sites and the use of representative sampling methods within them. The sites may be chosen according to specific criteria designed to enable comparative analysis between settings, or they may be chosen randomly from a universe of possible sites in order to represent a population of interest. The latter procedure yields a representative cluster sample that generates unbiased statistical estimates. Whether chosen randomly or according to *a priori* specifications, however, both internal and external validity are greatly enhanced by multiple field sites. A variety of sites also enhance the strength of inference in qualitative as well as quantitative analyses.

Parallel Sampling. Whenever a social process transcends distinct geographic or cultural areas, parallel sampling is recommended. Parallel sampling involves the gathering of contemporaneous samples in the different geographic locations that serve as loci for the social or economic process under study. In the case of migration, representative samples of respondents are surveyed in both sending and receiving areas.

This strategy is necessary because migration, like most social and economic processes, is selective. The population of people with U.S. migratory experience contains two very different classes of beings: those who have returned home and those who have remained abroad. Because the decision to stay or return is highly selective of different characteristics and experiences, neither class is representative of all those with migrant experience. The use of origin or destination samples alone produces biased statistical analyses and misleading statements about migratory processes (Lindstrom & Massey, 1994).

Multiplicity Sampling. Parallel sampling raises certain troubling technical issues, however. Whereas it is straightforward to design a representative sample of returned migrants who live in a particular sending community, it is more difficult to generate a representative sample of settled emigrants from that community who reside elsewhere. The main difficulty lies in constructing a sampling frame that includes all out-migrants from a community because they are typically scattered across a variety of towns and cities, both domestic and foreign. New techniques of multiplicity sampling, however, solve the main problems of parallel sampling (Kalton & Anderson, 1986).

In a multiplicity sample of out-migrants, respondents in sending communities provide information not only about themselves and others in the household, but also about some well-defined class of relatives—usually siblings—who live outside the community. When the survey of households in the sending community is complete, a sampling frame for settled out-migrant siblings will have been compiled and a random sample of emigrants may be chosen from it. Researchers then return to households containing relatives of the sampled siblings to obtain information necessary to locate them in destination areas. Then they go to these destination areas to administer the interview schedule, yielding a representative sample of the out-migrant community.

Qualitative Components: Life Histories

In an ethnosurvey, qualitative life histories, or case studies, are compiled along with the quantitative event histories. These in-depth stories provide a basis for exploratory analysis and induction and serve to illustrate the results of statistical analyses. Important patterns not readily deducible from prior theory often emerge in the compilation of case studies and lead to novel re-considerations and innovative quantitative analyses. Case studies also have considerable value as heuristic devices; complex statistical analyses typically have little meaning for members of the general public because they are poorly understood and too abstract to remember. Case studies that are well-chosen to illustrate a point established by more objective research can significantly enhance communication and memory by presenting findings in a way that makes sense in light of people's ordinary knowledge and experience.

Selecting Case Studies. It is important, of course, to choose case studies judiciously so that they are representative of patterns that have already been well-established through detailed ethnographic and statistical work. Case studies presented in a research report do not themselves establish the validity of findings; rather, they illustrate results established through other, more systematic methods and make the findings come alive in a deeper and more concrete way.

One way of selecting candidates for a qualitative life history is to use results from the quantitative survey. In conducting the survey and analyzing the resulting numerical data, interviewers and investigators remain alert for particularly interesting cases that typify certain patterns well. Of course, subjects for in-depth interviews should not be limited to respondents from the quantitative survey alone. It is also important to locate and interview informants from outside the representative sample, using chain-referral methods to locate people who have specialized knowledge or information that is relevant to the study. Life histories gathered from outside the sample can later be used as exemplary case studies. Sometimes, however, meaningful behavioral categories only become clear after the project has left the field, in which case it may be necessary to return to gather additional case studies.

The Interview Guide.   The flow of a qualitative interview is organized by an interview guide, which is basically a list of questions or topics that need to be covered in the course of an extended, naturalistic conversation. These items need not be covered in any particular order. Unlike a structured or even a semi-structured interview, qualitative interviews have no typical length and no set format. Although they may be guided by certain questions the researcher seeks to pose, the interviewer is free to decide when to ask each question, how to pose it, how much detail to request, and when to follow leads not anticipated in the interview guide.

Interview Setting.   Being naturalistic conversations, ethnographic interviews may occur at different times and in different settings, and they need not be completed in one sitting. In carrying out a qualitative interview, researchers take jottings and notes on a small pad, trying to be as unobtrusive as possible. The interviews may be taped, but often taping is not possible, and sometimes the best interviews occur spontaneously at unanticipated times or in places where taping is infeasible.

Focus Groups.   In recent years, focus groups have become popular as a tool for qualitative data collection. The technique grew originally out of market research but has increasingly been applied in academic studies as well. A focus group is a collective interview orchestrated by a skilled rapporteur who attempts to achieve a group dynamic that allows respondents to reveal thoughts and behaviors they would normally be reluctant to disclose. Step by step, the focus group interviewer poses questions relevant to the subject under discussion, and, in small increments, gets respondents to reveal attitudes and behaviors that ordinarily they would find difficult to discuss. The goal is to use the small group setting to construct a supportive social context within which respondents feel free to reveal insightful things about themselves and their community. Focus groups are particularly useful in generating information about salient behaviors that are widely diffused but rarely talked about (e.g. sex, childbearing, male–female relations, illegal migration).

Data Log. As soon as the interview or focus group is over, the investigator writes up a data log while memories are still fresh. In preparing the write-up, jottings and notes are used to reconstruct conversations and to write down salient quotes or to transcribe particularly salient parts of the conversation. If available, tape recordings can be used to aid in the write-up, but investigators should not attempt a complete transcription of an entire interview. Much, if not most, of what is said in an unstructured conversation is extraneous or irrelevant to the study, and transcription is an extremely burdensome and time-consuming activity that slows down fieldwork and sacrifices broader coverage of respondents. Focus-group sessions are typically taped or videotaped, and the encounter is reviewed later to create a log that summarizes the principal findings to emerge from the group interview, together with supporting quotes and observations.

Given the widespread availability of inexpensive laptop computers, qualitative data should be entered immediately into a machine-readable text file while still in the field. The entry can be done using simple word processing programs, and a surprising amount of analysis can be carried out using them alone (using search functions or word frequency counters). If necessary, once it has been entered, textual material can be ported to more sophisticated bibliographic or analytic packages that are specifically designed for text processing and qualitative analysis.

Qualitative Components: Ethnographic Fieldwork

Before, during, and after quantitative and qualitative interviewing, investigators should be actively engaged in gathering other information. Although the most intense periods of fieldwork occur before and after the administration of the representative sample survey, investigators should keep notes about their observations and activities throughout their time in the field. In general, this additional fieldwork occurs in three forms.

General Field Observation. As fieldworkers enter the field and gradually come to know it, they keep a record of their observations and emerging understandings. These data consist of descriptions of the geographical environment, the physical setting, the economy, the people, the daily activities, and key social groups in the community under study. Preliminary hypotheses, tentative explanations, and interesting patterns are generally noted.

Participant Observation. Fieldworkers also make an effort to participate in the life of the community by making friends, engaging in informal social activities, and by doing favors when asked. They generally attend all public events, town meetings, community celebrations, and sporting activities that draw people from the community into interactions that might be relevant to the subject of study. The resulting data consist of notes about social interactions in which the fieldworker has participated, providing information about four essential issues: who the actors involved in the interaction were, where the interaction took place, what events occurred, and why actors behaved and events transpired as observed. Such notes are compiled for any relevant social interaction in the community, including informal conversations, group discussions, and interviews with informants, as well as larger public events and activities. When possible, the accuracy of information should be cross-checked with reliable informants in the community.

Archival Research. In the course of a period in the field, investigators should attempt to reconstruct the history of the community and the process under investigation not only through event histories, case studies, and informal conversations, but, also, through the compilation of documentary evidence from newspapers, libraries, or official archives. Whenever possible, statements or generalizations made by respondents about conditions in the past should be confirmed by documentary evidence from census figures, government records, newspaper accounts, and books or pamphlets written by observers in the past. Documentary materials provide an invaluable point of reference in attempting to reconstruct the past and reconstitute the social processes that gave rise to the phenomenon under study.

Data Log. The data log for qualitative fieldwork consists of the daily notes growing out of general field observation, participant observation, and archival work. Like the qualitative interviews and focus group materials, these data should be entered into computerized text files on a regular basis. Separate text files should be maintained for general observations, participant observer notes, and notes on archival sources. Again, although sophisticated bibliographic and text processing packages are available, simple word processing programs will suffice for many purposes, and these text files can always be ported into more advanced programs should the need later arise.

THE MEXICAN MIGRATION PROJECT

The Mexican Migration Project (MMP) is supported by NICHD and directed by Douglas S. Massey of the University of Pennsylvania and Jorge Durand of the University of Guadalajara. Each year since 1987, they have gathered information from a representative sample of households in 4 to 6 Mexican communities using ethnosurvey methods. Communities are selected to represent a range of population sizes, political categories, economic structures, ethnic compositions, and geographical locations. Each Mexican survey is supplemented with a survey of settled out-migrants from the same community located in the United States and the Mexican and U.S. surveys are weighted to reflect their relative contributions to the total binational population.

To date, the MMP has completed surveys of 51 communities (5 in 1982 and 46 since 1987) yielding a database that includes some 70,000 persons enumerated in 10,000 households. The data set includes information on 16,000 current or former migrants to the United States, 55% of whom are undocumented. These data were compiled at a cost of roughly $18 per person or $77 per U.S. migrant. These figures compare quite favorably with costs achieved with standard survey methods, which can run $100 to $200 per subject for populations that are difficult to locate and interview. The low per-element cost indicates the relative efficiency of the ethnosurvey as a strategy for data collection.

Since the project's inception, data files have been made available to researchers on request and without restriction, but once the data set reached 30 communities, the project established a home page on the World Wide Web, thus facilitating the widest possible distribution of data (the Internet address is http://lexis.pop.upenn.edu/mexmig). As new communities are surveyed and the resulting data are entered, cleaned, and processed, they are progressively added to the database. The website offers data users the ability to download files directly from the Internet to their own computers. They can also click on icons to obtain a bibliography of publications based on the MMP data, a list of MMP personnel, copies of questionnaires in Spanish or English, code books for all data files, a data users' e-mail list, and a bulletin board for comments and queries.

These data have proved useful to investigators in a variety of research tasks, and the project currently supports 60 data users. In the task of demographic estimation, for example, the data were used by Massey and Singer (1995) to develop independent estimates of undocumented Mexican migration: a net figure of 1.9 million between 1980 and 1990. MMP data have also been used to estimate the amount of remittances into Mexico. Massey and Parrado (1994) found that at least $2 billion (U.S.) entered Mexico each year during the late 1980s, yielding a $6.5 billion effect on production and a $5.8 billion effect on national income once appropriate multipliers were taken into account (Durand, Parrado, & Massey, 1995). Migradollars play a key role in promoting productive investment and business formation in Mexico (Durand, Kandel, Parrado, & Massey, 1996; Massey & Parrado, 1997).

The MMP has also supported methodological research. Lindstrom and Massey (1994) examined how problems stemming from underenumeration, changing migrant selectivity, and emigration produce biases in models of immigrant assimilation estimated from census and CPS data. They found that underenumeration yields a downward bias in the estimated effects of human capital variables on wage rates and English ability, but that selective emigration did not significantly affect the estimates. They also found that period of last entry was a poor proxy for total migration experience among Mexicans.

The MMP data have also been used for theory construction and hypothesis testing. Based on a review of community studies, Durand and Massey (1992) argued that "a fruitful approach to developing general statements about Mexico-U.S. migration is to focus on the ways in which community variables interact with individual and household processes to produce the manifold [migration] outcomes that we observe" (p. 35). Drawing on this perspective, Massey, Goldring, and Durand (1994) specified a theory of social capital accumulation and used MMP data to show how common migratory processes are expressed differently in different locations because of structural factors operating at the community level. They concluded that future analyses had to use multilevel statistical models to examine the interplay of individual, household, community, and national-level factors.

Massey and Espinosa (1997) undertook just such an analysis using life history data from the MMP, systematically testing propositions derived from neoclassical economics, the new economics of labor migration, segmented labor market theory, social capital theory, and world systems theory (reviewed in Massey et al., 1993). Their analysis followed household heads year-by-year from age 15 onward and estimated event-history models to predict the odds of taking a first trip to the United States, the odds of taking an additional U.S. trip, and the odds of returning to Mexico. The authors found some support for all theories, but social capital theory and the new economics of labor migration were generally most efficacious in explaining initial migration, whereas social capital theory, neoclassical economics, and the new economics of migration together accounted for subsequent migration and return.

Over the years, the MMP data set has also become increasingly important as a tool in policy evaluation. Donato (1994), for example, used MMP data to trace the effects of U.S. immigration policy on the volume and composition of Mexican immigration. She has also studied how U.S. policies influence the rate and character of female immigration from Mexico (Donato, 1993).

Several studies have considered the consequences of the Immigration Reform and Control Act of 1986 (IRCA). An early analysis of MMP data by Massey, Donato, and Liang (1990) suggested that IRCA was not deterring Mexicans from making undocumented trips to the United States. Donato, Durand, and Massey (1992a) confirmed this conclusion with additional data and more sophisticated models, finding that IRCA had no effect on the odds of taking an initial or subsequent illegal trip to the United States. They also found that IRCA had few effects on the probability of apprehension, a fact later confirmed by Massey and Singer (1995), who found that the odds of apprehension actually fell from 1987 to 1990. Singer and Massey (1998) showed that new undocumented migrants were able to mobilize social ties to overcome the barriers erected by U.S. immigration authorities, whereas experienced migrants drew on their own knowledge and experience of border crossing. They found that probabilies of apprehension continued to fall through the early 1990s as Border Patrol officials shifted resources from immigration enforcement to drug interdiction.

Although it does not appear to have slowed undocumented migration from Mexico, IRCA has had other, unanticipated consequences. The enactment of employer sanctions, for example, led to a deterioration in the wages and working conditions of Mexican migrants in the United States (Donato, Durand, & Massey, 1992b; Donato & Massey, 1993; Phillips & Massey, in press). Massey, Donato, and Liang (1990) found that legal status was the strongest determinant of U.S. social service usage and argued that IRCA's massive legalization would eventually increase the demand for U.S. schooling, medical care, and welfare. Massey and Espinosa (1997) found, however, that the prospect of receiving public services was not a significant factor motivating the migration of Mexicans per se; rather, the demand for services was expressed after they had migrated and settled for other reasons.

Instead of deterring undocumented Mexican migration to the United States, IRCA appears to have increased it through its massive legalization program. Massey and Espinosa (1997) found that coming from a household containing someone who had legalized under IRCA was the strongest single predictor of later undocumented migration to the United States. Being related to someone who had received amnesty increased the odds of becoming an illegal migrant by a factor of nearly 10.

Thus, analysis of data from the Mexican Migration Project yields insights and conclusions that would be difficult to derive from standard data sources. Work based on its ethnosurvey data suggests that IRCA had powerful but largely unintended effects on the process of Mexican migration. Whereas the new law did little to deter Mexicans from crossing the border illegally, its employer sanctions undermined wages and working conditions in the United States while its massive legalization program increased the ultimate demand for U.S. public services and raised the likelihood of later undocumented migration by friends and relatives at home.

REFERENCES

Borus, M. E., & Wolpin, K. I. (1984). The National Longitudinal Surveys of labor market experience: Past and future uses to study labor market policy questions. *Vierteljahrshefte zur Wirtschaftsforschung, 4*, 428–438.

Donato, K. M. (1993). Current trends and patterns of female migration: Evidence from Mexico. *International Migration Review, 27*, 748–771.

Donato, K. M. (1994). U.S. policy and Mexican migration to the United States, 1942-94. *Social Science Quarterly, 75*, 705-729.

Donato, K. M., Durand, J., & Massey, D. S. (1992a). Stemming the tide? Assessing the deterrent effects of the Immigration Reform and Control Act. *Demography, 29*, 139-157.

Donato, K. M., Durand, J., & Massey, D. S. (1992b). Changing conditions in the U.S. labor market: Effects of the Immigration Reform and Control Act of 1986. *Population Research and Policy Review, 11*, 93-115.

Donato, K. M., & Massey, D. S. (1993). Effect of the Immigration Reform and Control Act on the wages of Mexican migrants. *Social Science Quarterly, 74*, 523-541.

Durand, J., Kandel, W., Parrado, E. A., & Massey, D. S. (1996). International migration and development in Mexican sending communities. *Demography, 33*, 249-264.

Durand, J., & Massey, D. S. (1992). Mexican migration to the United States: A critical review. *Latin American Research Review, 27*, 3-43.

Durand, J., Parrado, E. A., & Massey, D. S. (1995). Migradollars and Development: A reconsideration of the Mexican case. *International Migration Review, 30*, 423-444.

Kalton, G., & Anderson, D. W. (1986). Sampling rare populations. *Journal of the Royal Statistical Society A, 149*, 65-82.

Lindstrom, D. P., & Massey, D. S. (1994). Selective emigration, cohort quality, and models of immigrant assimilation. *Social Science Research, 23*, 315-349.

Massey, D. S., Alarcón, R., Durand, J., & González, H. (1987). *Return to Aztlan: The social process of international migration from western Mexico*. Berkeley: University of California Press.

Massey, D. S., Arango, J., Hugo, G., Kouaouci, A., Pellegrino, A., & Taylor, J. E. (1993). Theories of international migration: A review and appraisal. *Population and Development Review, 19*, 431-466.

Massey, D. S., Donato, K. M., & Liang, Z. (1990). Effects of the Immigration Reform and Control Act of 1986: Preliminary data from Mexico. In F. D. Bean, B. Edmonston, & J. S. Passel (Eds.), *Illegal immigration to the United States: The experience of the 1980s* (pp. 183-210). Washington, DC: Urban Institute Press.

Massey, D. S., & Espinosa, K. E. (1997). What's driving Mexico-U.S. migration? A theoretical, empirical and policy analysis. *American Journal of Sociology, 102*, 939-999.

Massey, D. S., Goldring, L., & Durand, J. (1994). Continuities in transnational migration: An analysis of 19 Mexican communities. *American Journal of Sociology, 99*, 1492-1533.

Massey, D. S., & Parrado, E. A. (1994). Migradollars: The remittances and savings of Mexican migrants to the United States. *Population Research and Policy Review, 13*, 3-30.

Massey, D. S., & Parrado, E. A. (1997). International migration and business formation in Mexico. *Social Science Quarterly, 79*, 1-20.

Massey, D. S., & Singer, A. (1995). New estimates of undocumented Mexican migration and the probability of apprehension. *Demography, 32*, 203-213.

Padilla, Y. C. (1996, August 21-23). *The effect of social background on the long-term economic integration of Mexican immigrants*. Paper presented at the Annual Meetings of the American Sociological Association, New York.

Passel, J. S. (1995, March 17). *Illegal migration: How large a problem?* Paper presented at the Conference on Latin American Migration: The Foreign Policy Dimension. Meridian International House, Washington, DC.

Phillips, J. A., & Massey, D. S. (in press). The new labor market: Immigrants and wages after IRCA. *Demography, 36*.

Portes, A. (1979). Illegal immigration and the international system: Lessons from recent legal immigrants from Mexico. *Social Problems, 26*, 425-438.

Singer, A., & Massey, D. S. (1998). The social process of undocumented border crossing. *International Migration Review, 32*, 561-592.

U.S. Immigration and Naturalization Service. (1992). *1991 statistical yearbook of the Immigration and Naturalization Service*. Washington, DC: U.S. Government Printing Office.
U.S. Immigration and Naturalization Service. (1995). *1994 statistical yearbook of the Immigration and Naturalization Service*. Washington, DC: U.S. Government Printing Office.

10

Assessing Protocols
for Child Interviews

Johnny Blair
University of Maryland

The variety of available pretesting methods has increased with the growing attention and resources devoted to this crucial stage in designing a survey. These methods, each with their own individual strengths, may be more effective when used in concert (Presser & Blair, 1994). Their combined use may extract more information from a given sample. This effect may be of particular importance if the sample size is small.

Different pretest methods make different demands on respondents. In conventional pretesting, the respondent simply answers the interview questions. Other methods require respondents to do things such as describe how they arrived at their answers, what they understood questions to mean, or why they had difficulty answering a particular question. The effectiveness of a pretest method depends on the respondent's ability to do the requested tasks. If some of these tasks pose difficulties for adults, they may be even more apt to do so for child respondents. In a study to develop interview protocols for a USDA Continuing Survey of Food Intakes by Individuals (CSFII), several pretesting methods were used with children age 6 to 11 and their parents. The CSFII asks about the foods the child ate on the day prior to an interview.

Survey information about children's behaviors quite often is collected by proxy. But, in some cases, children must be interviewed directly about their behaviors. This often happens because the parents are not aware of some of the behaviors being studied, as is frequently the case once children enter school. Although other proxies, such as teachers, might be available, they are unlikely to observe some behaviors, such as eating, in sufficient detail for survey purposes. In addition, logistical obstacles may prohibit the use of teachers as proxies. It is important to note that the parent may have information about some of the behaviors of interest. At the time of this research, CSFII reports for children under age 12 were collected by proxy. As the levels of missing data for children of school age were unacceptably high, it was decided to investigate the feasibility of collecting these data directly from them.

We learned in interviewer debriefings preceding this research that children were already contributing to some interviews informally. The children often volunteered information that their parents did not know, even though that was not part of the interview protocol. This anecdotal evidence encouraged the view that one could obtain this kind of information from children.

This small research project was intended only to help suggest directions that one might consider in the development of protocols to collect dietary intake data from children. The research objectives were to determine how well children age 6 to 11 could report the foods they ate and drank, understood these particular survey tasks and surveys in general, and understood relevant concepts such as the one-day reference period.

This chapter's focus is less on the results in terms of how the protocols worked and how they compare to each other, which has been reported elsewhere (Blair, Mack, & Ryan, 1994; Mack, Blair, & Presser, 1993, 1996; Presser, Blair, Mack, Ryan, & Van Dyne, 1993), as on the development of the protocols as instruments for child respondents, on the pretesting methodology, and on the performance of children as pretest and survey respondents (Scott, 1997).

THE DEVELOPMENT OF THE PROTOCOLS

We developed three protocols for use with children. The interview protocol being used by USDA at the time, the "Day One" interview, was slightly modified for children and used as a control. This was done because one USDA option was to simplify the current instrument so that it would be usable by children.

Based on a literature review (Presser et al., 1993), several issues and potential problems in interviewing children were considered in the development of the protocols. Some of these, of course, also would be concerns for adults as respondents, such as simply being able to completely remember the foods that were eaten the day before. Limiting reports to a specified reference period is something that is sometimes difficult for adult respondents; therefore, there was a concern that it would prove even more problematic for children.

Another issue considered was the limited verbal facility of children, both in their vocabulary and in their ability to handle moderately complex sentence construction. During these developmental years, children's vocabularies expand rapidly, by, on average, 300 words a month (Aitchison, 1997). However, considerable variation also exists between children. A survey instrument for children needs to be developed with this diversity in mind. There are myriad additional factors that could introduce response error in child reporting.

There were concerns about social desirability, the tendency both to overreport foods one is supposed to eat and underreport those foods that are considered unhealthy. In the case of children, these underreported items might be candy and other sweets or between-meal snacks. Even with young children, such social desirability constraints might have already developed. Related to social desirability is the authority differential between an adult interviewer and a child respondent. This could produce attempts by the child to please the interviewer by responding in ways the child thinks the interviewer wants or that they feel adults expect.

For both reasons of social desirability and the power differential, it is important to minimize the prompting of the child's suggestibility. This is mainly an issue of the use of probes. It is very easy inadvertently to use probes such as "Did you have anything to drink with the sandwich?" Although one might not consider such a question leading (or if so, only mildly so), the child might interpret it to mean that he or she should have had something to drink with the sandwich, and then report as much.

The question–answer process may be seen by children as a kind of test and lead to anxiety and tension in the interview situation. From the literature review, we learned that children may report less the more frequently they are questioned, and that they give less information on later questions than on earlier ones (Wood & Wood, 1983). This issue was explicitly addressed in one of the protocols. To minimize the potential test-like atmosphere in considering pretest methods, we considered how engaging the required tasks might be, which is probably also related to the respondents' interest in survey tasks and topics.

If respondents are interested in the survey topic, they may be motivated to expend more effort to provide their answers. This can be especially important when the response task is a difficult one. The literature suggested that this may be even more of a concern with children. In designing the protocols, we tried to lean toward including things to help maintain the child's interest and keep him engaged.

Finally, the literature supports the common sense intuition that for many types of survey reports, younger children are less reliable than older children (Hess & Torney, 1967; Zill, 1981). Because of difficulty understanding survey tasks, lack of relevant knowledge structures that can aid in encoding and recall, and greater suggestibility, younger children would be expected to perform less well than older children. However, smaller differences by age might occur if the survey reports are about recent and conceptually simple behaviors. Providing reports of foods recently eaten should meet these criteria.

Knowledge structures related to recall of foods eaten might include elements such as meal times, types of meals, types of foods that "go together" (e.g., milk and cereal), and locations and events that are often linked to eating (such as school lunchrooms, going to movies, or watching television). Such knowledge structures provide a framework for encoding memories about foods eaten recently. Features of those same structures might also be used as natural aids to recall. Because eating and drinking are among the most natural and frequent behaviors at any age, one might expect that these structures are relatively well developed even in young children. Some of the protocols developed were based on these assumptions about knowledge structures.

THE PROTOCOLS

Three protocols were designed: Open, Meals, and Locations. Preceding the administration of each protocol was a general introduction that went to some length and repetition to frame the reason for the interview and the tasks. Many of the issues of concern in interviewing children began to be addressed in the introduction, prior to the administration of the particular protocol. These issues included simple language, creating a conversational rather than test context, repeated emphasis, by repetition rather than directives, on the importance of completeness of reports, and similar repetition of the reference period.

Introduction:

Before we get started, could you tell me what you were told about what we're going to do today?

We're going to be talking about the things that you eat and drink. I'm trying to learn how children remember what they eat and drink. I also want to find out EVERYTHING children remember about the things they eat and drink.

I'd like you to help me with this.

We'll be talking about the things you ate or drank *yesterday.*

I'd like to find out what you ate and drank and also as much as you remember about *each thing* you ate and drank.

I'd like to find out *everything* you ate or drank yesterday, even if you *only* tasted or had part of something.

In addition to meals, I also want to know about *any* snacks you had.

I want to know about all the kinds of things you ate or drank *yesterday*, including candy, soda, gum or other snacks.

Do you have any questions about this?

The open protocol was completely unstructured. The child was simply asked to report all of the foods eaten or drunk on the previous day. The general introduction was used with all of the protocols, but the heart of this protocol was simply "Now tell me all the things you ate *yesterday*." This protocol addresses the concern in the literature about repeated questions possibly producing progressively fewer or shorter responses (Wood & Wood, 1983). Furthermore, there is evidence that young children may have a less-structured sense of their day and that imposing a structure on their reporting might make the response task more difficult.

The second protocol used a meals/nonmeals structure, which required starting at the beginning of the day and going through it chronologically. The children were asked about each meal they had and what they ate at that meal. This also served to frame between-meal eating, such as between breakfast and lunch, between lunch and dinner, and so forth. This protocol was motivated mainly by the idea, noted earlier, of developed knowledge structures based on the routine of different meals. Memory may be organized by structure of the schedule of regular meals and what happens at those meals. This would provide a logical structure for the child that would perhaps aid recall and keep the child focused on the point of the survey, which was to collect information about food intake.

Specifically, the interviewer asked the following questions:

- What was the first meal that you had?
- Did you eat anything prior to that meal?
- What was the next meal you had?
- Did you eat anything in between the first and second meals, for example, between breakfast and lunch?
- After going to bed, did you get up and eat or drink anything?

The third protocol was based on location. It was structured similarly to the meals/nonmeals protocol, but instead of asking about meals, it asked in chronological order about locations and activities from the previous day. This required the child recalling in sequence the places that he went to and then reporting for each location whether anything was eaten there and, if so, what it was. In addition to calling on a different knowledge structure, this protocol also sought to be more engaging by permitting the children to talk about things they did, which might be of more interest than simply reporting what they ate and drank. If the child is more engaged in the interview, he or she will probably produce better information and feel more at ease. Also, this may reduce the tendency of reporting or thinking about good foods versus bad or unhealthy foods.

As noted, the Day One interview served as a control. In this protocol, respondents are required to report, in chronological order, all foods eaten on the reference day. There are additional reporting requirements, such as how foods were cooked, which were eliminated from the modified Day One instrument used in this project.

THE USE OF MULTIPLE TESTING METHODS

This research was conducted under an agreement with limited participant approval, which precluded using more than nine respondents for any single protocol. Given these very small sample sizes, any statistical analysis would be severely limited and subject to large sampling error. Therefore, we expected that much of our data would have to be examined qualitatively.

The use of multiple pretest methods had two objectives: to obtain as much information as possible out of small sample sizes and to gain different perspectives on children's understanding of the role and performance of survey respondents. As will be seen, the multiple methods also provide information of different types, providing a richer qualitative data set to use to evaluate the protocols. The success of some of these methods, of course, depended on the respondent being able to provide certain kinds of information about how the instrument worked and difficulties they had.

It should also be kept in mind that some of the test methods were aimed at learning about children as survey respondents, in addition to testing these particular protocols.

These multiple methods led to multiple components in the research design. First, there was a standard experimental comparison of the four protocols, with an equal number of children and their parents randomly assigned to each protocol. Second, validation data were collected for a subset of the children. Third, based on findings from the experimental comparison of protocols, a second round of interviews was conducted that included a "reconciliation interview." Finally, in addition to the administration of the protocols, several other laboratory methodologies were used to gain insight into how well children understood the survey tasks asked of them.

The sample consisted of 9 children and their parents recruited through telephone screening of households and 27 children and parents recruited from nearby child-care centers. For those children recruited from the child-care centers, on the day prior to the interview, a Survey Research Center staff member observed the child (in a group setting) eating a meal at the center. The foods eaten were listed and used to validate the part of the interview report pertaining to that meal. The parents were paid $20 for participation, the children were paid $5. The children understood and liked the $5 much more than other incentives we had considered (in the small pretest), such as McDonald's coupons or toys. Child-care and community centers were paid $50 for permitting access to the children.

The 36 child–parent pairs were randomly assigned to each of the four protocols. The administration of the protocols averaged 17 minutes each. The Day One protocol was the longest and the Open the shortest.

ADDITIONAL METHODS

This list of test methods is quite extensive. However, they fit together well and there were few indications that they turned out to be terribly burdensome. These are described in the order they were used.

Preinterview Questions. The children were asked initially a couple of questions: first, what they had been told about what was going to happen in the interview and, second, what their understanding was about polls and surveys. Before the administration of each protocol each child was asked, "Could you tell me what you were told about what we're going to do today?" and "Tell me a little about what you've heard about polls and surveys. Why do you think polls and surveys are done?"

Videotaping. All of the child interviews were videotaped and the interaction between the child and the interviewer was coded as a way to possibly indicate places during the interview where the child was having difficulty. We also coded nonverbal behaviors of the children. Nonverbal behaviors include facial expressions, smiling, laughing, crying, body movements (e.g., fidgeting), which might be indicators of difficulties at particular points in the interview.

Think Aloud. During pretest development of the protocols, we conducted a small number of pretest interviews using think-aloud instructions. Children were given the relatively standard think-aloud instruction: "Tell us what you are thinking as you answer the questions." This method proved very difficult for most children and interfered with the main task of reporting. It was not used during the main data collection.

Drawing and Listing Foods. As an aid to recall, during the administration of the protocol, the children were asked either to draw or to list the foods and beverages eaten or drunk the previous day. Children ages 6 and 7 were asked to draw, children ages 10 and 11 were asked to list, and children ages 8 and 9 were given a choice of drawing or listing.

Sorting Food Models. Forty National Diary Council cardboard models of foods and beverages were supplemented with five pictures clipped from magazines of junk or snack foods. The children were asked to categorize these 45 foods into groups and to decide on a name for each group. They were permitted to use any groupings they wanted with no restrictions on the number or types of groups.

These data were coded into nine category types:

1. Foods liked or disliked
2. Meals (e.g., breakfast or lunch foods)
3. Food groups (e.g., dairy, meat, fruit)
4. Color (e.g., green foods)
5. Foods eaten on particular days (e.g., a Sunday group)
6. Foods that are healthy or unhealthy
7. Foods that "go together" such as "bread and butter"
8. The child could not decide on a name for the group
9. Other

Interview. The randomly assigned protocol was administered simultaneously by different interviewers to both the parent and the child in separate rooms.

Clean-Up Probes. Immediately after the administration of the protocol, both parents and children were asked these additional questions:

Is there anything that [you/child's name] tasted yesterday that you haven't mentioned?

Is there anything that [you/child's name] ate part of yesterday that you haven't mentioned?

Are there any snacks [you/child's name] had yesterday that you haven't mentioned yet?

Were there any other things [you/child's name] ate or drank that you didn't mention?

Did [you/child's name] eat anything yesterday that [you/he/she] had never had before?

Did [you/child's name] eat anything yesterday that [you/he/she] really liked?

Did [you/child's name] eat anything yesterday that [you/he/she] really did not like?

Debriefing of Child, Parent, and Interviewer. Debriefings with the child were done by another interviewer, not the interviewer that originally interviewed the child. In the child debriefings, the videotape of the child interview was played back as a recall aid. Children were asked about how well they liked or did not like the interview, which instructions were hard to understand, which things were hardest to remember, whether they reported foods they usually ate or drank, and whether they guessed at answers.

The parent debriefing paralleled that of the child but without the use of the videotape. The interviewer used a debriefing guide to do a self-debriefing, which included assessments of how at ease the child was and how much attention the child paid, along with how well the probes worked, among other questions.

Joint Parent–Child Reconciliation Interview. In a second round of interviewing, after administration of the protocol and the standard debriefings, the parent and child were brought together with a third interviewer to go through the foods and beverages that had been each listed in each individual interview. In this round of interviewing, the debriefing interview was done after the reconciliation interview so that the child could be asked about the reconciliation interview as well.

DISADVANTAGES OF THE PROTOCOLS

Each protocol also had possible disadvantages. For example, the Day One instrument as it stood at that time was very complex and, although it was simplified, it would probably still be difficult for children.

The completely unstructured Open protocol might lead to underreporting because of the lack of memory cues or aids to recall. It also might be difficult, at least for the children, in that it may be less interesting and therefore less engaging than some other methods.

The meals/nonmeals might bring to mind the notion of things that their parents have told them they should eat at meals and things that they should not eat. It might also be somewhat less engaging.

The locations protocol might depend greatly on the activities for that particular day. If it was a school day where the activities are fairly routine, it might be a relatively easy reporting task. On the other hand, if it was a day that was very atypical with a lot of unusual or different things happening, then it might be very difficult.

Finally, of the various supplemental methods, the one of most concern was the joint reconciliation interview. As mentioned, in the reconciliation interview, we brought the child and parent together in a room to go over the lists of foods that had been reported and to discuss the reasons for the reporting mismatches. There were concerns about how this procedure might affect the child, and that the situation may seem like an extreme testing situation or confrontational.

A great deal of time was spent testing different procedures and language to try to diffuse that concern. One of the main methods was to ask the parents and children brought together about *all* of the things that were reported, rather than just focusing on mismatched reports (i.e., when one person reported a food that the other did not). When the interviewer came to an item that had only been reported by one of the pair, she probed to try to find the reason for the misreporting.

RESULTS AND DISCUSSION

The Protocols

The analysis focused on the completeness of reports in terms of the amounts and numbers of food items reported. The Day One protocol yielded the lowest number of child reports and the Locations protocol the highest. There were no significant differences by child's age in the amount of reporting.

In all of the protocols except Day One, the children on average reported as many or more items than did the parents. However, this is dominated by the amount of reporting by the older children. The younger children reported slightly fewer items than did their parents. In comparing the actual items reported by children and parents, there were many mismatches. The Open and Meals protocols yielded the most matches. When comparing the child and observer reports, the Locations protocol had the highest accuracy.

It was expected that sometimes the child would report items of which the parent was not aware. That expectation was the main reason for considering interviewing children. One interesting finding was that many times the parents reported items that were not reported by the child. To investigate reasons for this, a second round of interviews was conducted.

In that second round of interviewing with nine child–parent pairs, after the protocol had been administered, a joint child–parent "reconciliation interview" was conducted to investigate reasons for this finding. The Locations protocol was used for these nine cases. The main reason for the discrepancy was the assumption by parents that the children had eaten food taken with them to school.

The Multiple Methods

The pre-interview questions served the function of putting the child at ease and also learning their expectations about the interview. In general, they had been given only very general information along the lines of "they're going to be asking you some questions about things you do." Fortunately, the parents had not said things that would raise the child's anxieties or lead them to expect a difficult or test-like atmosphere. None of the children seemed to have problems remembering what had been told to them or were reluctant to report it.

In trying out think-aloud procedures, as noted, it was found that the children were often distracted from the reporting task. It seemed that, at least for this small group of children, the cognitive burden of thinking aloud in addition to reporting was too much. But it should be noted again that the sample sizes were extremely small.

The analysis of nonverbal videotaped behaviors was not productive. Although it was possible to code at least very overt behaviors, the interpretation of them was problematic. The literature in nonverbal behaviors was not particularly helpful in these analyses. Although the coding of the behaviors themselves can be done with high reliability (Baesler & Burgoon, 1987), there is little work on the interpretation of the coded behaviors. For example, staring off past the interviewer into the distance might indicate distraction or concentration. Looking into or showing awareness of the camera might indicate anxiety or interest and engagement. The frequency of such ambiguities made this analysis unproductive.

The children were engaged by the drawing and listing tasks. However, frequently the interviewer had to remind them of the central reporting tasks. This again suggests that for many children of these ages handling multiple tasks is burdensome. However, unlike the think-aloud task, this additional task was interesting to the children.

Similarly, the sorting task was enthusiastically accomplished. The children were able, in almost all cases, to understand the required task and to provide sensible names or rationales for the food groupings they used.

The clean-up probes were very effective. Significant additional reports resulted from these probes. The children were not bothered by the repetition of the probes right after the interview, perhaps because the probes did not take very much time.

The debriefing interviews provided confirmation about the child's engagement and interest in the interviews. They did not hesitate to report their feelings. The use of a different interviewer seems to have been effective; there were no difficulties in establishing a conversation with the new person.

The reconciliation interviews were very effective in uncovering the reasons for the mismatches in parent–child reports. The steps taken to avoid discomfort of the children appeared effective. The children were not reluctant to simply say, in some instances, they just "forgot" to report a particular food, or that they did not eat something that was put in their lunch at home. Last, in these interviews the children frequently reported things that had been eaten on another day, which supported the concerns about the difficulty of children handling the reference period.

In the debriefing interview that followed, the children generally reported that they were not ill at ease with reviewing their reports with their parents. However, several children did report (both in this and the earlier round) that they would not like to have done the original interview with their parent present.

Additionally, in both the main and reconciliation interviews, parents were often quick to say that even though the reported foods were eaten the day previous to the interview, this was not what the child "usually" ate; according to several parents, their child usually ate far more healthy things than reported for the previous day. Unfortunately, as in many instances, the sample sizes were too small to try to compare the amount of social desirability in parent versus child reporting.

The validation proved very effective although there were problems in matching the foods reported because we had only observed one meal—the day before—at the summer camp. The child debriefings worked well. We found that the children could talk about their interview experiences and tell us about parts of the interview that were difficult or easy for them.

Children as Survey and Pretest Respondents

As noted at the outset, one neglected issue in survey research concerns not just children as respondents, but children as *pretest* respondents. It is often overlooked that in some types of pretesting, we sometimes ask much more of respondents than in typical surveys. Because a variety of pretest methods were used, this project afforded a rare opportunity to observe children's response to alternative pretest methods.

Some of these methods require additional tasks of the child respondents such as reporting on difficulties that they may have had in understanding questions or problems they had generating answers to the questions. There was little reporting about problems with specific questions. This may have resulted because the questions were of such a natural conversational style that the child could not recall specific questions as such.

In this research, the examination of the children's knowledge structures, their ability to organize or at least report events in terms of when they occurred, and their ability to understand particular concepts was done simultaneously with the testing of the specific protocols. It may have been more effective to separate the examination of these cognitive fundamentals from the design and testing of the protocols, which, in fact, already incorporated assumptions about them.

Few of the children knew what polls or surveys were. There were no differences by age. Only one of the children had any idea "why . . . polls and surveys are done." Children's understanding of their role as survey respondents may affect their performance. It is often forgotten how much prior knowledge the researcher assumes the respondent is bringing to the interview situation. Adult respondents typically know something about what surveys are, even if they have never participated in one. They have usually been in situations where they have had to provide survey-like information, as when filling out forms or answering questions in a doctor's office. Through various means, adults bring considerable prior information to the interview. This is far less true with children. The implication is that much more introduction and explanation is likely to be necessary for children to be good survey respondents. However, on the evidence of this study, when that information is provided, even in a laboratory setting, children are very good at providing certain types of behavioral information.

This sample of children included some who are very young, 6 to 7 years old, but even with the older 8- to 11-year-olds, the development of the children, as expected, varied greatly. The level of development relates directly to the cognitive ability of the children to perform many survey and pretest tasks. One implication of this is that the variance one would expect in small samples may be especially large because of variance in cognitive abilities within this population. So the results of this research should be taken only as indicative of possible results of further research with larger samples.

ACKNOWLEDGMENT

The research reported here was conducted as part of a cooperative agreement between the University of Maryland Survey Research Center and the USDA Human Nutrition Information Service. Stanley Presser was principal investigator and Johnny Blair was project director.

REFERENCES

Aitchison, J. (1997). *The language web: The power and problem of words.* Cambridge, England: Cambridge University Press.
Baesler, E. J., & Burgoon, J. K. (1987). Measurement and reliability of nonverbal behavior. *Journal of Nonverbal Behavior, 11,* 205–233.

Blair, J., Mack, K., & Ryan, C. (1994, May). *Memory for dietary intake by young children: The effects of alternative interview structures.* Paper presented at the Fourth Conference on Practical Aspects of Memory, University of Maryland, College Park, MD.

Hess, R., & Torney, J. (1967). *The development of political attitudes in children.* Chicago: Aldine.

Mack, K. A., Blair, J., & Presser, S. (1993). *An experimental comparison of alternative 24-hour diet recall questionnaire protocols for children.* Proceedings of the American Statistical Association winter meetings.

Mack, K. A., Blair, J., & Presser, S. (1996). Measuring and improving data quality in children's reports of dietary intake. In R. B. Warnecke (Ed.), *Proceedings of the Sixth Conference on Health Survey Methods* (pp. 51–55). DHHS Pub. No. (PHS) 96-1013. Hyattsville, MD: U.S. Department of Health and Human Services.

Presser, S., & Blair, J. (1994). Do different pretest methods produce different results? In P. V. Marsden (Ed.), *Sociological methodology* (pp. 73–104). Oxford, England: Blackwell.

Presser, S., Blair, J., Mack, K., Ryan, C. M., & Van Dyne, M. A. (1993). *Final report on the University of Maryland–USDA Cooperative Agreement to Improve Reporting for Children in the Continuing Survey of Food Intakes by Individuals Project.*

Scott, J. (1997). Children as respondents: Methods for improving data quality. In L. Lyberg, P. Biemer, M. Collins, E. De Leeuw, C. Dippo, N. Schwarz, & D. Trewin (Eds.), *Survey measurement and process quality* (pp. 331–350). New York: Wiley.

Wood, H., & Wood, D. (1983). Questioning the pre-school child. *Educational Review, 35,* 149–162.

Zill, N. (1981). *American children happy, healthy and insecure.* Unpublished report of the Foundation for Child Development's national survey of children.

11

Do I Do What I Say?
A Perspective on Self-Report Methods
in Drug Dependence Epidemiology

James C. Anthony
Yehuda D. Neumark
Michelle L. Van Etten
Johns Hopkins University

THREE TRADITIONS OF ASSESSMENT IN DRUG DEPENDENCE EPIDEMIOLOGY

The origins of drug dependence epidemiology can be traced to a large number of prenumerate and pre-ethnographic descriptions of drug-taking practices in various parts of the world, logged by world travelers, explorers, and merchants (e.g., see Sonnedecker, 1962). These descriptions are based on direct or indirect observation of drug users. They serve as important historical accounts of opium-taking, smoking of hashish and tobacco, coca leaf-chewing, and drinking of coffee, tea, chocolate, and alcoholic beverages.

A more numerate developmental period emerged from 19th century census procedures. During the 1800s, it became customary to have U.S. census-takers count up the number of known "inebriates," "lunatics," "insane" persons, and "idiots" while they also enumerated the nation's citizenry. This was accomplished not only by direct observation during routine door-to-door census-taking but also by queries to knowledgeable key informants within households and communities. For example, as part of the 1880 U.S. census, nearly 100,000 physicians in all parts of the country were contacted, furnished with blank forms, and asked to report to the Census Office all idiots and lunatics "within the sphere of their personal knowledge" (Wines, 1888, pp. ix–x).

During 1916, psychiatrist Aaron Rosanoff completed an often-neglected classic field survey of citizens living in Nassau County, New York. Rosanoff perfected a two-stage ascertainment method to detect the prevailing cases of mental disorders, including those affected by alcohol and drug problems. In the first stage, Rosanoff had social workers and other nonpsychiatrist staff members go door to door, seeking information about all of Nassau County's citizens. Their methods included direct face-to-face assessments as well as collection of data from key informants within each household. These unscheduled interviews included a brief cognitive mental status screening procedure (e.g., test items on orientation to place and time; arithmetic tasks, proverb interpretations), as well as more or less standardized probes about disturbances of the mental life and behavior. When the first-stage assessment nominated a case within a household, Rosanoff and a psychiatrist colleague returned to the household for an in-depth assessment. On this basis, primarily drawing from self-report or key informant data, Rosanoff was able to sort the disturbances into specific fine-grained diagnostic categories of his time. Thereafter, he was able to produce the first disorder-specific estimates for the prevalence of these disturbances in an American community population (Rosanoff, 1917).

Dating from the 1920s, we have a long-standing tradition of U.S. Public Health Service-supported and other social and psychological research on seriously involved drug users. A great body of clinical and epidemiological evidence in this tradition was created by investigators who were affiliated with federal correctional facilities and hospitals, to which officially detected drug users were referred. For the most part, these investigators used anamnestic self-report methods to study the background and history of seriously involved drug users who had been incarcerated for drug-related offenses (e.g., see Kolb, 1925; Pescor, 1939). In these investigations, as well as later research on both treated and untreated, incarcerated and nonincarcerated drug users, there often was a blend of the strengths of clinical research and field survey research (e.g., see Ball & Chambers, 1970; Ball, Shaffer, & Nurco, 1983; Chein, Gerard, Lee, & Rosenfeld, 1964; Nurco et al., 1991). These studies tended to emphasize accuracy or fidelity of information derived from the personal narratives or life stories of seriously involved drug users versus reliability of assessment. From these and other early studies (e.g., see Becker, 1963; Dai, 1937; Lindesmith, 1947), there emerged many of strengths now seen in modern ethnographic studies of drug users (Carlson, Harvey, & Falck, 1995; Feldman & Aldrich, 1990).

During the 20th century, we also can see emergence of strengths of a second and more psychometrically oriented tradition of field research, which sought to surpass traditional clinical research methods in standardization and reliability. Aided by advances in factor analyses contributed by Thorndike and others, this tradition fostered development of the Minnesota Multiphasic Personality Inventory and the Army Neuropsychiatric

Screening Adjunct used to evaluate recruits for the Armed Services in WWII (Starr, 1950), as well as development of the Addiction Research Center Inventory (ARCI) at the Public Health Service facility in Lexington—the ARCI seeking to differentiate and discriminate between effects of different drugs (e.g., see Hill, Haertzen, Wolbach, & Miner, 1963). The influence of this psychometric tradition can be seen in some recent studies to assess social psychological constructs such as socially desirable responding and psychiatric illness (Goldberg, 1972; Latkin, Vlahov, & Anthony, 1993; Paulhus, 1984). This tradition continues to motivate use of standardized multiple-item assessments of latent constructs of drug involvement, the determinants of HIV infection, and progression to AIDS.

A third tradition influencing drug survey assessment methods can be traced back to advances in sociology, social psychology, and applied public opinion research prior to WWII, with influences from a post-WWII emergence of standardized assessment in clinical psychiatry. In this tradition, there is a blend of careful attention to the wording of interview questions, the validity of survey response, and the reliability of responses to interview questions. As compared to the more psychometric tradition within psychology, in its earlier years this more sociological tradition involved somewhat greater interpretation of the manifest content of responses to individual items. There was somewhat less emphasis on formal psychometrics and latent variable analyses (e.g., see Cantril, 1944; Hyman et al., 1954; Payne, 1951; Suchman, Phillips, & Streib, 1958). This distinction has changed since midcentury (e.g., see Clogg, 1979; Goodman, 1978; Lazarsfeld & Henry, 1968) but the sociological tradition's increasing attention to latent variables has not displaced its ever-strong concern about the individual items used for assessment (e.g., see Converse & Presser, 1986; Schuman & Presser, 1981; Sudman & Bradburn, 1982).

Robins, Helzer, Cottler, and their research groups in the Washington University at St. Louis have been the major contributors in the development of drug-dependence assessments in this tradition. As one of the pioneers in efforts to devise standardized criteria and standardized assessments of psychiatric disorders generally, Robins crafted a field interview assessment of narcotics addiction for use in her classic investigation about childhood deviance and later risk of crime and psychiatric disturbances in adulthood (Robins, 1966). Later refinements were incorporated as part of follow-up studies of Vietnam veterans' drug experiences before, during, and after their foreign service, and for the NIMH Epidemiologic Catchment Area (ECA) surveys (e.g., see Anthony & Helzer, 1991; Robins et al., 1985). The resulting drug dependence assessments in the Diagnostic Interview Schedule (DIS) and Composite International Diagnostic Interview (CIDI) have been applied not only in the ECA surveys but also in the National Household Survey on

Drug Abuse and the National Comorbidity Survey and elsewhere (e.g., see Anthony, Warner, & Kessler, 1994; Cottler et al., 1997; Ensminger, Anthony, & McCord, 1997; Kandel, Grant, Kessler, Warner, & Chen, 1997).

Notwithstanding the strengths of these several traditions, it now is time to do more in epidemiologic field surveys of drug use and drug dependence. What now is needed is an added strength from new approaches such as computer-assisted assessments, drug assays developed in toxicology laboratories (e.g., sweat patch assays), experience sampling methods, ethnographic assessments of survey procedures, and cognitive evaluation of interview items. By combining these strengths, it will be possible to gain more information from assessments in future investigations with special attention to information that will help us resolve issues that now remain perplexing (such as quantification of dose). In part, these issues are perplexing because there is little knowledge about the accuracy and reliability of our assessments about drug use and related risk behaviors.

COMPUTER-ASSISTED AND COMPUTERIZED ADAPTIVE TESTING AND SAMPLING IN EPIDEMIOLOGY

With respect to the three traditions of drug dependence assessment methodology, those most aligned with computerized assessments are the psychometric tradition and the more recent survey-oriented tradition, perhaps best exemplified by a computer-assisted adaptive testing paradigm. In adaptive testing, the computational power of a desktop or laptop computer can be harnessed to evaluate a subject's early responses to initially presented sets of test items and to use the observed pattern of responses to select an appropriate sample of subsequent sets of test items. More than a simple computer-controlled logical branching sequence within interviews, adaptive testing actually can be used to grade a subject in relation to some underlying dimension of performance. It then can draw down the most appropriate item sets to refine the evidence on the subject's position relative to that dimension (Green, 1988).

The value of computerized assessments has been recognized outside of the formal psychometric research tradition and has extended into the realm of clinical research on psychiatric disturbances and sensitive behaviors. Drug and alcohol dependence scales and even the DIS and the CIDI have been converted to computer-assisted assessment and compared with conventional paper-and-pencil methods (e.g., see Erdman, Klein, & Greist, 1983; Greist et al., 1987; Skinner & Allen, 1983). In fact, the current question for our field is not whether the large-sample National Household Survey on Drug Abuse will be converted to computer-assisted assessment but rather how the conversion will be made with minimum distortion of trend data from each successive survey. The background to these current decisions has been discussed by Turner, Lessler, and Groeferer (1992).

In many current survey research applications, the power of the computer now is not harnessed for adaptive testing as just described. Nonetheless, the computer is used to reduce the burden on interviewers who otherwise must recall complicated instructions about when and how to ask probing questions. As summarized elsewhere (Turner et al., 1992), there are important methodological advantages and opportunities when traditional paper-and-pencil instruments are converted to computerized assessments. It is possible to implement computer-controlled branching through complex questionnaires, and there can be automated consistency checks with feedback to reconcile inconsistencies and to check for out-of-range values such as we sometimes see when respondents report on the frequency of their drug-injecting behavior (e.g., see Fendrich, Mackesy-Amiti, Wislar, & Goldstein, 1997; Johnston & O'Malley, 1997; Lyles et al., 1997). In this mode of computer-assisted assessment, data files are produced efficiently, less expensively, and more accurately than when hardcopy must be turned over to data-entry clerks or when optical forms must be scanned.

In addition, applied within the framework of a standardized system with analog or digitized recordings of an interviewer reading interview questions, the stimulus (e.g., sex, voice, and physical appearance of the interviewer) can be standardized for greater experimental control over sources of measurement error (e.g., see Lessler & O'Reilly, 1997). This Audio Computer-Assisted Self-Interviewing methodology (ACASI) can be used for any respondent who can hear and type on a keyboard, with no need for multilingual members of the research team except for whoever is hired to translate and dictate the questions for recording. In light of current overseas research on HIV, AIDS, and drug use, as well as the growing ethnic diversity within our local population, this is a consideration of increasing importance.

Keyboard proficiency is not a critical element in this line of methodological innovation. Reliance on keyboarding can be reduced with a response interface via touch-sensitive screens, optical character recognition for handwriting, or use of a microphone to record spoken replies. It now is recognized that the computer interface can be an important characteristic of computerized assessment. For example, in their review of computerized assessment of self-disclosure, Weisband and Kiesler (1996) argued that computerized assessments are multidimensional, with options for animation, speech and speech recognition, talking to people on-screen, embedded emotional responses, feedback through auditory and kinesthetic channels, and virtual reality.

By way of example, consider one recent study in which two computer-assisted methods were compared. One involved having the subjects interact with a female computer counselor (an on-screen talking face), whereas the other involved simply corresponding with her via text on the screen (i.e., by typing information and reading responses from the off-screen counselor, with no on-screen talking face). The subjects were found to disclose more to the off-screen counselor and to disclose less to the talking face of the on-screen counselor, who was not evaluated as favorably as the never-seen counselor who interacted via text only (Weisband & Kiesler, 1996).

Another experiment with ACASI methods, planned by our research group but not yet initiated, actually finesses a need to have the respondent acknowledge drug-taking but still allows for estimation of the prevalence of illicit drug use and may yield new evidence about the causes and consequences of drug-taking. Here, ACASI is used to present respondents with a sequence of lists, each containing five activities in a standard behavioral repertoire (Johanson, Duffy, & Anthony, 1996). At the end of each list, respondents are asked to record the number of activities engaged in but are not asked to say whether they engaged in any specific activity. For some of the lists, we substitute a drug-taking activity (e.g., smoking marijuana, injecting cocaine, smoking ice) in place of a nonsensitive topic such as riding a bicycle, selecting respondents and lists at random for this substitution. The substituted item causes a perturbation in frequency distributions and covariances for the listed activities, and comparison of the observed perturbed evidence with the expected unperturbed results yields information to derive an estimated prevalence of the drug-taking activity. With an elaboration of this basic method and calling on the powers of computerized adaptive testing, it becomes possible—during the interview session—to estimate the respondent's position on a dimensional scale: for example, predicted probability of having smoked ice at some point during the 2 days prior to assessment. Although not necessarily known with certainty, this estimated position or predicted probability can be used as a size measure within the framework of regression-based sampling, helping the investigator to draw and recruit an especially informative but much smaller second-stage sample for more intensive scrutiny (e.g., bioassay for recent drug use).

For more than 15 years, our research group (and others) have been using concepts such as size measures and regression-based sampling in order to conduct sequenced multistage sampling (SMSS) for field studies of mental and behavioral disturbances, including drug dependence (e.g., see Anthony et al., 1985). These involve a relatively simple elaboration of the two-stage field survey approach devised by Rosanoff in 1917, the primary difference being that our approach involves sampling along the entire range of values on the dimension for predictive probability of being a case. In contrast, Rosanoff introduced the second-stage clinical examination only for cases nominated by the first-stage assessment.

We now have harnessed computer-assisted telephone interviewing (CATI) in a continuing protocol to investigate aging, brain structure, and cognition, with first-stage sampling (via random-digit dialing) and assessment to guide sampling and recruitment for a second-stage, 5-hour magnetic resonance imaging session, neuropsychological and personality testing, and standardized clinical psychiatric examinations. However, we are not making full use of computerized adaptive testing as described within the framework of SMSS designs. To our knowledge, no one else is doing so.

Without gainsaying these advantages of computerized assessment, we also must acknowledge the possibility that computerization will get in the way of making valid or accurate assessments. Some observers have voiced concern that a computerized assessment might be less reliable than an interviewer-mediated assessment—for example, if the participant became disengaged from the assessment task and began to respond at random, rather than with focused attention. We must take concerns such as these seriously. A sensible plan is to make these issues part of an overall research program on measurement of drug experiences, with comparative reliability and validity studies. In this fashion, we might learn when a Computer-Assisted Personal Interview (CAPI) is needed (e.g., when an interviewer is needed to help develop and maintain trust, rapport, and attention to the tasks at hand). And, we can learn when it is preferable to apply Computer-Assisted Self-Interviewing (CASI) (e.g., when presence of an interviewer might induce or reinforce socially desirable responding).

In this context, before closing this section on ways to improve self-report of drug experiences via computerization, it might be important to mention the results of a recent meta-analysis of 39 publications on experimental studies. In these studies, computer-assisted assessments were compared to standard paper-and-pencil methods, as completed between 1969 and 1994. Drawing from studies in the social science, computer science, and medical literatures, the authors adopted a broad definition of self-disclosure and included studies of questionnaires that solicited highly sensitive information such as a person's criminal record. They also included studies of forms on which consumers were asked to disclose their complaints. Across the 39 studies using 100 measures, computer administration increased self-disclosure as compared to conventional methods. Effect sizes were larger comparing computer administration with in-person interviews, when forms solicited sensitive information, and when medical or psychiatric patients were the subjects (Weisband & Kiesler, 1996).

DRUG EXPOSURE TESTING

As originally envisaged, many of the specific aims and hypotheses in epidemiological research on drug use and drug dependence could be addressed by using information solely based on self-report interview. For example, the original ALIVE Study protocol on the natural history of HIV infection among injecting drug users was specified in relation to a recruitment plan for individuals who had injected drugs at any time since the start of the HIV epidemic in Baltimore (Vlahov et al., 1991). In our most recent work, we are investigating transitions from initial opportunities to try marijuana until the initial actual use of marijuana, with a focus on the age or timing of an individual's first opportunity to try a drug (Van Etten, Neumark, & Anthony, 1997). Drug dependence and drug injection histories over a span of decades, initial opportunities to try drugs—these are aspects of personal behavioral history and experience for which there are no good bioassay methods and most likely never will be.

Self-report methodology also has meshed well with large-sample longitudinal research designs. For example, the ALIVE study protocol called for recruitment of almost 3,000 injecting drug users as subjects, with an initial baseline visit and with 6-month intervals between each follow-up visit. The research questions were focused on aspects of the injection history that might promote HIV infection (e.g., frequency of injections, frequency of needle-sharing, location of injections in shooting galleries or elsewhere). There was an emphasis on what had happened during the 6 months prior to assessment, or before that. These are variables not well-measured by available bioassays, although we did have physician assistants make ratings for injection stigmata (e.g., see Anthony et al., 1990).

Notwithstanding these circumstances, there are many reasons to begin an integration of drug exposure bioassay methods in large-sample longitudinal research on drug-taking and drug dependence. For example, research progress on HIV infection in relation to drug-taking and the natural history of the HIV infection has started to place stress on a more fine-grained measurement of drug exposures and drug-taking behavior. In relation to our studies of how continuous and intermittent drug-taking might influence the slope of CD4+ lymphocyte cell decline among HIV-infected drug users, there is a need to reduce measurement error in our field studies on this hypothesized influence (e.g., see Lyles et al., 1997). In particular, bioassays to confirm recent self-reported abstinence among generally active heroin and cocaine users would have strengthened that work, even if relatively inexpensive qualitative EMIT assays for recent opioid and cocaine exposure had been applied. Although still controversial and limited in some respects (e.g., when used for employee drug testing), the use of bioassay methods to detect drug exposures now warrants closer scrutiny in relation to our epidemiological studies of drug-taking.

For many epidemiological studies on drug-taking and drug dependence, it is both possible and useful to apply methods now widely used in many other clinical studies (e.g., enzyme-linked immunoassay techniques). For example, available assays for cocaine, opioids, and other drug classes of

interest can be included as part of the laboratory protocol for serum specimens. These specimens typically must be gathered in studies of infections
among injecting drug users (e.g., to test for HIV seropositivity or for lymphocyte assays), and the already available specimen can be analyzed via
drug immunoassay methods with or without confirmation (e.g., via chromatography). Alternately, in some instances, it might be appropriate to institute a suitable and secure urine specimen collection protocol.

These bioassays for urine and serum specimens have proven to be quite
effective for qualitative assays of recent drug use in research, and there is
growing interest in quantitative assays as well (e.g., see Cone, 1997; Preston,
Silverman, Schuster, & Cone, 1996, 1997). These methods would complement
the self-report data and provide a means to confirm or falsify self-report
information about quite recent drug exposures. Many observers have voiced
concern about self-report misrepresentation of recent drug use even when
the participants already are known to be active drug users (e.g., see Greenfield, Bigelow, & Brooner, 1995; Hser, 1997). Because of concerns such as
these, immunoassay screening of specimens with followup confirmatory gas
chromatography–mass spectrometry (GC–MS) remains the standard protocol for treatment program and workplace drug testing (Cone, 1997; Dupont
& Baumgartner, 1995). Confirmation with GC-MS also should be considered
when any protocol has hypotheses that demand the highest level of accuracy about recent drug exposures.

Although still subject to reservations (e.g., see Bost, 1993; Cone, 1997;
Holden, 1990; Kidwell & Blank, 1995), some field researchers have formed a
consensus about the value of analyses to detect drug exposure via hair
specimens (e.g., see Gropper, 1995; Magura, Freeman, Siddiqi, & Lipton, 1992;
Magura & Kang, 1997). Drugs or their metabolites are absorbed into hair
and can be detected in the hair for extended periods following use (e.g., see
Cone, 1997; Cone, Darwin, & Wang, 1993). Furthermore, it seems that drugs
are retained in the hair for weeks or even months as compared to the much
shorter periods during which certain drugs such as cocaine and heroin can
be detected in blood or urine (e.g., see Gropper, 1995). Although more
controversial, use of hair samples to provide quantitatively detailed information about patterns of use over time has been reported. There are open
questions about detecting very recent drug use in hair. Nonetheless, hair
analysis tends to provide a wider window of detection of drug exposures
and allows for less frequent specimen collection procedures that are more
acceptable to many research participants when compared with alternative
procedures to obtain serum and urine (e.g., see Cone, 1997).

Answers to some important toxicological questions about hair assays
remain unknown. Mechanisms by which externally applied drugs are incorporated into the hair remain unresolved, as does the degree to which
absorbed drugs can be removed by washing and the extent to which hair

treatment may influence test results (Cone et al., 1993; Kidwell & Blank, 1995; McBay, 1995). This, in part, is what accounts for a continuing controversy about widespread use of hair testing to detect illicit drug use when administrative actions are intended (e.g., employee termination). Fortunately, these controversial issues are less pronounced in a research context when the harm of falsely positive or falsely negative results can be constrained (e.g., see Holden, 1990). It seems that the time has come to introduce hair testing on a limited scale within some of the ongoing epidemiological studies that involve assessment of drug exposures. A primary goal of these initial studies must be to evaluate the fieldworthiness and complexities of taking hair samples within the framework of large-sample research on subjects recruited from households. Another goal is to identify any special problems or aspects of the hair bioassay methods that should be known to our field generally.

Another promising drug exposure methodology involves detection of drugs and their metabolites in sweat. Experimental studies have long and consistently shown that drugs (including cocaine, amphetamines, and PCP) can be detected in sweat (Henderson & Wilson, 1973; Smith & Liu, 1986; Suzuki, Inoue, Hori, & Inayama, 1994). A recently developed nonocclusive adhesive sweat patch allows for the collection and retention of drugs present in sweat and has been evaluated in small-sample studies. For example, Cone, Hillsgrove, Jenkins, Keenan, and Darwin (1994) applied these patches to a limited number of subjects who then received known doses of cocaine. The sweat patch tests proved capable of detecting the drug along a dose-response curve beginning at 1 to 5 mg administration. Trace amounts of intravenous, intranasal, and smoked cocaine were detectable in sweat 2 hours postdose, with the majority of the drug being excreted within 24 hours. Similar results were found in a separate small-sample ($n = 18$) controlled cocaine-administration experiment (Burns & Baselt, 1995). In a larger study of 290 subjects, immunoassay of cocaine captured in sweat patches revealed a sensitivity of 95% and specificity of 99% when compared to the GC–MS gold standard at a 10 mg/L cutoff (Spiehler, Fay, Fogerson, Schoendorfer, & Niedbala, 1996). Intersubject differences were observed in the amount of cocaine captured by the patches, as well as some intrasubject differences that seemed to depend on the location of the patch (Burns & Baselt, 1995; Cone et al., 1994).

As with hair testing, there are concerns about environmental contamination, particularly during application and removal of the patch. Subject to the resolution of these concerns, the sweat patch will likely prove itself as a fairly noninvasive method for illicit drug exposure testing, providing a window of detection between that of urine testing and hair testing (Cone, 1997). As such, this approach merits evaluation for large-sample epidemiological studies and for smaller-scale intervention studies, possibly in complement with computerized adaptive testing or SMS sampling methods described in the prior section of this chapter, or in relation to experience sampling methods to be discussed in a later section.

Rapid advances in development of monoclonal and polyclonal antibodies for a variety of controlled substances have created new opportunities for development of drug exposure assays (e.g., Devine et al., 1995). There is some hope for the study of neurotransmission and second messenger systems via biochemical signals in peripheral blood cells and other peripheral body fluids (Manzo et al., 1996), which might provide insights about neuroadaptation and drug dependence. Most apparent in cancer epidemiology, occupational medicine, and genotoxicity studies, there also is a new line of biomonitoring research that involves study of DNA and mRNA changes after toxic exposures. It remains to be seen whether CYP1A1 mRNA levels, methods for DNA adduct determination in humans, alkaline single cell gel electrophoresis (the comet assay for detecting DNA strand breaks), or other genotoxicity assays will be sensitive and specific with respect to tobacco or other psychoactive drug exposures. It also remains to be seen whether these methods can distinguish time-limited versus chronic exposure as a manifestation of neuroadaptive changes (Hellman, Vaghef, Friis, & Edling, 1997; Hemminki, 1997; Manzo et al., 1996; Rumbsy, Yardley-Jones, Anderson, Phillimore, & Davies, 1996).

Finally, given our difficulty recruiting subjects in general population studies for invasive blood-drawing bioassay procedures, it is important to explore possibilities that saliva and buccal cell analyses might be adequate for exposure assays and cytogenetic studies (e.g., see Cone, 1997; Surralles et al., 1997). In the epidemiological context, our experience shows that it is relatively easy to secure participation in studies that involve no more than a light scrape of buccal cells from inside the mouth, plus self-report methods. It is far more difficult to maintain adequate general population sample response rates when blood must be drawn or urine specimens must be obtained outside the settings of clinical research centers or study offices.

Recent growth in NIDA's bench science research budget should accommodate a translation of new research findings on this front into stages of evaluation for clinical and epidemiological testing. These frontiers will become an important part of our research in the 21st century, as the growing field of molecular epidemiology intersects with the ongoing traditions of drug-dependence epidemiology.

EXPERIENCE SAMPLING METHODS AND EPIDEMIOLOGY

Starting in the 19th century, William James conducted formal studies of consciousness and refined diary methods used to record details of human experience. This tradition of research now has evolved toward what is known as the Experience Sampling Method (ESM). This method was developed primarily by Csikszentmihalyi and Larson at the University of Chicago Department of Psychology in response to a need for more accurate assessment of the subjective experience of individuals in their natural environments (Csikszentmihalyi & Larson, 1987; Larson & Csikszentmihalyi, 1983). In more recent applications, an adaptation of ESM has been described with the term Ecological Momentary Assessment (EMA). EMA can be characterized in relation to four traits: (a) phenomena are assessed as they occur; (b) assessments are dependent on careful time-sampling, (c) assessment protocols involve repeated longitudinal observations of individual subjects, and (d) assessments are made in the environment inhabited by the research subject (Stone & Shiffman, 1994).

In its current form, ESM works by having research participants carry signaling devices that prompt them to make an immediate and systematic record about their experience(s) as sampled at these randomized points in time. Thus, in contrast to many self-report interview or questionnaire methods, ESM circumvents many of the biases that can distort individuals' retrospective reports of their daily behavior and experiences. Often, ESM studies schedule 7 to 10 random signals per day over the course of 15 to 18 target hours, for a 1-week period. However, some studies have used other schedules such as four signals per day over a 3-month period.

Signaling devices used to elicit the respondents' recording behavior have ranged from electronic pagers to programmed pocket calculators to programmed wrist watches, with sound or vibration signals. Respondents are asked to reply to the signal as soon as possible. They do so by making marks on standardized experience-sample forms (ESFs), typically designed to take no more than 2 minutes to complete, but sometimes data entry is via handheld computers or data storage devices. The ESFs can include open questions about location, social context, activities, thought content, time of signal and form completion, as well as analog or Likert scales measuring a variety of dimensions of the respondent's perceived situation (e.g., affect, motivation, concentration). In many contexts, compliance with ESM is generally good. Reliability and validity have been well within acceptable ranges in a limited number of evaluations. But, as mentioned later in this chapter, there is no substantial body of experience with ESM as applied in the study of seriously involved drug users, nor to our knowledge in the study of HIV or other infectious diseases among drug users (Csikszentmihalyi & Larson, 1987).

There is no need for pioneers to demonstrate that ESM can work in the study of alcohol and drug use. This application of ESM already has been carried out, not only in early samples of adolescent drug users (Larson, Csikszentmihalyi, & Freeman, 1992), but also in samples of cases with alcohol or drug problems (Filstead, Reich, Parella, & Rossi, 1985), and seriously involved heroin users (Kaplan, 1992; Kaplan & Lambert, 1995). For example, Kaplan and the Maastricht research group in the Netherlands used ESM to characterize the amount of time spent craving heroin in relation to other activities and to examine the situational determinants of craving in dependent heroin users. They found that heroin-dependent cases spent more time in self-care and caring for the symptoms of others than in the acquisition or use of drugs. The authors contrasted these findings with reports about heroin users in the United States, where the heroin-dependent cases have been characterized as spending a disproportionate amount of time in drug-related behaviors at the expense of self-care. These important studies, however, do not answer all of the logistical and other methodological questions about using ESM with samples of injecting drug users in America nor in studies of HIV risk behaviors and progression from HIV infection to AIDS among drug users.

Several publications have outlined considerations necessary when using ESM in general (Csikszentmihalyi & Larson, 1987; Larson & Csikszentmihalyi, 1983). More recently, Kaplan and Lambert (1995) made suggestions on using ESM in drug abuse and HIV research. To offer some brief examples, they noted that:

1. a strong research alliance between participants and researchers may be particularly important when ESM is used in drug abuse and HIV research;
2. methods to safeguard confidentiality are particularly important;
3. prompt response to ESM signals is a concern (e.g., with drug dealers); and
4. illiteracy can be a problem when written cues or prompts are used to elicit responding, or when experience sampling forms are used.

It also is important to anticipate some ethical considerations that deserve more detailed scrutiny, including the possibility that the ESM signal might cue drug-seeking or drug-taking behavior.

Notwithstanding these challenges, there is a considerable information value to be gained by adapting ESM in epidemiological prospective studies of drug users, especially to strengthen and extend the information provided by self-reports at the time of a periodic assessment. Even if the ESM methods cannot be adapted readily to studies of seriously involved drug users, recently completed ESM studies (Kaplan, 1992; Kaplan & Lambert, 1995; Shiffman et al., 1996) show great potential for their application when drug dependence is less severe or not present, and with comparison samples of nondrug-using participants. Due to the focus of this chapter on self-report data about drug taking, emphasis has been given to the value of using ESM in the study of drug-taking behavior and drug-dependence issues. However, there also are clear advantages to using ESM in the study of HIV risk behaviors and AIDS and in evaluation of new medication or other intervention strategies for drug dependence. This is a methodological innovation that can help us to understand the successes and the failures of interventions at various stages of the progressions and transitions that lead toward serious drug involvement—adding to other evaluative evidence from periodic self-reports and bioassays.

ETHNOGRAPHIC FIELD METHODS AND EPIDEMIOLOGY

As reflected in our general introduction, anthropological field studies and ethnography have played important and sustained roles in the development of understanding about drug use and drug dependence. Complementing other scientific disciplines, ethnography brings formal concepts and methods to the problem of learning the diversity of human perspectives on individual and shared behavior. In shedding light on these perspectives, it has helped to advance research on the processes by which assessments and interventions work or do not work, the unanticipated features or consequences of assessments or interventions, and the results of assessments or interventions in terms of participants' lives and the environments they experience and shape.

The contributions of formal ethnographic field methods to this research field had their origins in the classic studies cited previously (e.g., Dai, 1937). These contributions have expanded over the years (e.g., see Agar, 1973, 1986; Akins & Beschner, 1980; Carlson et al., 1995; Feldman & Aldrich, 1990). Most recent, there has been a deliberate effort to build bridges between epidemiology and ethnography as part of NIDA's Community Epidemiology Work Group and AIDS research program (e.g., see Adler, 1993; Wiebel, 1988). The National AIDS Demonstration Research (NADR) Projects have demonstrated the value of ethnography and qualitative data analysis methods in research on HIV, AIDS, and drug use, including the evaluation of interventions in natural settings (e.g., see Carlson et al., 1995). To date, our own work with these methods in the context of the ALIVE study and related investigations at Hopkins have not tapped all of the strengths of ethnography and ethnographic field methods. Our research team's experiences have been limited to the use of focus groups and detailed individualized interviews as part of our interview and intervention development process (e.g., as described by Anthony et al., 1990).

By drawing on the strengths of both classic and more recent ethnographic studies (e.g., Booth, Koester, Reichardt, & Brester, 1993; Wiebel, 1993), self-report methodology can be improved. Specific concepts, principles, and methods of ethnography are used to guide individualized assessment and intervention debriefing sessions as well as focus groups. From their origins in market research, the techniques of individualized debriefing sessions and focus groups have come to be widely applied as a qualitative data collection technique within the behavioral sciences. Whether conducted with individuals or in groups, these sessions are used to inform the content and language of survey questionnaires, to examine unexplained variation or to confirm findings, to monitor the research process itself, and to cross-validate data collected by other methods.

In the context of epidemiological research with a bridge to ethnography, the question is not whether self-report methods are needed, but only how the self-report evidence will be made most strong (e.g., see Adler, 1993). One readily appreciated way to strengthen epidemiologically derived self-report data on drug experiences in the population involves the SMSS sampling approach. Namely, sequenced multi-stage sampling already has been used to select the most informative participants for additional invasive procedures or more intensive scrutiny. SMSS also can be used to select, from a large epidemiological sample, those participants who will be most informative when seeking to draw inferences about substantive ethnographic research questions. This yoking of epidemiology with ethnography yields a benefit in the form of greater understanding of responses to self-report answers in the first-stage epidemiological assessment, and in addition, there is a benefit of securing a better sample for ethnographic observation. Thompson (1997) provided a useful discussion of these benefits of improved sampling for ethnographic studies.

COGNITIVE EVALUATION METHODS

Starting about 25 years ago, there was a confluence of research in the cognitive sciences with those of survey methodology. In response to this multidisciplinary interaction, and to stimulate new interactions, several meetings were held for cognitive scientists and social survey methodologists to discuss common interests. One influential meeting was a 1-day seminar in the United Kingdom, jointly sponsored by the U.K. Social Science Research Council and the Royal Statistical Society (Moss & Goldstein, 1979). There was a subsequent lengthier advanced research seminar and follow-up meeting sponsored by the U.S. National Research Council's Committee on National Statistics (Fienberg, Loftus, & Tanur, 1985; Jabine, Straf, Tanur, & Tourangeau, 1984). In brief, the cognitive science perspectives drew on the work of Tulving and others for theoretical models of information processing and memory. These models consist of a central processor for thinking, a short-term memory corresponding to a consciousness or focus of attention

(STM), and a long-term memory corresponding to an encoded and retrievable representation of past experience and learning.

Approached from this perspective, the assessment tasks for health research are regarded somewhat differently than has been traditional for investigators trained in public opinion polls or social surveys. The distinction between cognitive science and social science research on survey methodology was at the heart of discussions during the NRC seminars in 1983 and 1984. As summarized in the final seminar report, the main distinctions can be framed succinctly:

> Survey researchers typically focus on properties of the stimulus (questions) that might affect the valid processing of information. These properties can be classified into three categories: (a) wording of the question; (b) structure of the response alternatives; and (c) context of question (e.g., other questions asked, the instructions to the respondent, the setting in which the interview is conducted). The concern here is that the meaning of the question be the same to all respondents, and, of course, be the same meaning as that intended by the investigator. We might rephrase this concern by saying that survey researchers are concerned that they are setting the same cognitive task for all of the respondents. There is relatively less attention paid to whether or not a particular cognitive task is possible for the respondent or whether it is an easy or difficult task.
>
> Cognitive researchers, however, typically focus on properties of the processing system that affect the way in which information is handled. These may also be classified into three categories: (a) encoding strategies; (b) retrieval strategies; and (c) stores (lexical, semantic, episodic or archival). Experimental cognitive research is oriented toward studying microprocesses of information processing. Survey methodological research is oriented toward studying macroprocesses of comprehension and information retrieval. (Jabine et al., 1984)

Subsequent to these influential meetings, there has been a dramatic increase in the number of studies that have applied the theories and methods of cognitive science to improvement of standardized health research and survey methodology. Recent examples include Jobe and Mingay (1989), who used cognitive evaluation methods to improve the reliability and validity of reports from elderly respondents; Jobe and Mingay (1989) who tested methods to improve the reporting of medical visits; and Dilorio, Holcombe, Belcher, and Maibach (1994) who evaluated self-reported sexually transmitted disease histories. Much of this work in the United States has been carried out as part of the work of a new laboratory for research on cognitive aspects of survey methodology created at the National Center for Health Statistics (Willis, 1997).

In large part, these studies have extended the social scientists' traditional concerns about some of the most central features of the standardized assessment:

- Question Wording, which might involve different comprehension of the same term in a standardized item (e.g., "piggy-backing" in research on drug injections), different questions on the same topic, questions that ask about general versus specific topics, and how attention is focused by the words used in the question;
- Response Categories, whether coarse or fine-grained;
- Contextual Meaning, including question order effects;
- Questions about Time (e.g., when was the last time you . . . ?); and
- Questions about Frequency (e.g., how many times have you . . . ?).

With respect to questions about frequency, the cognitive evaluation (CE) of standardized survey questions has led to some important advances in our understanding of: (a) characteristics determining ability to make frequency judgments accurately, (b) constraints hindering abilities to make frequency judgments, and (c) strategies to improve accuracy of frequency judgments. In addition, CE has clarified how respondents use what cognitive scientists sometimes term *the availability heuristic*—the extent to which frequency judgments are influenced by recent thinking or hearing about an event or having some personal involvement with an event (Bradburn & Danis, 1983).

Based on the more than 10 years of work since the NRC advanced seminar (e.g., see Jabine et al., 1984), still-relevant research directions from the perspective of cognitive sciences can be based on the following questions:

- To the extent that interpretation and memory of experience is governed by higher-level knowledge structures such as scripts, do certain interview situations evoke the structures, which subsequently determine responding to interview items?
- If such a structure or script can be identified in the context of interviewing about sensitive drug use or sexual behaviors, can recall for events be improved by having the order of the questions follow the order of the relevant script?
- What are the general strategies or heuristics used by respondents in research on HIV, AIDS, and drug use when they generate answers to questions about the frequency and recency of sensitive behaviors? Would a "think-aloud" protocol on these topics disclose similarities or differences in the strategies and heuristics used to assess one domain (e.g., drug use) versus another domain (e.g., sexual behavior) versus other domains (e.g., nutritional intake)? Can accuracy and reliability of response be promoted by suggesting specific strategies or heuristics to the respondents?
- Based on observations about part–set cueing, which involves using some members of a class of experiences in an attempt to prompt

retrieval of other members of that class, and the evidence that part–set cueing actually can reduce recall performance, what is the optimal number of examples to provide respondents when they are asked to report on sensitive behaviors such as problems and complications or symptoms associated with infectious diseases or drug use?

CONCLUSIONS AND RECOMMENDATIONS

Epidemiologists who study drug taking and drug dependence take it on the chin for their heavy reliance on self-report data about these sensitive topics. The cognitive evaluation laboratory is one avenue for achieving dramatic improvements in the quality of self-report evidence. Indeed, as argued in this chapter, for much of what drug-dependence epidemiologists wish to study, self-report methods provide the only logistically feasible source of data (e.g., age at first opportunity to try a drug; a subjectively felt compulsion to smoke ice). We have no alternative but to seek better self-report methods.

In addition to the fact that much of our subject matter now must be measured by self-report, there are two other reasons for a heavy reliance on self-report methods in epidemiology:

1. Epidemiologists work hard to secure broadly representative population samples, less subject to known and suspected distortions that suffuse evidence based on treatment-seeking patients, arrestees, or volunteers solicited via advertising campaigns or chain-referral methods.

2. Large samples are required for much epidemiological research. As a society, we have marshaled resources and capability to draw locally or nationally representative samples of literally tens of thousands of Americans and to launch successful recruitment efforts to secure participation of 80% or more of the designated respondents. Costs will skyrocket and participation rates will plummet if burdens of participation are changed to replace self-report methods with either bioassays, ethnographic observations of behavior, or experience-sampling methods.

For this reason, this chapter has stressed how epidemiologists can use SMSS methods to draw the best subsamples for more invasive, more intensive, and ultimately more informative scrutiny. Looking to other branches of epidemiology (e.g., dementia, cancer), drug-dependence researchers will find many examples of sequenced two-stage and multistage sampling plans. In these other branches of epidemiology, there is pertinent experience about how to recruit successfully for these more intensive assessment protocols (e.g., with bioassays), and also how to use the first-stage information in order to probe whether and how nonparticipation might have distorted the evidence.

The current situation in drug-dependence research is clear: Epidemiologists have the best achievable population samples but lack measurement methods with the best possible resolving power; other scientists have measurements with more resolving power, but they generally take these measurements on catch-as-catch-can samples of study participants. SMSS designs provide a bridge between these drug dependence research groups and laboratories. SMSS designs give epidemiologists access to the best possible measurement methods and give the other sciences access to the best achievable samples with an opportunity to check distortions introduced when some participants at one stage of measurement will not consent to the next stage of measurement.

In the past, our research group has made the observation that much would be gained if self-report epidemiological field study assessment were made part of clinical research protocols, even when these protocols actually have better measurements. That is, if the clinical research protocol involves superior drug exposure and drug dependence assays, then also administer the DIS or CIDI questions in order to provide the field with solid evidence about the interrelationships between the assay data and the self-report data. This recommendation would tend to strengthen our body of evidence on the self-report data.

To close this chapter, a different recommendation is made. Namely, epidemiologists should seek out opportunities to use SMSS designs in order to yoke their first-stage assessments (self-report and otherwise) with standard clinical research protocols (bioassays, ESM), as well as ethnographic research protocols that would be crushed if the sample size ran to the thousands. In this fashion, we can marry the best of epidemiology with the best of the other scientific disciplines that can contribute evidence about drug dependence and its borderlands.

ACKNOWLEDGMENTS

This chapter is a reworking and extension of material written as part of an assessment core segment of a center proposal for research on drug-taking, HIV/AIDS, and other infectious diseases. Final preparation of the chapter for this volume was supported in part by active NIDA research grant awards for which the author is Principal Investigator (R01DA10502, R01DA09897). Thanks to Marsha Rosenberg and Carolyn Furr, who provided library and bibliographic research assistance.

REFERENCES

Adler, P. A. (1993). Ethnography and epidemiology: Building bridges. In *National Institute on Drug Abuse. Epidemiologic trends in drug abuse* (NIH Publication No. 93-3645, pp. 531–543). Rockville, MD: National Institute on Drug Abuse.

Agar, M. (1973). *Ripping and running: A formal ethnography of urban heroin users.* New York: Academic Press.

Agar, M. (1986). *Speaking of ethnography.* Newbury Park, CA: Sage.

Akins, C., & Beschner, G. (Eds.). (1980). *Ethnography: A research tool for policymakers in the drug and alcohol fields.* DHHS Pub. No. (ADM)80-946. Washington, DC: U.S. Government Printing Office.

Anthony, J. C., Folstein, M. F., Romanoski, A. J., VonKorff, M. R., Nestadt, G. R., Chahal, R., Brown, C. H., Shapiro, S., Kramer, M., et al. (1985). Comparison of the lay Diagnostic Interview Schedule and a standardized psychiatric diagnosis: Experience in Eastern Baltimore. *Arch Gen Psychiatry, 42,* 667–675.

Anthony, J. C., & Helzer, J. E. (1991). Syndromes of drug abuse and dependence. In L. N. Robins & D. A. Regier (Eds.), *Psychiatric disorders in America: The Epidemiologic Catchment Area Study* (pp. 116–154). New York: The Free Press.

Anthony, J. C., Vlahov, D., Nelson, K. E., Cohn, S., Astemborski, J., & Solomon, L. (1990). New evidence on intravenous cocaine use and the risk of infection with human immunodeficiency virus type 1. *American Journal of Epidemiology, 134,* 1175–1189.

Anthony, J. C., Warner, L. A., & Kessler, R. C. (1994). Comparative epidemiology of dependence on tobacco, alcohol, controlled substances, and inhalants: Basic findings from the National Comorbidity Survey. *Experimental & Clinical Psychopharmacology 2,* 244–268.

Ball, J. C., & Chambers, C. D. (1970). *The epidemiology of opiate addiction in the United States.* Springfield, IL: Thomas.

Ball, J. C., Shaffer, J. W., & Nurco, D. N. (1983). The day-to-day criminality of heroin addicts in Baltimore—A study in the continuity of offence rates. *Drug and Alcohol Dependence, 12,* 119–142.

Becker, H. (1963). *Outsiders: Studies in the sociology of deviance.* New York: The Free Press.

Booth, R., Koester, S., Reichardt, C., & Brester, T. (1993). Qualitative and quantitative methods to assess behavioral change among injection drug users. In D. Fisher & R. Needle (Eds.), *AIDS and community-based drug intervention programs.* New York: Haworth.

Bost, R. O. (1993). Hair analysis—Perspectives and limits of a proposed forensic method of proof: A review. *Forensic Science International, 63,* 31–42.

Bradburn, N., & Danis, C. (1983). Potential contributions of cognitive sciences to survey questionnaire design [Appendix A]. In T. B. Jabine, M. L. Straf, J. M. Tanur, & R. Tourangeau (Eds.), *Cognitive aspects of survey methodology: Building a bridge between disciplines.* Washington, D.C.: National Academy Press.

Burns, M., & Baselt, R. C. (1995). Monitoring drug use with a sweat patch: An experiment with cocaine. *Journal of Analytical Toxicology, 19,* 41–48.

Cantril, H. (1944). *Gauging public opinion.* Princeton, NJ: Princeton University Press.

Carlson, R. G., Harvey, A. S., & Falck, R. S. (1995). Qualitative research methods in drug abuse and AIDS prevention research: An overview. In E. Y. Lambert, R. S. Ashery, & R. H. Needle (Eds.), *Qualitative methods in drug abuse and HIV research* (DHHS Publication No. 95-4025). Rockville, MD: National Institute on Drug Abuse.

Chein, I., Gerard, D. L., Lee, R. S., & Rosenfeld, E. (1964). *The road to H.* New York: Basic Books.

Clogg, C. C. (1979). Some latent structure models for the analysis of Likert-type data. *Social Science Research, 8,* 287–301.

Cone, E. J. (1997). New developments in biological measures of drug prevalence. In L. Harrison & H. Hughes (Eds.), *The validity of self-reported drug use: Improving the accuracy of survey estimates* (NIH Publication No. 97-4147, pp. 108–129). Rockville, MD: U.S. Department of Health and Human Services.

Cone, E. J., Darwin, W. D., & Wang, W-L. (1993). The occurrence of cocaine, heroin and metabolites in hair of drug abusers. *Forensic Science International, 63,* 55–68.

Cone, E. J., Hillsgrove, M. J., Jenkins, A. J., Keenan, R. M., & Darwin, W. D. (1994). Sweat testing for heroin, cocaine, and metabolites. *Journal of Analytical Toxicology, 18,* 298–305.

Converse, J. M., & Presser, S. (1986). *Survey questions: Handcrafting the standardized questionnaire.* Newbury Park, CA: Sage.

Cottler, L. B., Grant, B. F., Blaine, J., Mavreas, V., Pull, C., Hasin, D., Compton, W. M., Rubio-Stipec, M., & Mager, D. (1997). Concordance of DSM-IV alcohol and drug use disorder criteria and diagnoses as measured by AUDADIS-ADR, CIDI and SCAN. *Drug and Alcohol Dependence, 47*(3), 195–205.

Csikszentmihalyi, M., & Larson, R. (1987). Validity and reliability of the experience sample method. *Journal of Nervous and Mental Disease, 175,* 526–536.

Dai, B. (1970). *Opium addiction in Chicago.* Montclair, NJ: Patterson Smith. (Original work published 1937)

Devine, P. J., Anis, N. A., Wright, J., Kim, S., Eldefrawi, A. T., & Eldefrawi, M. E. (1995). A fiber-optic cocaine biosensor. *Analytical Biochemistry, 227,* 216–224.

DiIorio, C., Holcombe, J., Belcher, L., & Maibach, E. (1994). Use of the cognitive assessment method to evaluate the adequacy of sexually transmitted disease history questions. *Journal of Nursing Measurement, 2,* 107–116.

Dupont, R. L., & Baumgartner, V. A. (1995). Drug testing by urine and hair analysis: Complementary features and scientific issues. *Forensic Science International, 70,* 63–76.

Ensminger, M. E., Anthony, J. C., & McCord, J. (1997). The inner city and drug use: Initial findings from an epidemiological study. *Drug and Alcohol Dependence, 48,* 175–184.

Erdman, H., Klein, M. H., & Greist, J. H. (1983). The reliability of a computer interview for drug use/abuse information. *Behavior Research Methods and Instrumentation, 15,* 66–68.

Feldman, H. W., & Aldrich, M. R. (1990). The role of ethnography in substance abuse research and public policy: Historical precedent and future prospects. *NIDA Research Monograph, 98,* 12–30.

Fendrich, M., Mackesy-Amiti, M. E., Wislar, J. S., & Goldstein, P. (1997). The reliability and consistency of drug reporting in ethnographic samples. In L. Harrison & H. Hughes (Eds.), *The validity of self-reported drug use: Improving the accuracy of survey estimates* (NIH Publication No. 97-4147, pp. 81–107). Rockville, MD: U.S. Department of Health and Human Services.

Fienberg, S. E., Loftus, E. F., & Tanur, J. M. (1985). Cognitive aspects of health survey methodology: An overview. *Milbank Memorial Fund Quarterly. Health and Society, 63,* 547–64.

Filstead, W., Reich, W., Parella, D., & Rossi, J. (1985). *Using electronic pagers to monitor the process of recovery in alcoholics and drug abusers.* Paper presented at the 34th International Congress on Alcohol, Drug Abuse and Tobacco, Calgary, Alberta, Canada.

Goldberg, D. P. (1972). The detection of psychiatric illness by questionnaire (Maudsley Monograph No. 21). London: University Press.

Goodman, L. A. (1978). *Analyzing qualitative/categorical data: Log-linear models and latent structure analysis.* Cambridge, MA: Abt books.

Green, B. F. (1988). Construct validity of computer-based tests. In H. Wainer & H. I. Braun (Eds.), *Test validity* (pp. 77–86). Hillsdale, NJ: Lawrence Erlbaum Associates.

Greenfield, L., Bigelow, G. E., & Brooner, R. K. (1995). Validity of intravenous drug abusers' self-reported changes in HIV high-risk drug use behaviors. *Drug and Alcohol Dependence, 39,* 91–98.

Griest, J. H., Klein, M. H., Erdman, H. P., Bires, J. K., Bass, S. M., Machtinger, P. E., & Kresge, D. G. (1987). Comparison of computer- and interviewer-administered versions of the Diagnostic Interview Schedule. *Hospital and Community Psychiatry, 38,* 1304–1311.

Gropper, B. A. (1995). Historical overview: Research and development on drug testing by hair analysis. In E. J. Cone, M. J. Welch, & M. B. G. Babecki (Eds.), *Hair testing for drugs of abuse: International research on standards and technology* (NIH Publication No. 95-3727, pp. 7–18). Rockville, MD: U.S. Department of Health and Human Services.

Hellman, B., Vaghef, H., Friis, L., & Edling, C. (1997). Alkaline single cell gel electrophoresis of DNA fragments in biomonitoring for genotoxicity: An introductory study on healthy human volunteers. *International Archives of Occupational & Environmental Health, 69*(3), 185–192.

Hemminki, K. (1997). DNA adducts and mutations in occupational and environmental biomonitoring. *Environmental Health Perspectives, 105*, 823–827.

Henderson, G. L., & Wilson, B. K. (1973). Excretion of methadone and metabolites in human sweat. Research Communication in Chemistry. *Pathology and Pharmacology, 5*, 1–8.

Hill, H. E., Haertzen, C. A., Wolbach, A. B., Jr., & Miner, E. J. (1963). The Addiction Research Center Inventory: Standardization of scales which evaluate subjective effects of morphine, amphetamine, pentobarbital, alcohol, LSD-25, pyrahexyl and chlorpromazine. *Psychopharmacologia, 4*, 167–183.

Holden, C. (1990). Hairy problems for a new drug testing method. *Science, 249*, 1099–1100.

Hser, Y-I. (1997). Self-reported drug use: Results of selected empirical investigations of validity. In L. Harrison & H. Hughes (Eds.), *The Validity of self-reported drug use: Improving the accuracy of survey estimates* (NIH Publication No. 97-4147, pp. 320–343). Rockville, MD: U.S. Department of Health and Human Services.

Hyman, H., Cobb, W. J., et al. (1954). *Interviewing in social research.* Chicago: University of Chicago Press.

Jabine T. B., Straf, M. L., Tanur, J. M., & Tourangeau, R. (Eds.). (1984). *Cognitive aspects of survey methodology: Building a bridge between disciplines.* Washington, DC: National Academy Press.

Jobe, J. B., & Mingay, D. J. (1989). Cognitive research improves questionnaires. *American Journal of Public Health, 79*, 1053–1055.

Johanson C. E., Duffy F. F., & Anthony J. C. (1996). Associations between drug use and behavioral repertoire in urban youths. *Addiction, 91*(4), 523–534.

Johnston L. D., & O'Malley, P. M. (1997). The recanting of earlier reported drug use by young adults. In L. Harrison & H. Hughes (Eds.), *The validity of self-reported drug use: Improving the accuracy of survey estimates* (NIH Publication No. 97-4147, pp. 59–80). Rockville, MD: U.S. Department of Health and Human Services.

Kandel, D., Grant, B., Kessler, R. C., Warner, L. A., & Chen, K. (1997). Prevalence and demographic correlates of symptoms of last year dependence on alcohol, nicotine, marijuana and cocaine in the U.S. population. *Drug and Alcohol Dependence, 44*(1), 11–29.

Kaplan, C. D. (1992). Drug craving and drug use in the daily life of heroin addicts. In M. W. DeVries (Ed.), *The experience of psychopathology: Investigating mental disorders in their natural settings* (pp. 193–218). Cambridge, England: Cambridge University Press.

Kaplan, C. D., & Lambert, E. Y. (1995). The daily life of heroin-addicted persons: The biography of specific methodology. *NIDA Research Monograph, 157*, 100–116.

Kidwell, D. A., & Blank, D. L. (1995). Mechanisms of incorporation of drugs into hair and the interpretation of hair analysis data. In E. J. Cone, M. J. Welch, & M. B. G. Babecki (Eds.), *Hair testing for drugs of abuse: International research on standards and technology* (NIH Publication No. 95-3727, pp. 19–90). Rockville, MD: U.S. Department of Health and Human Services.

Kolb, L. (1925). Types and characteristics of drug addicts. *Mental Hygiene, 9*, 300–313.

Larson, R., & Csikszentmihalyi, M. (1983). The experience sampling method. *New Directions for Methodology of Social & Behavioral Science, 15*, 41–56.

Larson, R., Csikszentmihalyi, M., & Freeman, M. (1992). Alcohol and marijuana use in adolescents' daily lives. In M. V. deVries (Ed.), *The experience of psychopathology: Investigating mental disorders in their natural settings* (pp. 180–192). Cambridge, England: Cambridge University Press.

Latkin, C. A., Vlahov, D., & Anthony, J. C. (1993). Socially desirable responding and self-reported HIV infection risk behaviors among intravenous drug users. *Addiction, 88*, 517–526.

Lazarsfeld, P. F., & Henry, N. W. (1968). *Latent structure analysis*. Boston: Houghton-Mifflin.

Lessler, J. T., & O'Reilly, J. M. (1997). Mode of interview and reporting of sensitive issues: Design and implementation of audio computer-assisted self-interviewing. *NIDA Research Monograph, 167*, 366–382.

Lindesmith, A. R. (1947). *Opiate addiction*. Bloomington, IN: Principia Press.

Lyles, C. M., Margolick, J. B., Astemborski, J., Graham, N., Anthony, J. C., Hoover, D., & Vlahov, D. (1997). The influence of drug use patterns on the rate of CD4+ lymphocyte decline among HIV-1-infected injecting drug users. *AIDS, 11*, 1255–1262.

Magura, S., Freeman, R. C., Siddiqi, Q., & Lipton, D. S. (1992). The validity of hair analysis for detecting cocaine and heroin use among addicts. *International Journal of the Addictions, 27*, 51–69.

Magura, S., & Kang, S. Y. (1997). The validity of self-reported cocaine use in two high-risk populations. *NIDA Research Monograph, 167*, 227–246.

Manzo, L., Artigas, F., Martinez, E., Mutti, A,. Bergamaschi, E., Nicotera, P., Tonini, M., Candura, S. M., Ray, D. E., & Costa, L. G. (1996). Biochemical markers of neurotoxicity. A review of mechanistic studies and applications. *Human & Experimental Toxicology, 15*, S20–S35.

McBay, A. J. (1995). Comparison of urine and hair testing for drugs of abuse. *Journal of Analytical Toxicology, 19*, 201–202.

Moss, L., & Goldstein, H. (Eds.). (1979). *The recall method in social surveys*. London: NFER Publishing.

Nurco, D. N., Hanlon, T. E., Balter, M. B., Kinlock, T. W., et al. (1991). A classification of narcotic addicts based on type, amount, and severity of crime. *Journal of Drug Issues, 21*, 429–448.

Paulhus, D. L. (1984). Two-component models of socially desirable responding. *Journal of Personality and Social Psychology, 46*, 598–609.

Payne, S. L. (1951). *The art of asking questions*. Princeton, NJ: Princeton University Press.

Pescor, M. J. (1939). The Kolb classification of drug addicts. *Public Health Reports, 155*(10).

Preston, K., Silverman, C., Schuster, C., & Cone, E. (1996). Improving outcome measures. II Application of urine drug testing rules in a cocaine trial. *NIDA Research Monograph, 162*, 144.

Preston K. L., Silverman, K., Schuster, C. R., & Cone, E. J. (1997). In L. Harrison & H. Hughes (Eds.), *The validity of self-reported drug use: Improving the accuracy of survey estimates* (NIH Publication No. 97-4147, pp. 130–145). Rockville, MD: U.S. Department of Health and Human Services.

Robins, L. N. (1966). *Deviant children grown up*. Baltimore: Williams & Wilkins.

Robins, L. N., Helzer, J. C., Orvaschel, H., et al. (1985). The Diagnostic Interview Schedule. In W. W. Eaton & L. G. Kessler (Eds.), *Epidemiologic field methods in psychiatry: The NIMH Epidemiologic Catchment Area Program*. New York: Academic Press.

Rosanoff, A. J. (1917). Survey of mental disorders: In Nassau County, NY. *Psychological Bulletin, 2*, 105–231.

Rumsby, P. C., Yardley-Jones, A., Anderson, D., Phillimore, H. E., & Davies, M. J. (1996). Detection of CYP1A1 mRNA levels and CYP1A1 Msp polymorphisms as possible biomarkers of exposure and susceptibility in smokers and non-smokers. *Teratogenesis, Carcinogenesis, & Mutagenesis, 16*(1), 65–74.

Schuman, H., & Presser, S. (1981). *Questions and answers in attitude surveys: Experiments on question form, wording, and context*. New York: Academic Press.

Shiffman, S., Paty, J. A., Gnys, M., Kassle, J. A., & Hickcox, M. (1996). First lapses in smoking: Within-subjects analysis of real-time reports. *Journal of Consulting and Clinical Psychology, 64*, 366–379.

Skinner, H. A., & Allen, B. (1983). Does the computer make a difference? Computerized versus face-to-face versus self-report assessment of alcohol, drug, and tobacco use. *Journal of Consulting and Clinical Psychology, 51*, 267–275.

Smith, F. P., & Liu, R. H. (1986). Detection of cocaine metabolite in persperation stain, menstrual bloodstain, and hair. *Journal of Forensic Sciences, 31*, 1269–1273.

Sonnedecker, G. (1962). Emergence of the concept of opiate addiction. *Journal Mondial de Pharmacie, 3*, 286–287.

Spiehler, V., Fay, J., Fogerson, R., Schoendorfer, D., & Niedbala, R. S. (1996). Enzyme immunoassay validation for qualitative detection of cocaine in sweat. *Clinical Chemistry, 42*, 34–38.

Star, S. A. (1950). The screening of psychoneurotics: Comparison of psychiatric diagnoses and test scores at all induction stations. In S. A. Stouffer, L. Guttman, & E. A. Suchman (Eds.), *Measurement and prediction.* Princeton, NJ: Princeton University Press.

Stone, A. A., & Shiffman, S. (1994). Ecological momentary assessment (EMA) in behavioral medicine. *Annals of Behavioral Medicine, 16*, 199–202.

Suchman, E. A., Phillips, B. S., & Streib, G. F. (1958). An analysis of the validity of health questions. *Social Forces, 36*, 223–232.

Sudman, S., & Bradburn, N. M. (1982). *Asking questions.* San Francisco, CA: Jossey-Bass.

Surralles, J., Autio, K., Nylund, L., Jarventaus, H., Norppa, H., Veidebaum, T., Sorsa, M., & Peltonen, K. (1997). Molecular cytogenetic analysis of buccal cells and lymphocytes from benzene-exposed workers. *Carcinogenesis, 18*(4), 817–823.

Suzuki, S-I., Inoue, T., Hori, H., & Inayama, S. (1994). Analysis of methamphetamine in hair, nail, sweat, and saliva by mass fragmentography. *Journal of Analytical Toxicology, 18*, 298–305.

Thompson, S. K. (1997). Adaptive sampling in behavioral surveys. In L. Harrison & H. Hughes (Eds.), *The validity of self-reported drug use: Improving the accuracy of survey estimates* (NIH Publication No. 97-4147, pp. 296–319). Rockville, MD: U.S. Department of Health and Human Services.

Turner, C. F., Lessler, J. T., & Groeferer, J. C. (Eds.). (1992). *Survey measurement of drug use.* DHHS Publication No. (ADM) 92-1929. Washington, DC: U.S. Government Printing Office.

Van Etten, M. L., Neumark, Y. D., & Anthony, J. C. (1997). Initial opportunity to use marijuana and the transition to first use: United States, 1979–1994. *Drug and Alcohol Dependence, 49*(1), 1–7.

Vlahov, D., Anthony, J. C., Munoz, A., Margolick, J., Nelson, K. E., Celentano, D. D., Solomon, L., & Polk, B. F. (1991). The ALIVE study, a longitudinal study of HIV-1 infection in intravenous drug users: description of methods and characteristics of participants. *NIDA Research Monograph, 109*, 75–100.

Wiebel, W. W. (1988). Combining ethnographic and epidemiologic methods for targeted AIDS interventions. In R. J. Battjes & R. W. Pickens (Eds.), *Needle-sharing among intravenous drug abuses. NIDA Research Monograph 98*, DHHS Publication No. (ADM)88-1567.

Wiebel, W. W. (1993). *The indigenous leader outreach model: Intervention manual* (DHHS Publication No. 93-3581). Rockville, MD: National Institute on Drug Abuse.

Weisband, S., & Kiesler, S. (1996, April). *Self disclosure on computer forms: Meta-analysis and implications.* Paper presented at Conference on Human Factors in Computing Systems, Vancouver, British Columbia.

Willis, G. B. (1997). The use of the psychological laboratory to study sensitive survey topics. In L. Harrison & H. Hughes (Eds.), *The validity of self-reported drug use: Improving the accuracy of survey estimates* (NIH Publication No. 97-4147, pp. 416–438). Rockville, MD: U.S. Department of Health and Human Services.

Wines, F. H. (1888). *Report on the defective, dependent, and delinquent classes of the population of the United States as returned at the Tenth Census (June 1, 1880).* Washington, DC: Government Printing Office.

V

SELF-REPORT OF
DISTANT MEMORIES

Jaylan S. Turkkan
The National Institute on Drug Abuse,
The National Institutes of Health

Consider the difficulty of determining whether your friend or loved one has accurately described his or her past traumatic experiences. After all, these are persons for whom you have a framework for interpreting their answers based on your knowledge of their other behavior. The difficulty is multiply compounded for behavioral and social scientists who have no outside knowledge of research volunteers and must rely on what they say in research settings fraught with anxiety and distrust around extremely sensitive matters. In many cases, the answers to such sensitive questions have a direct bearing on the well-being, indeed, freedom, of others who may be implicated in the traumatic experiences. Nowhere has this issue been brought more into focus and hence controversy than memories of childhood abuse. Chapters by Elizabeth Loftus and Linda Williams and her colleagues are testimony to the complexities surrounding any situation in which volunteers are asked about their past. If you repeatedly and strongly urge and guide the volunteer to answer, do you encourage confabulation and manufacture of answers, or do you get closer to the truth? It must be emphasized that when research volunteers—whether children or adults—are strongly urged to respond, they will respond with *something*. Whether that something is true or not is the special research province of Loftus and Williams. Loftus' chapter describes the conditions under which research volunteers come to report having experienced events that never occurred. Williams and her colleagues are determining the conditions under which subjects fail to report events that did occur. The current controversy will be much benefitted from rigorous research approaches such as these.

12

Suggestion, Imagination, and the Transformation of Reality

Elizabeth F. Loftus
University of Washington

When people answer questions about the past, they obviously can be quite accurate in their recounting, but sometimes they are quite inaccurate. They fail to remember things that, if accuracy and completeness are desirable, should be reported. And they sometimes remember and report things that did not happen.

One of the ways in which people can be led to remember something that did not happen is when they are provided with misinformation about the past. The misinformation studies can be traced back to the early 1970s. These studies repeatedly showed that when people witness an event and are later exposed to new and misleading information about that event, their recollections often become distorted. The misinformation can sometimes invade a person's mind, like a Trojan horse, precisely because the person does not detect its influence.

The kinds of studies that investigators have conducted to show how memory can become skewed when people are fed misinformation utilize a simple procedure. Subjects first see a complex event, such as a simulated automobile accident. Next, half of the subjects receive misleading information about the accident while the others get no misinformation. Finally, all subjects try to remember the original accident. In one actual study using this paradigm, subjects saw an accident and later some of them received misinformation about the traffic sign used to control traffic. The misled subjects got the false suggestion that the stop sign that they had actually seen was a yield sign. When asked later what kind of traffic sign they remembered seeing at the intersection, those who had been given the false suggestion tended to adopt it as their memory and claimed that they had seen a yield sign. Those who had not received the phony information had more accurate memories.

Literally hundreds of experiments have now been published documenting memory distortion induced by exposure to misinformation (see Ayers & Reder, 1998, for a useful summary of this line of research). In these studies, people have recalled not only stop signs as yield signs, but they have also recalled nonexistent broken glass and tape recorders, a blue vehicle used in a crime as white, Minnie Mouse when they really saw Mickey Mouse, and even something as large and conspicuous as a barn in a country setting that happened to have no buildings. Taken together, these studies show that misinformation can change an individual's recollection in predictable, and sometimes very powerful, ways. Misinformation has the potential for invading our memories when we talk to other people, when we are interrogated in a suggestive fashion, or when we see biased media coverage about some event that we may have experienced ourselves. After more than two decades exploring the power of misinformation, we have learned a great deal about the conditions that make people especially susceptible to its damaging influence. We have learned, for example, that memories are more easily modified when the passage of time allows the original memory to fade. Those faded, weakened memories—like disease-ridden bodies—become particularly vulnerable to infection from outside contamination. One misinformation takes hold, many subjects appear to genuinely believe in the created memories. Psychophysiological measures designed to detect deception cannot even penetrate their new truth (Amato-Henderson, 1996).

Later studies extending the misinformation effect showed that people can be led to develop entirely false memories for things that never happened (see Loftus, 1997, for a summary of this research). A common method of planting false memories was to enlist the help of a relative of the subject who essentially said, "I saw this happen." Using this type of methodology, people have been led to believe and remember that they were lost in a shopping mall for an extended time at age 5 (Loftus & Pickrell, 1995), that they were hospitalized for a probable ear infection as a young child (Hyman, Husband, & Billings, 1995), that they knocked over a punch bowl at a family wedding (Hyman & Pentland, 1996), that they got their hand caught in a mousetrap and had to go to the hospital to get it removed or fell off a tricycle and had to get stitches in their leg (Ceci, Huffman, Smith, & Loftus 1994; Ceci, Loftus, Leichtman, & Bruck, 1994). Many of these created memories are about personal experiences that, had they happened, would have been at least mildly traumatic when they occurred.

HOW FALSE MEMORIES COME ABOUT

As the number of independent investigations of false memory creation grow, there is an increased understanding of how it is that adults create false memories of complete, emotional, and self-participatory experiences. In the lost-in-the-mall type of study, implantation occurs when another individual, usually a family member, claims to have seen the event happen. This can be a powerful suggestive technique. In fact, false claims to have seen a subject do something have even led to false confessions to wrongdoing. This was shown in one study that explored the reactions of individuals who were accused of damaging a computer by pressing the wrong key (Kassin & Kiechel, 1996). These innocent subjects initially denied the charge, but when a confederate then said that she saw the subject behave incorrectly, many subjects signed a confession, internalized guilt for the act, and went on to confabulate details that were consistent with that belief. These findings show powerfully that false incriminating evidence can lead people to accept guilt for a crime they did not commit and even to develop memories to go along with their new-found beliefs.

False memory creation is a constructive enterprise that combines personal knowledge about the past with the content of the suggestions received from others. During this constructive process, individuals face a difficult source-monitoring task as they struggle to decide whether their constructed memory is the product of genuine memory or whether it arises from suggestion or some other process. In the studies on false memory creation, several ingredients have been identified. First, there are social demands to remember. The researchers exert some pressure on the subjects to come up with memories. Second, memory construction is sometimes explicitly encouraged when people are having trouble remembering. And finally, subjects are often discouraged from explicitly monitoring whether their constructions are real or not. Memory creations are most likely when these ingredients are present, whether this occurs in an experimental setting, in a therapeutic setting, or in other common life activities. If respondents have acquired false memories by these means, they may report those memories to others who inquire into their past.

IMAGINATION AS SUGGESTION

Strong suggestions that mislead people about their past can occur when one individual deliberately or unwittingly influences another individual. Although these may not occur all that often, more subtle interventions can also mislead people about the past. One of those involves the sheer act of imagination.

It is commonplace for people to have the experience of confusing whether they actually did something or whether they only imagined doing that thing. In fact, "Did I Do It or Did I Only Imagine Doing It?" was the title of a provocative publication by Anderson published in 1984. In several studies, subjects traced a line drawing that was given to them, or they imagined tracing it. When tested later, subjects thought that they actually traced an item that they had only imagined tracing sufficiently often that the investigator was prompted to conclude that, "Memories of doing are readily confused with memories of imagining doing" (p. 609).

Would confusions between imaginations and memory occur in more complex settings? We know that imagination exercises are used in a variety of unusual settings. People sometimes imagine themselves winning lotteries or becoming king. Therapists sometimes ask their patients to imagine a counterfactual past. Police interrogators sometimes ask suspects who deny committing crimes to imagine someone doing it. Is it possible that such imaginations, like line tracings, could later be confused with reality? Several paradigms have recently been used to investigate this question, and they have led to the conclusion that imagination can affect memory. It can sometimes lead people to have memories for things that never happened—things that never happened in their recent past and things that never happened in their childhood.

IMAGINING CHILDHOOD EVENTS

To explore what happens to memory when people imagine events that did not occur, one study used a three-stage procedure (Garry, Manning, Loftus, & Sherman, 1996). Subjects were first asked about 40 possible events from their childhood, and they indicated the likelihood that these events happened to them on a scale of responses ranging from definitely did not happen to definitely did happen. Two weeks later, the subjects were asked to imagine that they had experienced some of these events. The events included falling and breaking a window with their hand, getting in trouble for calling 911, finding a $10 bill in a parking lot, or being pulled out of the water by a lifeguard. Different subjects were asked to imagine different events.

Consider a typical 1-minute imagination exercise, one in which subjects imagined breaking a window with their hand. They were told to picture it was after school and they were playing in the house when they heard a strange noise outside. They were told to imagine themselves running toward the window, tripping, falling, reaching out, and breaking a window with their hand. While imagining the scene, the subjects were asked several questions, such as, "What did you trip on?" and, "How did you feel?" After imagining several situations, the subjects again, some time later, were given the list of 40 childhood events to respond to.

Comparing the responses to the two questionnaires about possible child-hood experiences, it was found that a 1-minute act of imagination led a significant minority of subjects to say an event was more likely to have happened after previously identifying it as unlikely to have occurred. In the broken window scenario, 24% of the subjects who imagined the event showed an increase in confidence that the event had actually happened. For those subjects who did not imagine breaking the window, 12% showed a corresponding increase. In the "got in trouble for calling 911" scenario, 20% of the subjects who imagined the event showed an increase in confidence that the event had occurred to them as a child. For those subjects who did not imagine getting in trouble for calling 911, only 11% showed a correspond-ing increase.

Across the eight events that some subjects were asked to imagine, the researchers found that there was more positive change in the imagined scenarios, 34%, than in the nonimagined ones, 25%. There are a number of possible explanations for this imagination inflation, or why imagining an event led some people to change their minds about the likelihood of a fictitious event actually having happened. One reason is that an act of imagination simply made the event seem more familiar when the second assessment was made and that familiarity was mistakenly related to child-hood memories, rather than to the act of imagination.

Of course, it is also possible that the act of imagination reminded subjects of a true experience that they had. If this had happened, you might have expected to see many instances in which subjects initially gave a low score indicating the event probably had not happened to them, but the second time jumped to a high score, indicating that the event definitely did happen to them. Such big jumps were relatively rare and when removed from the analysis, did not change the conclusions. Still, it might be nice to have stronger evidence that the initial event did not happen in the first place so the power of imagination could more confidently be connected to the con-struction of a false memory rather than the elicitation of a true one. Such evidence can be found in a different paradigm in which subjects were asked to imagine recent experiences rather than childhood ones.

IMAGINING RECENT EXPERIENCES

Imagination can also make people believe that they have done things in the recent past that they did not in fact do. This was shown in a pair of studies by Goff and Roediger that involved multiple sessions (Goff, 1996; Goff & Roediger, 1996). During the initial encoding session, subjects listened to a list of action statements as they were read aloud. For each statement, subjects were instructed to do the stated action, to imagine doing it, or simply to listen to the statement but do nothing else. The actions were simple ones such as: knock on the table, lift the stapler, break the toothpick, cross your fingers, roll your eyes. During a second imagination session, subjects had to imagine various actions. Finally during a test session, they had to answer questions about what they actually did during the initial session. The investigators found that, after imagination, subjects sometimes claimed that they had actually performed an action on the first occasion when they had not. The more times they imagined an unperformed action, the more often they made this mistake. So, for example, in one study, after five imaginings, subjects claimed they had performed a nonperformed action 13% of the time.

Why do people think they did something that they only imagined? The answer cannot be that imagination reminded them of a true event that they actually did because the investigators had recorded exactly what the subject did and did not do. In this paradigm, subjects were clearly remembering events that did not happen. The investigators offered a number of possible explanations for these findings. Perhaps imagining an action many times makes the statement itself seem very familiar, and subjects may think it was familiar because it occurred during the first session even if they do not actually remember performing that action.

Of course, familiarity is not the total answer here. Another finding from this research was that when the imagination session was very close to the test session, as opposed to separated by a week, subjects were not as likely to claim that imagined experiences were previously performed. Presumably if subjects were trying to make a source monitoring judgment (did I do it or did I just imagine doing it?), they would have an easier time knowing that they imagined it if the imaginations had very recently been performed. They could readily attribute any experienced familiarity to the recent imagination rather than to a real experience from weeks earlier.

DIARY STUDIES

One might be tempted to dismiss the finding that people can be led to falsely remember having recently broken a toothpick after imagining it because of the relative artificiality of the paradigm. After all, a subject who experiences a huge array of mini-events in an experimental laboratory and later misre-members some imagined mini-events as if they were part of that huge array is a far cry from showing that imagination can influence your own personal autobiography. A very different paradigm, involving autobiographical diary recordings and rememberings, however, shows that the power of imagination to lead to false memories is far from restricted to mini-laboratory events. One such diary study worked like this: Two diarists wrote down events and thoughts from their lives over a period of 5 months (Conway, Collins, Gath-ercole, & Anderson, 1996). As they recorded these true experiences, they also recorded false events that had not occurred but could plausibly have occurred on the day of the recording. The false events, therefore, were only imagined. Some 7 months after completion of the diaries, the two individuals were tested. For items that were judged as true, the subjects indicated whether they consciously remembered the event, or, if not, whether the item simply evoked feelings of familiarity or whether there was no sense of familiarity but simply a guess.

The diarists occasionally reported their earlier imaginations as if they were real experiences. A total of 55 imagined experiences were later re-ported as real. The false memories were less likely than the true ones to be accompanied by conscious feelings of recollection, but over 40% of the false memories were of this type. A forced choice test, in which diarists had to choose between a true and false memory and say which was which, pro-duced lower false memory rates. However, it should be kept in mind that the particular diary method used in this research may overestimate the accuracy of everyday memories because the diary method is one that gives preferential rehearsal to certain true memories. Unrehearsed and randomly selected everyday events may be recalled less accurately. Setting aside the matter of how the diary results might generalize to the larger population of memories, these results were sufficiently impressive to warrant the conclu-sion: "False memories can be a common occurrence" (Conway et al., 1996, p. 93). The value of this research lies in part in its rather clever method for showing that people will sometimes erroneously accept as true, and even occasionally recollectively experience, descriptions of their past that are in fact completely false but were previously imagined.

PRACTICAL IMPLICATIONS

The 1990s brought with it tremendous controversy over the issue of repres-sion of memories of childhood trauma, particularly sexual abuse (Lindsay & Read, 1995; Loftus, 1993; Loftus & Ketcham, 1994). Some mental health professionals, even if only a minority of them, decided they needed to discover child sexual abuse in their patients' past, even when the patient had denied it. For some, the recommended method for finding that abuse began by asking the patient to imagine the abuse. In her book on sexual abuse, therapist Maltz (1991) directed her clients to:

> spend time imagining that you were sexually abused, without worry about accuracy, proving anything or having your ideas make sense. As you give rein to your imagination, let your intuition guide your thoughts. . . . Ask yourself

... these questions: What time of day is it? Where are you? Indoors or out-
doors? What kind of things are happening? Is there one or more person with
you? (pp. 50–51)

Maltz further recommended that therapists continue asking: "Who would
have been likely perpetrators? When were you most vulnerable to sexual
abuse in your life?" (pp. 50–51). In another book on surviving abuse, therapist
Dinsmore (1991) encouraged writing exercises as a way of reclaiming memory:

> I suggest that all my clients maintain journals. The journal may be used for
> free writing or for responses to specific exercises that I suggest. I may ask the
> client to write a letter to an imaginary child who is currently being sexually
> abused. This letter ... may trigger a memory from the survivor's own child-
> hood. I may ask another client to write a description of her life at age ten as
> she imagines it might have been. This, too, may trigger a memory. (p. 70)

Besides the individual therapist who recommends such imagination exercises for this purpose, there are also surveys of reputable mental health
professionals that confirm their use. In one survey, psychologists with doctoral degrees were asked about techniques that they had used with abuse
victims to help them remember sexual abuse, and 11% said they have
instructed their clients to let the imagination run wild. In another survey,
22% of psychologists had instructed their clients to "give free rein to the
imagination." (Poole, Lindsay, Memon, & Bull, 1995, p. 432). What impact
might these imagination exercises have on the client? Is it possible that
imagining an event might lead some clients to falsely believe that they had
experienced an event that they had not experienced?

The power of imagined experiences to cause people to later believe that
they had these experiences has important implications for professionals
who use self-report as a means of knowing about the past of an individual
or group of individuals. To the extent that imagined experiences are being
reported as if they were true experiences, estimates of the occurrence of
events will be inflated.

These empirical findings also raise a question about repeated interviews
with individuals. In numerous surveys, people are repeatedly interviewed
about some past activity. For example, they might be repeatedly interviewed
about their use of cigarettes, alcohol, marijuana, or other substances (O'Malley, Bachman, & Johnston, 1988). What impact does an initial interview have
on the follow-up? If some of the respondents try to answer questions by
imagining themselves in particular situations involving the use of those
substances, perhaps the imaginings could later be reported as actual experiences.

THEORETICAL IMPLICATIONS

These findings provide further examples of a truth about mental awareness. Namely, humans can be led to make source-monitoring errors of a particular kind. We have known for some time that we sometimes confuse imaginations with perceptions, at least for rather simple experiences (Johnson, Raye, Wang, & Taylor, 1979). However, the newer paradigms show us that we imaginations can even distort our autobiographies, making us believe we had a past that we did not have. With this work, we have located yet one more hole in that very thin curtain that separates imagination and memory. And perhaps, to borrow a little from Salman Rushdie, the work is telling this: Imagination is like everything else; live with it for long enough and it becomes part of the furniture of memory.

The precise mechanisms by which false memories are constructed, either via strong suggestion or imagination-like activities, awaits further research. We still have much to learn about the degree of confidence and the characteristics of false memories that are created in these ways. We have more to learn about what types of individuals are particularly susceptible to these forms of suggestion and, conversely, who is resistant. As we are learning more, it is probably important to heed the cautionary tale in the data already obtained: Mental health professionals, interviewers, and others need to know how much they can potentially influence participants in research, clinical, and forensic contexts and take care to avoid that influence when it might be harmful. Periodic re-reading of Shakespeare's *Midsummer Nights Dream* (1594/1980, Act V, Scene 1, lines 13–23, p. 251), with a small substitution (change poet to biased interviewer) might help keep these important ideas in mind, reminding us how hard it can sometimes be to distinguished a bush from an imagined bear:

> The poet's eye, in fine fanciful rolling,
> Doth glance from heaven to earth, from earth to heaven;
> And as imagination bodies forth
> The forms of things unknown, the poet's pen
> Turns them to shapes and gives to airy nothing
> A local habitation and a name.
> Such tricks hath strong imagination, that if it would but apprehend some
> joy, it comprehends some bringer of that joy;
> Or in the night, imagining some fear,
> How easy is a bush supposed a bear!

REFERENCES

Amato-Henderson, S. L. (1996). *Effects of misinformation as revealed through the concealed knowledge test.* Unpublished doctoral dissertation, University of North Dakota, Grand Forks.

Anderson, R. E. (1984). Did I do it or did I only imagine doing it? *Journal of Experimental Psychology: General, 113,* 594–613.

Ayers, M. S., & Reder, L. M. (1998). A theoretical review of the misinformation effect: Predictions from an activation-based memory model. *Psychonomic Bulletin and Review, 5*, 1–21.

Ceci, S. J., Huffman, M. L. C., Smith, E., & Loftus, E. F. (1994). Repeatedly thinking about a non-event: Source misattributions among preschoolers. *Consciousness and Cognition, 3*, 388–407.

Ceci, S. J., Loftus, E. F., Leichtman, M. D., & Bruck, M. (1994). The possible role of source misattributions in the creation of false beliefs among preschoolers. *International Journal of Clinical and Experimental Hypnosis, 42*, 304–320.

Conway, M. A., Collins, A. F., Gathercole, S. E., & Anderson, S. J. (1996). Recollections of true and false autobiographical memories. *Journal of Experimental Psychology: General, 125*, 69–95.

Dinsmore, C. (1991). *From surviving to thriving*. Albany: State University of New York Press.

Garry, M., Manning, C., Loftus, E. F., & Sherman, S. J. (1996). Imagination inflation. *Psychonomic Bulletin and Review, 3*, 208–214.

Goff, L. M. (1996). *Imagination inflation: The effects of number of imaginings on recognition and source monitoring*. Unpublished master's thesis, Rice University, Houston, TX.

Goff, L. M., & Roediger, H. L. (1996, November). *Imagination inflation: Multiple imaginings can lead to false recollection of one's actions*. Paper presented at the annual meeting of the Psychonomic Society, Chicago.

Hyman, I. E., Husband, T. H., & Billings, F. J. (1995). False memories of childhood experiences. *Applied Cognitive Psychology, 9*, 181–197.

Hyman, I. E., & Pentland, J. (1996). The role of mental imagery in the creation of false childhood memories. *Journal of Memory and Language, 35*, 101–117.

Johnson, M. K., Raye, C. L., Wang, A. Y., & Taylor, T. H. (1979). Fact and fantasy: The roles of accuracy and variability in confusing imaginations with perceptual experience. *Journal of Experimental Psychology: Human Learning and Memory, 5*, 229–240.

Kassin, S. M., & Kiechel, K. L. (1996). The social psychology of false confessions: Compliance, internalization, and confabulation. *Psychological Science, 7*, 125–128.

Lindsay, D. S., & Read, J. D. (1995). "Memory work" and recovered memories of childhood sexual abuse. *Psychology, Public Policy, & the Law, 1*, 846–907.

Loftus, E. F. (1993). The reality of repressed memories. *American Psychologist, 48*, 518–537.

Loftus, E. F. (1997, September). Creating false memories. *Scientific American, 277*, 82–87.

Loftus, E. F., & Ketcham, K. (1994). *The myth of repressed memory*. New York: St. Martin's Press.

Loftus, E. F., & Pickrell, J. (1995). The formation of false memories. *Psychiatric Annals, 25*, 720–724.

Maltz, W. (1991). *The sexual abuse healing journey*. New York: HarperCollins.

O'Malley, P. M., Bachman, J. G., & Johnston, L. D. (1988). Period, age, and cohort effects on substance use among young Americans: A decade of change, 1976–1986. *American Journal of Public Health, 78*, 1315–1321.

Poole, D. A., Lindsay, D. S., Memon, A., & Bull, R. (1995). Psychotherapy and the recovery of memories of childhood sexual abuse: US and British Practitioners' opinions, practices, and experiences. *Journal of Consulting and Clinical Psychology, 63*, 426–437.

Shakespeare, W. (1594/1980). A Midsummer night's dream. In D. Bevington (Ed.), *The complete works of Shakespeare*. London: Scott Foresman.

13

Validity of Women's Self-Reports of Documented Child Sexual Abuse

Linda M. Williams
Wellesley College

Jane A. Siegel
Widener University

Judith Jackson Pomeroy
California Lutheran University

Most of our current knowledge about the prevalence of child sexual abuse comes from studies such as those of Russell (1986), Finkelhor (1979, 1984), Kilpatrick (1992), Bagley and Ramsay (1985), and Wyatt (1985). These studies survey adults in the community and ask them to report whether they were sexually abused as a child. Based on these retrospective studies, we know that child sexual abuse is more common than was once believed: The best community surveys indicate that at least 1 in 4 girls and 1 in 6 boys are sexually abused before the age of 18.

Despite their usefulness in providing information about child sexual abuse, community studies raise questions about the validity of adult retrospective reports of childhood trauma. Although some skeptics dismiss such studies as seriously distorted overreporting resulting from women's fantasies about sexual abuse or leading questions posed by researchers, it is more likely that figures from retrospective studies underestimate the size of the problem. This underestimate may be due to lack of recall of the abuse (Williams, 1994) because some may choose not to tell about the abuse (Femina, Yeager, & Lewis, 1990), or because adults are not asked about their abuse history in a manner likely to generate an accurate report (Koss, 1993). Improved methods for the conduct of retrospective research are needed both to increase the accuracy of calculations of the prevalence of victimization and to enhance our understanding of the scope and nature of child sexual abuse. Furthermore, methodological problems associated with generating accurate reports of child sexual victimization in retrospective research have implications for our knowledge of the long-term consequences of abuse. If some adults do not disclose their abuse histories in retrospective surveys or if they disclose only a truncated account of such abuse, then comparisons made of the social and psychological functioning of victims and nonvictims may underestimate or overestimate the true effect of the abuse.

The percentage of adults who report sexual abuse in retrospective studies ranges from 6% to 62% for females and 3% to 31% for males (Finkelhor, 1994, p. 7). Some portion of this variation is no doubt attributable to the population surveyed (i.e., a "true" difference in prevalence among different populations); some is accounted for by the method used to elicit the information (e.g., self-completed questionnaire or telephone vs. face-to-face interview; Martin, Anderson, Romans, Mullen, & O'Shea, 1993; A. Urquiza, personal communication, 1993), and some may be attributable to the definition of abuse used by the investigators (Wyatt & Peters, 1986). There is some evidence, however, that the number and wording of screening questions used to elicit a history of abuse may be the most important reason for variation in estimates of the prevalence of child sexual abuse (Peters, Wyatt & Finkelhor, 1986).

Of course, most researchers have no way of knowing whether the answers they receive in response to questions about histories of abuse in childhood are true or are false negatives, because nothing is known about the respondents' past history of victimization. The longitudinal design of this research provided a unique opportunity to learn more about the effectiveness of questions used to elicit adults' reports of sexual abuse in childhood. This study has the advantage of access to contemporaneously collected information on the initial reports of the abuse suffered by girls in the 1970s. All of the women who were interviewed for this study had reported sexual abuse before the age of 13. This paper presents the results of an analysis of the women's responses to questions about child sexual abuse asked in face-to-face interviews from 1990 to 1992. The findings provide evidence about the questions that were most successful in eliciting reports of child sexual abuse and have important implications for those interested in improving retrospective research on child abuse.

METHODS

Subjects

One hundred thirty-six women were interviewed from 1990 to 1992 as part of a study of recovery from child sexual victimization (Williams, Siegel, Hyman, & Jackson-Graves, 1993; Williams, 1994, 1995; Banyard & Williams,

1996). These women were initially seen 17 years earlier in the early 1970s when the sexual abuse was reported. At the time of the abuse they were examined and treated in a hospital emergency room where all sexual abuse victims in that city were taken. Details of the sexual assault were recorded contemporaneous to the report of the abuse and documented in both hospital medical records and research interviews with the child and/or her care giver (see McCahill, Meyer, & Fischman, 1979).

At the time of abuse, the girls ranged in age from 10 months to 12 years. At the time of reinterview, the women ranged from age 18 to 31. The majority of the women (86%) are African American. The sexual abuse these women reported in childhood ranged from sexual intercourse to touching and fondling. In three fifths of the cases, sexual penetration had been reported. Sexual abuse was defined as sexual contact that was against the child's wishes, involved force or coercion, or involved a perpetrator who was 5 or more years older than the victim. Some type of physical force (pushing, shoving, slapping, beating, or choking) was used by the perpetrator in a majority of the cases. All of the perpetrators were males. In one third of the cases, the offender was a member of the immediate or extended family, in one fourth a stranger.

Data Collection

From 1990 to 1992, the women were located and asked to participate in a follow-up study of women who, during childhood, received medical care at the identified hospital. Informed consent following human subjects' guidelines was obtained. The women were not informed of their victimization history although some women connected the hospital visit to their experiences with child sexual abuse. Procedures for protection of human subjects were carefully followed and the women were assured of confidentiality.

All of the data were collected in face-to-face interviews. Two women (one White and one African American), blind to the circumstances of the sexual abuse reported in the 1970s, were trained to conduct interviews on sensitive and potentially upsetting, personal topics. All but a few of the 136 interviews were conducted in a centrally located office that was set up to insure privacy and comfort. On some occasions, a woman was interviewed at her home or at another office closer to her home. Thus, for nearly all the cases, the woman spoke in complete privacy.

The interview was structured to build rapport and ease the discussion of increasingly personal and potentially upsetting topics. The interview began with a focus on aspects of the woman's life with less potential to evoke memories of trauma, such as her education, employment situation, and family of origin composition. These initial questions were not intended to elicit any reports of child abuse, but on occasion did so. For example, the women were asked if they were ever separated from their mother or father for more than 2 months. If they responded affirmatively, they were asked about the reason for the separation. Some women reported separations due to sexual abuse by a family member. Such unsolicited responses of child sexual abuse experiences are not part of the analysis presented in this chapter.

Measures

A series of questions specifically designed to elicit reports of child sexual abuse were asked in two separate parts of the interview. After sufficient rapport had been established via questions about family, work, and social life, a series of questions about some specific and potentially stressful life events were posed. These included whether the woman had ever been arrested, whether any relatives had died, information about a major career change, and residence changes and relocations. As part of this section on life events the women were asked some general questions about victimization experiences (see Appendix, questions 120–123). First, they were asked if they had ever been physically attacked by a stranger or by someone they knew. Then they were asked if they had ever been sexually assaulted by a stranger or by someone they knew. These general questions are similar to what have been referred to as "gate" questions (Koss, 1993) although they were not used for this purpose in this study. They are nonspecific questions that were subject to the respondent's definition of what constitutes a physical attack or sexual assault. If the women responded affirmatively to any of those questions, they were asked only to tell us the age at which the event occurred.

These questions were followed by a series of unrelated questions about other topics, such as drug and alcohol use and psychological functioning. Following those questions, the women were told that they would next be asked about their sexual experiences and love life. This section began with questions about dating experiences and then turned to more detailed questions about sexual experiences, from childhood to the present (Appendix, questions 192 to 205). These questions are what has been referred to as "behaviorally specific" questions (Koss, 1993), and were adapted from questions used by Russell (1986, 1988). Other research on adults' responses to questions about their child sexual abuse experiences has demonstrated the importance of asking such detailed questions in order to elicit reports (Martin, Anderson, Romans, Mullen, & O'Shea, 1993).[1] These questions differ from the gate questions in that they focus on specific sexual behaviors, the

---

[1]It is important to note that in the series of questions beginning with #192, the experience was not labeled sexual abuse nor were the words "sexual abuse" used.

relationship of the person who perpetrated the behavior, or a specific age difference that, for purposes of this research, defined the sexual contact between the older person and the child or adolescent as sexual abuse. During the interview, whenever any of these behaviorally specific screening questions were answered affirmatively, the women were asked the age at which the sexual contact occurred and the relationship of the other person involved. Questions were asked later to ascertain that the response was consistent with our definition of child sexual abuse that included only incidents that occurred before the woman was 18 years old and involved sexual contact (a) against her wishes or by force, (b) by someone in a position of authority, or (c) when the other person was 5 or more years older. Two raters reviewed the interviews to assess whether the woman had or had not recalled the index abuse and to document the differences between the 1970s and 1990s account of the abuse (Williams, 1995).

RESULTS

This analysis examines the women's response patterns for both the index abuse (i.e., the abuse documented in our research records that brought them into the hospital in the 1970s) and any other sexual victimizations reported to the interviewer. Although more than one third of the women did not report the index abuse (see Williams, 1994), the total number of child sexual abuse incidents the women reported to the interviewer far exceeded the number of index abuse experiences. In all, in response to these questions (see Appendix), 340 distinct incidents of child sexual abuse by different perpetrators were reported by the 136 women.

Reports of the Index of Child Sexual Abuse

Figure 13.1 is a graph of the proportion of reports elicited by each question. Line 1 represents the proportion of reports of the index abuse that each question elicited. Note that the N is 77 for the analysis represented by line 1 because it includes only those who actually reported the index abuse. Thus, for example, 19% of the women who told us about the index abuse did so in response to the very first gate question asked, 23% to the second, and so forth. By the time the first four gate questions (120 to 123) had been asked, fully 75% of the index abuse experiences had already been reported. However, nine more questions were needed to generate all of the reports of the index abuse that we received in response to our specific questions. (Three women told us about the index abuse in response to other questions from other parts of the interview.)

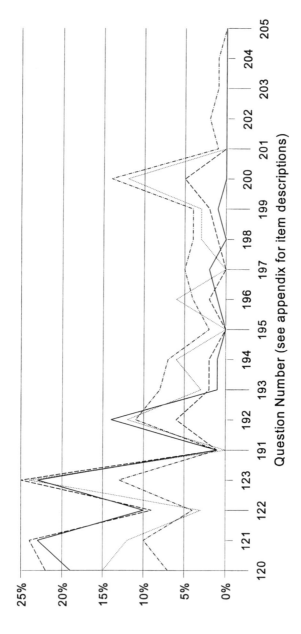

FIG. 13.1. Women's reports of child sexual abuse (CSA) elicited by interview questions (proportions).

1. Report of the index CSA (N=77, MV=3)
2. First report of any CSA (N=115, MV=5, no report=16)
3. First report of CSA (Of those who did not recall the index abuse) (N=33, no report=16)
4. Any child sexual abuse reports (N=340 reports)

Question Number (see appendix for item descriptions)

A large proportion of responses were elicited simply by asking about physical attacks, prior to any question about sexual abuse or sexual violence.[2] And fully three fourths of the women's reports of the index abuse (at least among those who reported the index abuse) came in response to the four, very general gate questions.

Question 191 was designed to begin to introduce the topic of sexual contact with others during childhood and to help put the woman at ease. It was not intended to elicit reports of child sexual abuse. Thus, the first behaviorally specific question asked was question 192. This behaviorally specific question elicited 14% of the index reports (Fig. 13.1). Therefore, after having asked just this one behaviorally specific question, plus the four gate questions, 90% of the index abuse experiences that would be recalled had been reported to the interviewer (Fig. 13.2). Each of the remaining questions drew only a small number of new reports of the index abuse.

First Report of Any Child Sexual Abuse

Line 2 in Figs. 13.1 and 13.2 shows the distribution of which questions elicited each woman's first mention to the interviewer of any child sexual abuse experience, regardless of whether it was the index abuse. For example, some of the women who did not recall the index abuse reported another clearly different abuse experience. Or, some women who had suffered more than one victimization first told the interviewer about a child sexual victimization other than the index abuse. Twelve percent of the women never reported a child sexual abuse experience and were not included in the analyses. Twenty-two percent of the women who reported any child sexual abuse did so for the first time in response to question 120, 24% in response to question 121, and so forth.

The cumulative pattern (Fig. 13.2) is quite similar to that for the index abuse reports, with a surprising 80% of all the women (including those who did not recall the index abuse) telling the interviewer about child sexual abuse in response to one of the four gate questions. Again, the questions about being physically attacked (questions 120 & 121) elicited more reports of child sexual victimization than did the next two questions about being sexually assaulted (Fig. 13.2). The first of the behaviorally specific questions (question 192) again evoked the greatest proportion of the remaining reports (6%). Thus, by the time these first five questions had been asked, 87%

---

[2]It is possible that some of the women were primed to talk about child sexual abuse because they had concluded that the focus of our research was on child sexual abuse when we told them that we were following-up women who were seen in the emergency room of the city hospital. Some women recalled that they were seen at this hospital following a report of sexual abuse. Therefore, they may have suspected that they would be asked about abuse experiences and were waiting for the first opportunity to mention such events.

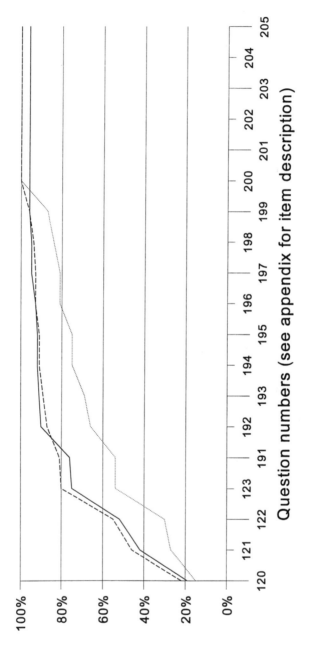

Question numbers (see appendix for item description)

1. Report of the index (documented) CSA (N=80, MV=3)
2. First report of any CSA (N=136, no report=16, missing=5)
3. First report of CSA (for women who did not recall the index abuse) (N=49, no report=16)

FIG. 13.2. Women's reports of CSA (cumulative figures).

of the women who told about any abuse were properly identified as having been sexually abused during childhood (prior to age 18). It should be noted that, due to the fact that 12% of the women never reported any child sexual abuse, after the first five questions only 73% of the women had been correctly identified as having been sexually abused during childhood.

In contrast to the response pattern that occurred when we considered only what questions elicited the index abuse, one of the later behaviorally specific questions (#200) elicited a number of first reports of any child sexual victimization. This question asked about sexual contact during childhood with someone 5 or more years older, even if the child or adolescent had agreed. Some women had not reported a sexual abuse incident prior to this question because they did not consider this type of sexual contact to have been coercive, assaultive, or unwanted. For example, one woman reported in response to question 200 that, when she was 15, she had a sexual relationship with a 23-year-old man. Although this fits our operational definition of abuse, the woman herself did not view this experience as abusive and, therefore, did not identify it in response to earlier questions about unwanted or coercive sex. Not all responses to this question reflected such ambiguity about how one should define child sexual victimization. One response shows how important behaviorally specific questions are in eliciting information on child sexual abuse experiences. This woman reported, in response to question 200, that she was a prostitute at the age of 10, at which time she had what she termed "consenting" sex with adult men.

Figure 13.2 reveals that although 87% of the women had reported child sexual abuse in response to the first five questions, an additional 15 women (13% of the women who reported any child sexual abuse) would have been misclassified as "not sexually abused" if the eight additional questions that followed had not been asked. And, 16 (12%) of the women in the sample never reported any child sexual abuse experience, including the abuse that had been documented in their hospital records. These women would comprise the false negatives (i.e., those who report no abuse when, in fact, they have a history of abuse) if this were a retrospective study.

First Report of Child Sexual Abuse by Women
Who Did Not Recall the Index Abuse

An examination of the questions that elicited the woman's first report of child sexual abuse to the interviewer was also made for only those 49 women who did not recall the index abuse (Fig. 13.1, line 3). Sixty-seven percent of these women reported some other child sexual abuse in response to these questions. Again, even for these women who did not report the index abuse, the majority of the reports were made in response to the first four gate questions. And, by the time the first behaviorally specific question (#192) was asked, abuse was reported by over two thirds of the 33 women who did not recall the index abuse but who reported some other abuse. As with the rest of the respondents, the age difference question (#200) drew new reports of abuse.

Reports of Any Child Sexual Abuse

Three-hundred-forty child sexual abuse incidents (by different perpetrators) were reported by the 136 women who were interviewed. Figure 13.1 (line 4) shows which questions were most successful in eliciting these reports of child sexual abuse; that is, the proportion of the 340 incidents that each question elicited. It is interesting to note that despite its apparent success in generating women's first mentions of any child sexual victimization, the first gate question (#120) only elicited 25 reports, that is, only 7% of all the child sexual abuse reported to us by the women. The question that elicited the largest proportion of all reports of child sexual abuse was question 200, about sexual contact during childhood with someone who was 5 or more years older.

In the Appendix, we have indicated after each questions the mean age of the victims at the time of all the sexual abuse uncovered by each question. Note that the gate questions elicited reports of abuse that occurred when the women were younger (ages 9–11), compared to the ages for some of the behaviorally specific questions. This suggests that these more behaviorally specific questions are needed to elicit information about abuse that occurred during adolescence, some of which might take the form of acquaintance rape. Similar types of behaviorally specific questions may also have been needed to elicit more reports from those who were abused at a very young age. For example, the 16 women (12% of the sample) who never told our interviewer about any child sexual abuse experience were, according to our hospital records, young at the time of the index abuse (average age = 7 years). Some of these women, particularly those who were very young at the time of the abuse, may not recall the index abuse in response to any question, but for others it is possible that different questions would have elicited a report.

In Fig. 13.3, we group the questions according to type. The four gate questions were grouped together and the behavior specific questions were categorized as: (a) sexual behavior oriented (sexbeh) questions that asked about specific sexual acts that may have occurred (4 questions); (b) relationship-oriented questions (relat) that focused on the relationship of the abuser to the respondent (2 questions); (c) age-related questions (age) that asked about sexual contact in the context of age differentials (2 questions); (d) unwanted sex (5 questions); and (e) questions about sexual experiences that evoked fear or involved violence or assault (2 questions). The key to Fig. 13.3 indicates which questions were included in each category.

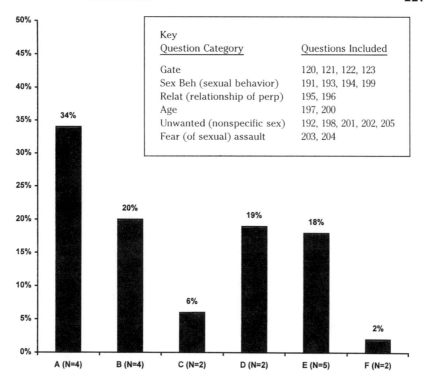

FIG. 13.3. Proportion of all child sexual abuse reports generated by question types (N = 340 incidents).

As can be seen from Fig. 13.3, the gate questions accounted for only 34% of all the abuse reported by the women. Thus, although a majority of first reports were elicited by the gate questions and we were able to correctly categorize 67% of the women as sexually abused after the first four gate questions were asked, the behaviorally specific questions were needed to evoke the majority of all the abuse reported.

DISCUSSION

These analyses show that a series of questions are required to generate women's reports of child sexual abuse on interview 17 years following a documented experience of child sexual abuse. Whereas a surprisingly high proportion of the women told of experiences of sexual victimization in childhood in response to the four initial gate questions, many women (33%) would have been falsely labeled as nonvictims if only the gate questions had been asked. Even if one additional question is asked about unwanted sex prior to age 18 (#192), only 73% of the women would have been properly identified as victims of child sexual abuse, leaving 27% of the women as false negatives. It should be noted that the proportion of false negatives found in this study may be a conservative estimate—lower than might be found in a community survey—because some of the women in this sample were undoubtedly aware of the focus of the study (on recovery from child sexual abuse) and may have been more likely to quickly mention experiences of child sexual abuse. Most important, even after extensive questioning, 12% of the women with documented histories of sexual abuse in childhood reported no experiences of child sexual victimization.

False negatives that would occur if only the gate questions were asked are likely to include many women who experienced abuse during pre- or early adolescence. After more behaviorally specific questions have been asked, the women who still do not report or, more likely, do not recall the abuse were younger at the time of the victimization and were likely to have been sexually abused by someone known to them (Williams, 1994). Of course, it is also possible that the questions posed here did not address the issue in a way that allowed the women to feel comfortable enough to answer. In those cases, additional or different questions might have evoked a report. For other women, however, there may not be any such questions: Their abuse experience may simply not be a topic they are willing to discuss.

These findings have implications for researchers who wish to ascertain the victimization status of adult respondents. For those who estimate the prevalence of child sexual abuse among adults, these findings underscore the necessity of asking questions that direct the respondent's attention to specific kinds of behaviors or relationships salient to her experiences.

The findings also have implications for those who use retrospective methodologies to estimate the incidence of child sexual victimization and to describe the nature and scope of child sexual abuse. The importance of asking behaviorally specific questions is highlighted by the fact that the gate questions evoked only a minority (34%) of all the child sexual victimization experiences reported during the course of the interviews.

Researchers who want to elicit reports of child sexual abuse in the context of a study that examines such abuse as one of many possible predictors of some outcome such as psychological, social, or economic problems may feel that they cannot afford to spend time asking so many questions. They should be aware, however, that a simple screener question such as "Were you ever sexually abused?" or even one or two more behaviorally specific questions will probably result in false assumptions about the actual victimization status of the respondents, which in turn could lead to erroneous conclusions about the outcome of interest.

The response pattern observed in this study may be attributable to several things that occurred when the interviewer asked more questions about experiences with sexual contact during childhood and asked more behaviorally specific questions. First, the women may have been encouraged by the question to rethink or to redefine experiences and respond affirmatively to our questions. In this way behaviorally specific questions help to provide a definitional framework for the respondent. Undoubtedly the long series of questions incrementally provided more detail on the definitions and types of sexual experiences that were of interest. Each new question added considerations of different sexual acts (grabbing, feeling, etc., not just intercourse) and the relationship to the person with whom the sexual contact occurred (an older relative, a person in a position of authority, a boyfriend). These questions then helped the woman to apply our definitions to her experiences and may have entered into her decision to report an experience.

In addition to providing a definitional framework, a long series of questions may actually trigger memories of child sexual abuse. Indeed, after answering "no" to many questions, several women volunteered that they now recalled an experience of child sexual victimization that they had forgotten or had not thought about for years. Other women may have had this same experience of memory triggered by questions, but we did not systematically collect this information. The extent of the questioning about sexual contacts in childhood and the amount of time that the women had to think back on childhood experiences with sex may have had an impact on the success of the later questions in generating new reports of child sexual abuse.

In addition to behaviorally specific questions, questions asked in different contexts may elicit additional reports of child sexual abuse (see Femina et al., 1990). As we noted, some of the women told about experiences with child sexual abuse in the context of other questions about their family constellation. Future investigation might explore the effectiveness of questions asked in other contexts. For example, researchers might ask, "Did anyone in your family ever get into any trouble for his or her sexual behavior or activity?" or, "Have you known anyone who got into trouble for sexual activities or who would have gotten into trouble if he or she had been caught?" and follow-up with probes about any sexual contact this person may have had with the respondent.

Adults who are being interviewed about childhood experiences and other life events may recall abuse experiences later during the interview but not mention them because the topic is no longer being discussed. We, therefore, recommend that surveys be designed to revisit these questions toward the end of the interview. For instance, the respondent could be asked if she has thought of any other abuse or other unwanted sexual experiences that she did not mention in response to earlier questions. The ability to revisit questions is inherent in mail surveys because when completing a mail or written questionnaire, the respondent can usually go back and correct answers or add information about child sexual abuse that has been recalled while answering subsequent questions or after further reflection. This may explain why at least one study found that such surveys elicited more reports of some types of child sexual abuse (Martin et al., 1993). Therefore, when possible, this option should be offered to respondents in face-to-face and telephone interviews.

The findings presented here suggest that concern of researchers is properly focused on reducing the incidence of false negatives in retrospective studies. It also suggests that although retrospective studies miss a significant proportion of child sexual victimization, additional behaviorally specific questions, questions about abuse asked in different contexts and procedures that would permit respondents to revisit the questions before ending the interview, may reduce the number of false negatives.

APPENDIX

Interview Questions About Sexual Abuse

Were you ever:

120. *physically* attacked by a stranger? (mean age = 11)
121. *physically* attacked by someone you knew? (mean age = 10)
122. sexually assaulted by a stranger? (mean age = 11)
123. sexually assaulted/molested by someone you knew? (mean age = 9)

Let's talk in more detail about sexual experiences you have had with others, starting with experiences you had as a child with other children from things like playing "doctor" to things that may have happened to you when you were on a date. Then we'll talk about sexual experiences which may have been forced on you. These things may have happened only once, or they may have happened over a long period of time.

191. Now think back to *before you were 13*, did you have any sexual experiences *with other children*, including friends or strangers, brothers or sisters? Most children have had experiences like these. This includes curiosity about sex and seeing sexual activities or the sex organs, genitals, or private parts of others or any sex "play". Please tell a bit about *the most important experience* and we may talk in more detail about this later. (mean age = 7)

Now let's talk about the experiences that occurred *anytime* when you were a child or adolescent but before you were 18:

192. When you were a child or anytime before you turned *18* did anyone, male or female, ever try or succeed in having any kind of sexual relations with you when you didn't want to? (In other words, intercourse or anything else?) (mean age = 11)

193. When you were a child or anytime before you were 18, did anyone (else) ever try or succeed in touching your genitals or sex organs or getting you to touch their genitals when you didn't want to? (mean age = 12)

194. When you were a child or anytime before you turned 18, did anyone (else) ever feel you, grab you, or kiss you in a way you felt was sexually threatening? (mean age = 13)

195. Some people have experienced sexual advances by someone who had authority or power over them, such as a doctor, teacher, employer, minister, therapist, policeman, or much older person. When you were a child or anytime before you were 18, did you have any kind of sexual experience with someone who had authority over you? (Besides anyone you've already mentioned.) (mean age = 15)

196. People often don't think about their relatives when thinking about sexual experiences, so this question is about relatives. When you were a child or anytime before you were 18 did you have any sexual contact with an uncle, brother, father, grandfather, or sister, mother or other male or female relative? (Besides anyone you've already mentioned.) (mean age = 12)

197. When you were a child or anytime before you turned 18, did you have any sexual experiences with an older person like a camp counselor, baby-sitter, older friend or person who picked you up while hitch-hiking, that you haven't mentioned yet? (mean age = 13)

198. When you were a child or anytime before you turned 18 did you ever have any other unwanted sexual experience with anyone, male or female? This could include a boyfriend or other male or female friends. (Besides anyone you've already mentioned.) (mean age = 14)

199. When you were a child or anytime before you turned 18, did someone else who was older than you ever purposely expose their genitals to you in a way that *was meant to upset you*? (mean age = 12)

200. When you were a child or anytime before you turned 18, did you have sexual contact or experience with someone who was *5 or more years older* than you, even if you agreed? (Besides anyone you've already mentioned.) (mean age = 15)

201. Before you turned 18, did you have any (other) upsetting sexual experiences that you haven't mentioned yet?

Now we will include the time since you turned 18.

202. How about as an adult? Have you *ever* had an unwanted sexual experience with any one male or female? This could have been sex forced by a date, a friend, a husband, someone you knew only casually, or a stranger. It could be a boss or a family member. (mean age = 17)

203. Have you ever been in any (other) situation where there was violence or threat of violence, where you were also afraid of being sexually assaulted (—again, other than what you have already mentioned?)

204. In general, have you narrowly missed being sexually assaulted by someone (other than what you have already mentioned)?

205. Can you think of any (other) unwanted sexual experiences (that you haven't mentioned yet)?

ACKNOWLEDGMENT

This research was supported by the National Center on Child Abuse and Neglect (NCCAN grant # CA-90-1406).

REFERENCES

Bagley, C., & Ramsay, R. (1985). Disrupted childhood and vulnerability to sexual assault: Long-term sequels with implications for counseling. *Social Work and Human Sexuality, 4*, 33–48.

Banyard, V. L., & Williams, L. M. (1996). Characteristics of child sexual abuse as correlates of women's adjustment: A prospective study. *Journal of Marriage and the Family, 58*, 853–865.

Femina, D. D., Yeager, C. A., & Lewis, D. O. (1990). Child abuse: Adolescent records vs. adult recall. *Child Abuse and Neglect, 14*, 227–231.

Finkelhor, D. (1979). *Sexually victimized children*. New York: The Free Press.

Finkelhor, D. (1984). *Child sexual abuse: New theory and research*. New York: The Free Press.

Finkelhor, D. (1994). Current information on the scope and nature of child sexual abuse. *The Future of Children, 4*(2), 31–53.

Kilpatrick, D. (1992). *Rape in America: A report to the nation*. Charleston, SC: Crime Victims Research and Treatment Center.

Koss, M. P. (1993). Detecting the scope of rape: A review of prevalence research methods. *Journal of Interpersonal Violence, 8*, 198–222.

Martin, J., Anderson, J., Romans, S., Mullen, P., & O'Shea, M. (1993). Asking about child sexual abuse: Methodological implications of a two stage survey. *Child Abuse and Neglect, 17*, 383–392.

McCahill, T., Meyer, L. C., & Fischman, A. (1979). *The aftermath of rape*. Lexington, MA: Lexington.

Peters, S. D., Wyatt, G. E., & Finkelhor, D. (1986). Prevalence. In D. Finkelhor (Ed.), *A sourcebook on child sexual abuse* (pp. 15–59). Beverly Hills, CA: Sage.

Russell, D. (1986). *The secret trauma: Incest in the lives of girls and women*. New York: Basic Books.

Russell, D. E. H. (1988). The incidence and prevalence of intrafamilial and extrafamilial sexual abuse of female children. In L. E. A. Walker (Ed.), *Handbook of sexual abuse of children: Assessment and treatment issues* (pp. 19–36). New York: Springer-Verlag.

Williams, L. M. (1994). Recall of childhood trauma: A prospective study of women's memories of child sexual abuse. *Journal of Consulting and Clinical Psychology, 62*(6), 1167–1176.

Williams, L. M. (1995). Recovered memories of abuse in women with documented child sexual victimization histories. *Journal of Traumatic Stress, 8*(4), 649–673.

Williams, L. M., Siegel, J. S., Hyman, B., & Jackson-Graves, J. (1993). *Recovery from sexual abuse: A longitudinal study 1973–1990*. Durham, NH: Family Research Laboratory.

Wyatt, G. (1985). The sexual abuse of Afro-American and white American women in childhood. *Child Abuse and Neglect, 10*, 231–240.

Wyatt, G. E., & Peters, S. D. (1986). Issues in the definition of child sexual abuse in prevalence research. *Child Abuse and Neglect, 10*, 231–240.

VI

SELF-REPORTING OF HEALTH BEHAVIORS AND PSYCHIATRIC SYMPTOMS

Howard S. Kurtzman
National Institute of Mental Health

Self-reports are a crucial—often the only—source of information about psychiatric symptoms and health behaviors. But until recently, the validity and reliability of self-reports in these domains have been inadequate. As the authors in this section show, improved methods for eliciting self-reports are now being developed that take into account the processes by which subjects understand and respond to self-report requests.

Kessler, Wittchen, Abelson, and Zhao aim to improve the design of structured interviews for detecting psychiatric disorders in large community samples. Their recommendations address four determinants of subjects' self-reports: (a) Question comprehension: Questions should be phrased carefully to minimize vagueness and complexity and to clarify relations with preceding questions; (b) Task comprehension: It should be made clear to subjects whether, for example, a question is calling for an effortful search of memory or is only requesting easily accessible information; (c) Motivation: Subjects should be informed of the rationale for the interview, asked for an overt commitment to cooperate, and given verbal reinforcement throughout the interview; and (d) Ability to answer accurately: Questions should be structured in ways that encourage retrieval of specific autobiographical information rather than potentially biased inference or estimation about life events; also, more difficult memory searches should be placed at the beginning of the interview, before subjects' energy wanes. As the authors describe, implementation of these recommendations in the U.S. National

Comorbidity Survey appears to have yielded more effective detection of mental disorders.

Rand focuses on self-reports of adherence to drug and other therapeutic regimens. She points out that self-reports have many potential advantages, such as providing detailed information about a patient's pattern of adherence and the personal and situational factors that determine that pattern. But the accuracy of self-reports can be compromised by such factors as memory distortions and motives to provide socially desirable responses. Rand calls for systematic research to develop improved self-report instruments for assessing adherence in adults and children; these instruments would include items about the patient's beliefs and attitudes concerning adherence and about specific barriers to adherence. She also points to research on physicians' communication skills that suggests that direct, specific, but nonjudgmental questioning can increase the accuracy of self-reports in clinical settings.

Shiffman presents a method for obtaining self-reports that bypasses problems of memory distortion. With Computerized Ecological Momentary Assessment, subjects are signaled throughout the day to provide immediate reports about their current state by using a palm-top computer. With this method, Shiffman and colleagues investigated temporal and contextual patterns of cigarette smoking. Their data indicate that previous results based on global retrospective self-reports are largely inaccurate. Those previous results seem to reflect smokers' beliefs and memory reconstructions about their behavior, rather than their actual behavior. Shiffman's work leads to better models of smoking—and to more sophisticated and informative uses of self-reports across all areas of behavioral research.

14

Methodological Issues in Assessing Psychiatric Disorders With Self-Reports

Ronald C. Kessler
Harvard Medical School

Hans-Ulrich Wittchen
Max Planck Institute of Psychiatry

Jamie Abelson
The University of Michigan

Shanyang Zhao
Temple University

This chapter discusses methodological issues involved in obtaining accurate self-reports about psychiatric disorders from respondents in general population surveys using methods that do not require clinician administration or clinician judgment. Such data are subject to greater error than clinician-administered research diagnostic interviews but are nonetheless favored over the latter in large community surveys because of the considerable expense and substantial logistic complications associated with using clinicians as survey interviewers. Indeed, our understanding of the distribution and correlates of psychiatric disorders in the general population is based largely on the results of surveys in which trained lay interviewers rather than clinicians have administered fully structured interviews (e.g., Kessler et al., 1994; Robins & Regier, 1991).

Validity studies reviewed by Wittchen (1994) show that diagnoses based on these fully structured interviews are strongly related to independent clinical evaluations. However, this relationship is far from perfect. If the degree of invalidity is known, then aggregate prevalence estimates and measures of association can be corrected using standard psychometric methods. Extreme invalidity, however, jeopardizes the logic of this approach. Lack of validity introduces errors at the individual level that make it hazardous to use structured interviews for treatment decisions. As a result, there is considerable interest in improving currently available structured instruments.

Two lines of work have been carried out to achieve this goal. The first is to refine available structured interviews in an effort to increase their consistency with clinical diagnoses. The second is to develop and refine short screening scales that can be used as the first stage in two-stage psychiatric evaluations that administer more expensive and in-depth clinical interviews to all screened positives and a random subsample of screened negatives in the second stage. The first line of work has resulted in the development of elaborate structured interviews, taking as much as 2 hours to administer, that attempt to reproduce clinician-based diagnoses as accurately as possible. The second line of work has resulted in the development of brief interviews taking no more than 10 minutes to administer that attempt to screen in all true psychiatric cases and as few noncases as possible. Developments in only the first of these two areas are reviewed in this chapter. See Newman, Shrout, and Bland (1990) and Kessler and Mroczek (1995) for discussions of the second area.

HISTORICAL OVERVIEW

Descriptive studies comparing admission and discharge rates to and from asylums were carried out as early as the 17th century (Hunter & Macalpine, 1963) and continued to be the mainstay of research on psychiatric disorders up to the middle of the 20th century (e.g., Faris & Dunham, 1939; Hollingshead & Redlich, 1958). However, these studies were hampered by the fact that the treatment statistics that were the focus of this work confounded information about help-seeking and labeling with information about illness prevalence. In the few cases where population data were used rather than treatment statistics, informants such as police and clergy were asked to nominate people they considered to have emotional problems. Although this method was useful in avoiding the help-seeking bias associated with treatment studies, these informants tended to miss people whose disorders were characterized more by private distress than public acting out, leading to an underestimation of the percent of people with a psychiatric disorder as well as to a distorted picture of disorders being much more prevalent among men, whose disorders tend to be visible (e.g., acting out disorders), than women, whose disorders tend to be more private (e.g., mood disorders; Dohrenwend & Dohrenwend, 1965).

The end of World War II brought with it a growing appreciation of these methodological problems as well as a growing concern about the prevalence of mental illness. This concern was caused by the fact that many selective service recruits for World War II were found to suffer from emotional disorders and to return from the War with traumatic stress reactions. One response was the initiation of a number of local and national surveys of psychiatric disorders based on direct interviews with representative community samples. The earliest of these post-War surveys were either carried out by clinicians or used lay-interview data in combination with record data as input to clinician evaluations of caseness (e.g., Leighton, 1959; Srole, Langner, Michael, Opler, & Rennie, 1962). In later studies, clinician judgment was abandoned in favor of less expensive self-report symptom rating scales that assigned each respondent a score on a continuous dimension of nonspecific psychological distress (e.g., Gurin, Veroff, & Feld, 1960). Controversy surrounded the use of these rating scales from the start, focusing on such things as item bias, insensitivity, and restriction of symptom coverage (e.g., Dohrenwend & Dohrenwend, 1965; Seiler, 1973). Nonetheless, they continued to be the mainstay of community psychiatric epidemiology through the 1970s.

There were at least three factors that accounted for the attraction of symptom rating scales in these studies. First, these scales were much less expensive to administer than clinician-based interviews. Second, as compared to dichotomous clinician caseness judgments, continuous measures of distress dealt directly with the actual constellations of signs and symptoms that exist in the population rather than with the classification schemes imposed on these constellations by clinicians. Third, the clinician-based diagnostic interviews available during this period of time did not have good psychometric properties when administered in community samples (Dohrenwend, Yager, Egri, & Mendelsohn, 1978).

However, there were also disadvantages of working with symptom rating scales. Perhaps the most important of these was that there was nothing in these scales themselves that allowed researchers to discriminate between people who did and did not have clinically significant psychiatric problems. This discrimination was less important to social scientists, whose main concern was to characterize the range of distress associated with structural variations in risk factors, than to clinicians and social policy analysts, who wanted to make decisions regarding such things as the number of people in need of mental health services. A division consequently arose that lingers to this day between some researchers who work largely with measures of dimensional distress and others who work largely with dichotomous caseness measures.

A middle ground between these two positions was sought by some researchers who developed rules for classifying people with scores above a certain threshold on distress scales as psychiatric cases (e.g., Radloff, 1977), making it possible to study both continuous and dichotomous outcomes with the same measures. The precise cutpoints used in this research were usually based on statistical analyses that attempted to discriminate optimally between the scores of patients in psychiatric treatment and those of people in a community sample. However, as noted previously, considerable controversy surrounded the decision of exactly where to specify cutpoints. Dichotomous diagnostic measures allowed this sort of discrimination to be made directly based on an evaluation of diagnostic criteria, but these interviews were not precise due to lack of agreement on appropriate research diagnostic criteria and absence of valid instruments for carrying out research diagnostic interviews.

It was not until the late 1970s that the field was able to move beyond this controversy with the establishment of clear research diagnostic criteria by research-oriented psychiatrists who were concerned that lack of diagnostic clarity was hampering the cumulation of their research (Feighner, Robins, & Guze, 1972). Systematic research diagnostic interviews aimed at operationalizing these criteria were developed shortly thereafter (Endicott & Spitzer, 1978). The third edition of the Diagnostic and Statistical Manual (*DSM–III*) of the American Psychiatric Association (APA, 1980) was influenced by these initiatives as well as by parallel developments in Europe (World Health Organization, WHO, 1977). Research based on the revised criteria in *DSM–III* led to refinements in subsequent editions of the *DSM* (American Psychiatric Association, 1987, 1994) as well as to the development of more elaborate research diagnostic interviews (Keller, Lavori, & Neilsen, 1987, SCALUP; Spitzer, Williams, Gibbon, & First, 1992, SCID).

Despite these advances, there are still important limitations in the precision of psychiatric diagnoses for research purposes due to the fact that these diagnoses must rely largely on patient self-reports. Although behavioral observations play some part in diagnosis and objective tests exist to subtype some disorders (e.g., Thase et al., 1997), most psychiatric diagnoses require the clinician to make decisions about the presence or absence of emotional experiences such as sadness and worry that cannot be observed directly. The necessity of relying on patient self-reports is not unique to psychiatry. Similar problems arise, for example, in the evaluation of pain. However, psychiatry is on less firm footing than most other areas of medicine when it comes to objective confirmation of diagnosis because there is no known biological basis for most psychiatric disorders and no way of carrying out objective tests either to confirm or disconfirm self-reported symptoms.

This is perhaps most clear in the evaluation of cases where there might be secondary gain from receiving a diagnosis, such as in the evaluation of functional disability caused by post-traumatic stress disorder (PTSD) brought on by an automobile accident. Diagnosticians have searched long and hard for objective tests that might provide some clear way of determining whether people who seek compensation for such purported disabilities are, in fact, disabled rather than dissembling. However, these efforts have thus far been unsuccessful, with the proposed tests either not always being positive for cases thought to have the disorder or not always being negative for cases thought not to have the disorder.

Aware of this problem, research-oriented clinicians now typically base their diagnoses of psychiatric disorders on complex patterns of data that include not only intake interviews but also informant reports, medical records, objective tests, and systematic observations of clinical course and treatment response. Furthermore, in an effort to move beyond reliance on patient reports of internal states, the diagnostic criteria on which these diagnoses are based now go beyond the core emotions of the disorders under study to include behaviors and cognitions often found to be associated with these core emotions. These elaborations do not negate the problem of the ultimate unobservability of intrapsychic experiences. Nor do they resolve the criticism that some syndromes characterized as psychiatric disorders in the *DSM* and ICD (International Classification of Diseases) systems might more accurately be conceptualized as social problems rather than as illnesses (Illich, 1975). However, the use of multiple information sources and elaborate diagnostic criteria to generate research diagnoses has been successful in bringing about enough consistency in the labeling of emotional problems to allow knowledge to cumulate about such things as risk factors, course, and treatment response. And this consistency, in turn, has made it possible to search in a systematic way for more objective indicators of pathological processes based on medical tests.

This rigor has also created problems for the development of self-report instruments to approximate the diagnoses made by clinicians. In some cases, these problems are insurmountable. It is impossible, for example, to ask a respondent to provide a self-report on whether they have an abnormal EEG sleep profile. Although in some cases it may be possible to use patient self-reports of behavioral correlates as a substitute for data of this sort, this is not always possible. Therefore, the focus of most work on self-reported assessment of psychiatric disorder has been on instruments that attempt to approximate the data obtained in clinician-administered research diagnostic interviews.

The first fully structured diagnostic interview of this sort was the Diagnostic Interview Schedule (DIS; Robins, Helzer, Croughan, & Ratcliff, 1981). The DIS was developed with support from the National Institute of Mental Health for use in the Epidemiologic Catchment Area (ECA) Study (Robins & Regier, 1991). The ECA Study is the first of two major community-based epidemiologic studies of psychiatric disorders that have been carried out in the United States during the past 15 years. The ECA was a landmark study that led to replications in other countries as well as to the development of other structured diagnostic interviews. Most of the latter are based on the DIS. The most widely used of these new instruments is the WHO Composite International Diagnostic Interview (CIDI; WHO, 1990). The CIDI was used in the second major psychiatric epidemiologic study carried out in the United States in the past 15 years, the NCS (Kessler et al., 1994). The CIDI will be the focus of the remainder of the chapter. Much of the methodological evaluation of the CIDI described next occurred in preparation for its use in the NCS.

Four main methodological issues have been the subject of concern about the accuracy of structured research diagnostic interviews of psychiatric disorders like the DIS and CIDI. One is that the respondent may not understand the questions being asked. A second is that the respondent may not understand the task implied by the questions. A third is that the respondent may not be motivated to answer accurately. And a fourth is that the respondent may not be able to answer accurately. A considerable amount of methodological research has been carried out by survey researchers on each of these topics as they apply to community surveys in general (e.g., Bradburn, Sudman, & Associates, 1979; Cannell, Miller, & Oksenberg, 1981; Moss & Goldstein, 1979). This research has advanced considerably over the past decade as cognitive psychologists have become interested in the survey interview as a natural laboratory for studying cognitive processes (e.g., Biderman, 1980; Jabine, Straf, Tanur, & Tourangeau, 1984; Tanur, 1992). A number of important insights have emerged from this work that suggest practical ways of improving the accuracy of self-reported psychiatric assessments. In our own work, which we review later this chapter, we have used these insights to refine the CIDI.

THE IMPORTANCE OF QUESTION COMPREHENSION

It is obvious that ambiguous questions are likely to be misconstrued. It is perhaps less obvious, however, just how ambiguous most structured questions are and how often respondents must "read between the lines." In the first systematic study of this issue, Belson (1981) debriefed a sample of survey respondents on a set of standard survey questions and found that more than 70% of respondents interpreted some questions differently from the researcher, leading Belson to conclude that subtle misinterpretations are pervasive in survey situations. Oksenberg, Cannell, and Kanton (1991) came to a similar conclusion in their debriefing of a nationally representative sample of respondents who were administered standard-health-interview survey questions. At least one key phrase in two thirds of the questions in their analyses were misinterpreted by respondents. Both Belson and Oksenberg et al. found, furthermore, that respondents generally believed that they understood what the investigator meant even when their interpretations of the questions were quite idiosyncratic. Our own debriefing studies of the CIDI in preparation for the NCS found much the same result—that a great many respondents misunderstood important aspects of key diagnostic questions.

How is it possible for there to be so much misunderstanding? As Oksenberg and her colleagues discovered, the answer lies partly in the fact that many terms in surveys are vaguely defined. But beyond this is the more fundamental fact that the survey interview situation is a special kind of interaction in which the standard rules of conversation—rules that help fill in the gaps in meaning that exist in most speech—do not apply. Unlike the situation in normal conversational practice, the respondent in the survey interview often has only a vague notion of the person to whom he is talking or the purpose of the conversation (Cannell, Fowler, & Marquis, 1968). The person who asks the questions (the interviewer) is not the person who formulated the questions (the researcher), and the questioner is often unable to clarify the respondent's uncertainties about the intent of the questions. Furthermore, the flow of questions in the interview is established prior to the beginning of the conversation, which means that normal conversational rules of give and take in question-and-answer sequences do not apply. This leads to more misreading than in normal conversations even when questions are seemingly straightforward (Clark & Schober, 1992). This problem is compounded further when the topic of the interview is one that involves emotional experiences that are in many cases difficult to describe with clarity.

Clinical interviews attempt to deal with this problem by being interviewer based (Brown, 1989). In interviewer-based instruments, the interviewer is trained to have a deep understanding of the criteria being evaluated. The interview guide provides a script for certain entry questions and suggestions for the types of follow-up questions the interviewer should ask to assess each criterion but allows the interviewer to query the respondent as much as necessary to clarify the meaning of questions. Furthermore, the ultimate judgment lies with the interviewer rather than the respondent. Indeed, one might say that the interview is, in some sense, administered to the interviewer rather than to the respondent in that the responses of interest are responses to interviewer-based questions of the following sort: "Interviewer, based on your conversation with the respondent, would you say that he definitely, probably, possibly, probably not, or definitely does not meet the requirements of Criterion A?"

Fully structured psychiatric interviews like the CIDI cannot use this interviewer-based approach because, by definition, they are designed so that interviewer judgment plays no part in the responses. These respondent-based interviews use totally structured questions that the respondent answers, often in a yes–no format, either after reading the questions to themselves or after having an interviewer read the questions aloud. When the criterion of interest is fairly clear, there may be little difference between interviewer-based and respondent-based interviewing. For example, Criterion A9 in the *DSM–IV* assessment of Major Depressive Episode requires "recurrent thoughts of death (not just fear of dying), recurrent suicidal ideation without a specific plan, or a suicide attempt or a specific plan for committing suicide" (APA, 1994, p. 327). Whereas there may be some minor confusion over some of these terms, validation studies show that there is generally quite good agreement between clinician evaluations and simple self-reports based on structured questions designed to operationalize this criterion (Blazer, Kessler, McGonagle, & Swartz, 1994).

It is a good deal more difficult, however, to assess conceptually complex criteria with fully structured questions. Consider Criterion A8 for the same *DSM–IV* diagnosis, which requires "diminished ability to think or concentrate, or indecisiveness, nearly every day (either by subjective account or as observed by others)" (APA, 1994, p. 327). Questions arise about whether or not a small diminution in ability to concentrate qualifies and, if not, how to determine when the decrement is not small. Clinical researchers have resolved problems such as this, at least for purposes of establishing inter-rater reliability, by developing rules based on clinical vignettes that are used to specify the levels needed to qualify for the criteria. This is the hallmark of interviewer-based interviewing; that the interviewer has expert knowledge of the criteria and can judge whether the respondent does or does not qualify by probing until the level of the criterion symptom is clear. In respondent-based interviewing, in comparison, it is necessary to rely on the wording of the structured question to be sufficiently clear to operationalize the criteria.

In an effort to investigate the problem of question misunderstanding in the CIDI as part of the pilot studies for the NCS, we carried out a series of debriefing interviews with community respondents who were administered sections of the CIDI and then asked to explain what they thought the questions meant and why they answered the way they did. As noted earlier, we found a great deal of misunderstanding. However, we also found enormous variation across questions in the frequency of misunderstanding. In comparing questions with high levels of misunderstanding to those with lower levels, four discriminating features were found.

First, some commonly misunderstood questions were simply too complex for many respondents to grasp. A good example is the question in version 1.0 of the CIDI designed to operationalize the part of Criterion A in the *DSM–III–R* diagnosis of agoraphobia that stipulates that the person has a "fear of being in places or situations from which escape might be difficult (or embarrassing) or in which help might not be available in the event of suddenly developing a symptom(s) that could be incapacitating or ex-tremely embarrassing" (APA, 1987, p. 241). This is a very complex concept that contains several components. Yet CIDI 1.0 attempted to assess it with only a single question:

> When you had this unreasonably strong fear [of being in a crowd, leaving home alone, traveling on buses, cars and trains, or crossing a bridge], were you afraid of collapsing, or of the occurrence of other incapacitating or em-barrassing symptoms when no help was available or escape possible? (WHO, 1990, p. 15)

Our debriefing study found that the majority of respondents failed to grasp all aspects of this complex question. Indeed, when we asked people who had just answered the question, "Can you repeat the last question I just asked you?" we found that fewer than 15% were able to reproduce all the major elements of the question. Based on this evidence, we unpacked this question into a series of component questions, each of which was less conceptually challenging for the respondent. The most recent version of the CIDI, Version 2.1 (WHO, 1997) also operationalizes this criterion with a series of component questions.

A second type of commonly misunderstood CIDI question found in our pilot work involved vaguely defined terms rather than complex concepts. The most common examples concerned experiences that are a matter of degree, such as having "trouble concentrating" (WHO, 1990, p. 26) or "talking or moving more slowly than is normal" (WHO, 1990, p. 23). The CIDI ques-tions generally do a good job of suggesting to respondents how extreme and persistent these experiences need to be to qualify, but in some cases, lack of clarity remains.

As noted earlier, clinicians resolve this type of uncertainty in interviewer-based research diagnostic interviews by beginning with working models about the level needed to qualify for a particular symptom and then probing for concrete examples to determine whether the respondent's experience qualifies. For example, rather than ask, "Did you have a lot more trouble concentrating than is normal for you?" a clinician-interviewer would ask a series of questions such as, "Did you have trouble thinking or concentrat-ing?"; "(If so) What was that like?"; "What kinds of things did it interfere with?"; "Were you unable to read things that usually interest you or watch television or movies you usually like, because you could not pay attention to them?"; "Did it affect your work?"; "Tell me a little more about the ways in which it affected your work." or, "How often did this occur?" Responses would be integrated across all these sorts of questions by the clinician-in-terviewer based on their working model of the diagnostic criterion to rate the responses as either qualifying or not.

Our pilot work suggests that expansion of the CIDI questions to include more concrete examples along the lines of the questions asked in clinical interviews could go a long way to resolve misunderstandings of this type. However, for this to happen it would be necessary for CIDI development to be coordinated with independent clinical validation interviews that define the thresholds we seek to approximate in developing the example questions. Work of this type has not yet been carried out.

A third type of commonly misunderstood CIDI question found in our pilot work involves questions about odd experiences that could plausibly be interpreted in more than one way. The most challenging examples are in the evaluation of psychosis, where respondents are asked about such things as seeing and hearing things that others do not, someone reading their mind, and special messages being inserted directly into their mind. Many respondents have a tendency to normalize these questions and respond that yes, they have quite good vision or hearing or that they are so close to their spouse that it is sometimes as if he could read their mind or that there was once a time when a television program they watched the night before contained themes that happened to come up in real life for them the very next day.

In cases of this sort, it is critical that interviewers clarify for respondents the actual meaning of the questions and probe for examples to make sure respondents are understanding the questions as they were intended. In recognition of these special problems in the evaluation of psychosis, the CIDI includes instructions for interviewers to provide clarifications of this type and to elicit examples for each positive response to a question about psychotic symptoms. However, our pilot work for the NCS found that lay interviewers have great difficulty doing this, leading to extremely low validity of the CIDI psychosis section in relation to clinical interviews. As a result, we used a two-stage screening method to assess psychosis in the NCS in which the CIDI was followed with an independent clinican-administered evaluation of psychosis. Consistent with the pilot study results, the clinical follow-up interviews found that the CIDI psychosis section substantially overdiagnoses psychotic symptoms. Only 17% of CIDI cases of nonaffective psychosis were confirmed in the clinical reinterviews (Kendler, Gallagher, Abelson, & Kessler, 1996). We have been unable as yet to devise structured questions or procedures that resolve this problem in the framework of the CIDI.

A fourth type of commonly misunderstood CIDI question found in our pilot work, finally, involves a contextual misunderstanding; that is, a misunderstanding that derives more from the position of the question in the flow of the interview than from lack of clarity in the question. A good example is the evaluation of Criterion A in the *DSM–III–R* diagnosis of simple phobia, which stipulates that the fear of circumscribed stimuli must be persistent.

CIDI 1.0 operationalized this criterion by asking, "Did this strong unreasonable fear continue for months or even years?" Although seemingly not ambiguous in itself, the pilot work found that this question was misunderstood by a great many respondents because of the location of the question in the instrument. Specifically, this question followed an open-ended question that asked the respondent to give an example of a specific fear. In many cases the respondent would respond to this open-ended question by describing the autonomic arousal symptoms that occur on exposure to the stimulus such as feeling dizzy or having trouble breathing. When the follow-up question was administered right after this description—asking whether this fear continued for months or even years—the question was sometimes misunderstood as asking about the duration of the arousal symptoms. The respondent would invariably answer no, the nausea or dizziness or other physiological symptoms typically lasted no more than a few hours and certainly never went on for as long as months. This confusion led to under-diagnosis in these cases because CIDI 1.0 required a positive endorsement of the persistence question for a diagnosis. Once the potential for this misunderstanding was recognized, however, it was an easy matter to correct it with minor changes in question wording and placement.

TASK COMPREHENSION

Respondents not only sometimes misunderstand survey questions, but they also sometimes misunderstand the fundamental task they are being asked to carry out. Our debriefing studies found that misunderstanding of this second sort is especially common with the diagnostic stem questions in the CIDI. These stem questions are the first questions asked in each diagnostic section. They are used to determine whether a lifetime syndrome of a particular sort might have ever occurred. The questions provide what are, in effect, brief vignettes and ask the respondent whether they ever had an experience of this sort. If so, additional questions assess the specifics of the syndrome. If not, the remaining questions about this syndrome are skipped. As an example, one of the two diagnostic stems for major depression in CIDI 1.0 is, "In your lifetime, have you ever had two weeks or more when nearly every day you felt sad, blue, depressed?" (WHO, 1990, p. 20). If the respondent says no to this question as well as to a second stem question assessing anhedonia, he is coded as never having been depressed and the remaining questions about depression are skipped. We found that substantial confusion arose from respondents' failure to understand the purpose of such stem questions. In particular, only about half of the pilot respondents interpreted these questions as they were intended by the authors of the CIDI; namely, as a request to engage in active memory search and report episodes of the sort in the question. The other respondents interpreted the question as a request to report whether a memory of such an episode was readily accessible. These latter respondents did not believe that they were being asked to engage in active memory search and did not do so. Not surprisingly, these respondents were much less likely than those who understood the intent of the question to remember lifetime episodes.

Why did so many respondents misinterpret the intent of these lifetime recall questions? As Marquis and Cannell (1969) discovered in their research on standard interview practice, respondents are generally ill-informed about the purposes of the research and poorly motivated to participate actively. Furthermore, cues from interviewers often reinforce this inclination to participate in a half-hearted way. For example, when an interviewer asks a question that requires considerable thought, the respondent is likely to assume in the absence of instructions to the contrary that the interviewer is operating under normal conversational rules and, as such, is really asking for an immediate and appropriate answer. The work of Cannell et al. (1981) shows that this conversational artifact can be minimized by explicitly instructing respondents to answer completely and accurately. The use of such instructions can substantially improve the quality of data obtained in surveys.

Our work with the CIDI built on this result by investigating the effect of adding clarifying statements throughout the interview aimed at informing respondents that accuracy was important. For example, we experimented with the following introduction to CIDI stem questions for lifetime recall of specific psychiatric disorders, "The next question might be difficult to answer because you need to think back over your entire life. Please take your time and think carefully before answering." The use of this introduction led to a significant increase in the proportion of respondents who endorsed the stem questions.

MOTIVATION

One problem with emphasizing the need to work hard at a series of demanding and potentially embarrassing recall tasks is that more respondents than otherwise may refuse the job. Recognition of this problem among survey methodologists has led to the development of motivational techniques intended to increase the chances that respondents will accept the job of answering completely and accurately. Three techniques that have proven to be particularly useful in this regard are the use of motivational components in instructions, the use of contingent reinforcement strategies embedded in interviewer feedback probes, and the use of respondent commitment questions.

Motivational Instructions

There is evidence that clarifying instructions and research aims can help motivate complete and accurate reporting (Cannell et al., 1981). Debriefing shows that respondents are more willing to undertake laborious and possibly painful memory searches if they recognize some altruistic benefit of doing so. Even such an uncompelling rationale as "It is important for our research that you take your time and think carefully before answering" has motivational force. This is even more so when instructions include statements that have universalistic appeal, such as, "Accuracy is important because social policy makers will be using these results to make decisions that affect the lives of all of us." Based on this evidence, we developed and presented a statement containing a clear rationale for administering the CIDI at the onset of data collection and emphasized the importance of the survey for social policy purposes.

Contingent Reinforcements

Consistent with research on behavioral modification of verbal productions through reinforcement (e.g., Centers, 1964), several survey researchers have demonstrated that verbal reinforcers such as "thanks" and "that's useful" can significantly affect the behavior of survey respondents. Marquis and Cannell (1969), for example, showed experimentally that the use of such reinforcers resulted in a significant increase in the number of chronic conditions reported in response to an open-ended question about illnesses. These feedback remarks are often used in an unsystematic way, however, as part of general procedures to build and maintain rapport rather than in a systematic way to reinforce good respondent performance.

Based on these observations, Cannell and his associates developed a method for training interviewers to use systematic feedback—both positive and negative—to reinforce respondent effort in reporting (Oksenberg, Vinokur, & Cannell, 1979b). The central feature of this method is the use of structured feedback statements coordinated with the content and timing of instructions aimed at reinforcing respondent performance. It is important to recognize that it is performance that is being reinforced rather than the content of particular answers. For example, a difficult recall question may be prefaced with the instruction, "This next question may be difficult, so please take your time before answering." In contingent feedback instruction, interviewers would issue some expression of gratitude whenever the respondent seems to consider his or her answer carefully, whether they remembered anything or not. Alternatively, the interviewer might instruct the precipitous respondent, "You answered that awfully quickly. Was there anything (else), even something small?" Such invitations to reconsider would occur whenever the respondent gave an immediate answer whether or not anything was reported. We developed procedures of this sort so that structured feedback was programmed periodically throughout our CIDI interviews in the NCS in order to maintain the focus on performance standards and to reinforce motivation.

Experiments carried out by Cannell and his associates (Miller & Cannell, 1977; Vinokur, Oksenberg, & Cannell, 1979) have documented that the combined use of these contingent reinforcement probes with instructions explaining the importance of careful and accurate reporting leads to substantial improvement in recall of health-related events in general population surveys, including validated dates of medical events. Their results also show that self-enhancing response biases are reduced when these strategies are used, as indicated by both a decreased tendency to underreport potentially embarrassing conditions and behaviors (e.g., gynecologic problems, seeing an X-rated movie) and a decreased tendency to overreport self-enhancing behaviors (e.g., number of books read in the last 3 months, read the editorial page of the newspaper the previous day).

Commitment Questions

Instructions that define the nature of interviewer expectations for respondent behavior help to establish a perspective on the interview that can have motivational force. The literature on cognitive factors in surveys contains many examples of the subtle ways in which perspectives established in questions subsequently influence respondent behaviors. For example, Loftus and Palmer (1974) showed respondents a film of an automobile accident and asked them to estimate the speed the cars were traveling prior to the accident. Respondents estimated the rates as significantly greater if they were asked how fast the cars were traveling "when they collided" rather than "when they contacted each other." This same literature shows that perspective can have motivational force when it implies a common purpose (Clark & Schober, 1992). That is, if a question is posed in such a way that it implies that hard work will be invested in arriving at an answer, it is incumbent on the respondent either to demur explicitly or tacitly to accept the task of working hard as part of the common understanding between interviewer and respondent. By answering the question, the respondent, in effect, makes a commitment to honor the injunction implied in the perspective of the question and this implied commitment, in turn, creates motivation to this task (Marlatt, 1972).

Cannell, Miller, and Oskenberg (1981), based on this type of thinking, showed that it is possible to motivate the respondent to accept the goal of serious and active reporting by asking an explicit commitment question as part of the interview. This was done by prefacing the section of the interview that asked a series of lifetime diagnostic stem questions with the following commitment question:

> This interview asks about your physical and emotional well-being and about areas of your life that could affect your physical and emotional well-being. It is important for us to get accurate information. In order to do this, you will need to think carefully before answering the following questions. Are you willing to do this?

Consistent with the results of previous studies using similar questions (Cannell et al., 1981), we found that only a small fraction of respondents answered negatively. These interviews were terminated, based on the decision not to invest interviewer time on respondents not willing to work seriously at the task. Experimental studies carried out by Cannell and his associates (Cannell et al., 1981; Oksenberg et al., 1979a, 1979b) have shown that commitment questions improve accuracy of recall. Furthermore, their studies indicate that the joint use of motivating instructions, contingent feedback, and a commitment question has an interactive effect that increases the intensity of memory search and accuracy beyond the effects of any one component separately. This extends not only to the proportion of respondents in different experimental conditions who recall and report past experiences but also to other indicators of commitment such as amount of detail reported and use of personal records and other outside information sources such as memory aids during the course of the interview.

THE ABILITY TO ANSWER ACCURATELY

Episodic and Semantic Memories

Research on basic cognitive processes has shown that memories are organized and stored in structured sets of information packages commonly called schemas (Markus & Zajonc, 1985). When the respondent has a history of many instances of the same experience that cannot be discriminated, the separate instances tend to blend together in memory to form a special kind of memory schema called a *semantic memory*, a general memory for a prototypical experience (Jobe et al., 1990; Means & Loftus, 1991). For example, the person may have a semantic memory of what panic attacks are like but, due to the fact that he has had many such attacks in his lifetime, cannot specify details of any particular panic attack. In comparison, when the respondent has had only a small number of lifetime experiences of a certain sort or when one instance stands out in memory as much different from the others, a memory can likely be recovered for that particular episode. This is called an *episodic memory.*

In the case of memories of illness experiences, memory schemas tend to include not only semantic memories of prototypic symptoms but also personal theories about causes, course, and cure (Leventhal, Nerenz, & Steele, 1984; Skelton & Croyle, 1991). Some of these theories will conceptualize the experience in illness terms and others as a moral failing, a punishment from God, or a normal reaction to stress (Gilman, 1988). These interpretations influence the extent to which different memory cues are capable of triggering the schemas.

The effects of memory schemas and the difference between semantic and episodic memories are central themes in research on autobiographical memory. Indeed, we must determine whether episodic memories can be recovered and whether the respondent is answering the questions by referring to episodic memories or by drawing inferences of what the past must have been like on the basis of more general semantic memories. Research shows that people are more likely to recover episodic memories for experiences that are recent, distinctive, and unique, whereas for experiences that are frequent, typical, and regular, people will rely more on semantic memories (Belli, 1988; Brewer, 1986; Menon, 1994).

Asking Questions Without Knowing the Limits of Memory

When a survey question is designed to ask about a particular instance of an experience, it must be posed in such a way that the respondent knows he or she is being asked to recover an episodic memory. The researcher must have some basis for assuming that an episodic memory can be recovered for this experience. If it cannot, a question that asks for such a memory implicitly invites the respondent to infer or estimate rather than remember and this can have adverse effects on quality of reporting later in the interview (Pearson, Ross, & Dawes, 1992). In comparison, when a question is designed to recover a semantic memory or to use semantic memories to arrive at an answer by estimation, that should be made clear.

One difficulty with these injunctions in the case of retrospective recall questions about lifetime psychiatric disorders is uncertainty about what level of recall accuracy to expect. We confronted this problem in our work with the CIDI when we asked the standard CIDI questions about first onset, such as the panic onset question, "When was the first time you had one of these sudden spells of feeling frightened or anxious and had these problems like (PREVIOUSLY ENDORSED SYMPTOMS OF PANIC)?" (WHO, 1990, p. 13). Debriefing of pilot respondents revealed that some people had very vivid memories of their first panic attack, whereas others had no such memory.

The problem posed by this variation was how to develop a method of asking the question that reinforced our overall commitment to collect complete and accurate information while simultaneously recognizing the limits of autobiographical memory and avoiding a request for a precise answer from the subsample of respondents who were unable to recover an episodic memory for their first episode.

We resolved this problem by adapting several of the principles discussed previously to a three-part question series designed to inform respondents that answers should be as precise as possible while still recognizing the limits of memory. The question sequence began with what has been referred to in the literature as a *prequest*, a question aimed at clarifying the nature of the request for information in subsequent questions. The prequest question was:

> Can you remember your EXACT age the VERY FIRST TIME you had a sudden spell of feeling frightened or anxious and had several of these other things ("other things" refers to a checklist of symptoms that respondents previously reported which was presented for visual review on a cue card) at the same time? (Cannell et al., 1981, p. 24; emphasis in original)

During the pilot work, we probed positive responses to determine the basis for exact recall and discovered that, in general, these respondents were either younger (i.e., the event was likely to have occurred more recently), had a smaller number of lifetime episodes, or had a distinctive context that allowed them to date the age of their vividly recalled first attack. Based on this information, the final question series simply followed this answer with the question, "How old were you?" In comparison, respondents who answered the prequest negatively were asked a different follow-up question phrased in such a way as to make it clear that we wanted an estimate, based on our understanding that the respondent could not provide an exact answer. This question was: "ABOUT [emphasis in original] how old were you (the first time you had one of these attacks)?" Interviewers were instructed to accept a range response (e.g., "sometime in my early 20s") without probing, as we were soliciting an estimate. This question was then followed by another that was designed to provide an upper bound on our uncertainty concerning age-of-onset and to permit the respondent to answer even when uncertain about the exact age of the first attack: "What is the earliest age you can CLEARLY REMEMBER [emphasis in original] having one of these attacks?"

The latter question is much less demanding than the original question about the exact age of the very first attack and, not surprisingly in light of this, virtually all respondents were able to provide an age in their answer. Interestingly, the age given in response to this question was often earlier than the lower bound of the age range given in response to the preceding question. Debriefing showed that this seemingly inconsistent result was due to the fact that estimation was typically used to arrive at the response to the question, "ABOUT how old were you . . . ?" while active memory search focusing on the part of the life span implied by the answer to the preceding question was used to arrive at the response to the subsequent question.

It is difficult to know what effect this approach had on the accuracy of age of onset reports because there is no clear way of validating such reports. It is possible, however, to make an indirect assessment of this matter by building on previous evidence of bias in age of onset reports based on responses to the standard CIDI age of onset question. This evidence comes from the work of Simon and Von Korff (1995), who showed that respondents in the ECA Study who reported lifetime episodes of major depression gave implausible age of onset reports that clustered about 5 years before the interview, no matter how old the respondents were at the time of interview. A pattern of this sort is totally inconsistent with what we know about the age of onset distribution of depression in clinical samples, which shows that depression tends to be an early-onset disorder for many people with peak age of risk in the late teens through the middle years of life. The age of onset pattern found in the ECA is much more consistent with the methodological interpretation that most respondents do not have a vivid memory of age of onset and give reports about the last episode they can remember rather than the first episode they might have remembered if they had engaged in a more active memory search. If the more elaborate procedures we developed to assess age of onset are an improvement over the standard procedure, we would expect this problem to be reduced. Knäuper, Cannell, Schwarz, Bruce, and Kessler (in press), in a comparative analysis of the ECA data and data from the NCS, found that this was the case. There was no evidence in the NCS of a concentration of reported onsets 5 years earlier than the age at interview of respondents.

CONSOLIDATING THE DATA QUALITY-IMPROVEMENT STRATEGIES

We have reviewed a number of strategies that we used to optimize data quality in the CIDI either by improving understanding, by enhancing respondent commitment, or by adjusting questions to recognize that some respondents will be less able than others to provide completely accurate responses. As discussed in more detail elsewhere (Kessler, Mroczek & Belli, in press), we developed some additional strategies to deal with two or more of these problems at once. The most important of the latter was the development of a life review section that we administered near the beginning of the interview in an effort to both motivate and facilitate active memory search in answering CIDI diagnostic stem questions. This section started out with an introduction that explained to respondents that the questions might be difficult to answer because they required respondents to review their entire lives. The introduction then went on to say that despite this difficulty, it was very important for the research that these questions be answered accurately. The introduction ended with the injunction to "please take your time and think carefully before answering." The diagnostic stem questions for all CIDI diagnoses were then administered. Our hope in developing this section was that we could both explain the nature of the task and motivate the active memory search we hoped to stimulate by combining all the stem questions after a fairly detailed motivational introduction. We also recognized, based on our debriefing studies, that CIDI respondents quickly learn the logic of the stem-branch structure after a few sections and recognize that they can shorten the interview considerably by saying no to the stem questions. This problem was removed by asking all the stem questions near the beginning of the interview before the logic of the stem-branch structure became clear. Furthermore, respondents told us in debriefing interviews that their energy flagged as the interview progressed, making it much more difficult to carry out a serious memory search later in the interview than at the beginning. Again, the creation of a consolidated life review section near the beginning of the interview helped resolve this problem.

An experimental evaluation of the impact of using the life review section was carried out by randomly assigning 200 community respondents either to the standard version of the CIDI or to a version that was identical except that it included the life review section. As reported in more detail elsewhere (Kessler et al., 1998), this experiment documented that the life review section led to a significant increase in the proportion of respondents who endorsed diagnostic stem questions. For example, although 26.7% of respondents in the standard CIDI condition endorsed the "sad, blue, or depressed" stem question for major depression, a significantly higher 40.6% did so in the life review condition.

EVALUATING THE EFFECTS OF THE MODIFICATIONS

The previous sections reviewed a number of results from NCS pilot studies and evaluations carried out in the wake of the NCS that documented significant effects of our various CIDI modifications. Such things as the use of the life review section, the decomposition of complex questions into less complex subquestions, and the use of feedback to encourage thoughtful responses were found to change the responses of people interviewed with the

CIDI. It is not clear from any of the results reported so far, however, whether these changes were for the better or worse. Did we, as we hoped, change responses to be more accurate? Or did we have the opposite effect? This question is perhaps most important when it comes to prevalence estimates. We know that the NCS obtained much higher prevalence estimates than the ECA study. The lifetime prevalence of major depression in the NCS, for example, was over 17% (Kessler et al., 1994) compared to approximately 7% in the baseline ECA (Weissman, Bruce, Leaf, Florio, & Holzer, 1991). Could it be that our efforts to facilitate and motivate complete reporting led to overreporting of clinically unimportant experiences that were incorrectly coded as disorders? Or did we learn about genuine disorders that were overlooked in the ECA Study?

A definitive answer is impossible to obtain because of the many differences between the NCS and ECA, including date of administration (early 1980s for the ECA and early 1990s for the NCS), sampling frame (five local areas in the ECA and a nationally representative sample in the NCS), age range of the sample (18 and older in the ECA and 15 to 54 in the NCS) and diagnostic system (*DSM-III* in the ECA and *DSM-III-R* in the NCS). It would be possible to carry out a validation experiment in which the different versions of the DIS-CIDI were administered to random subsamples of a general population sample and identical clinical reinterviews used to carry out a comparative validation, but such an investigation has not as yet been funded. However, three observations lead us to believe that the modifications we introduced into the CIDI are improvements.

The first of these three concerns the basic NCS-ECA comparison. Comparative studies were done by NCS and ECA investigators to learn about reasons for differences in the prevalence estimates in the two surveys. As reported in more detail elsewhere (Regier et al., 1998), the NCS data were recoded to *DSM-III* criteria (the criteria used in the ECA) and the samples in the two surveys were restricted to be as comparable as possible (urban, White respondents in the age range 18–54) for purposes of this comparison. These modifications had little effect on the between-survey difference. However, the ECA Study had two waves of data collection. An attempt was made to reinterview all ECA respondents 1 year after the baseline interview. When the diagnostic data are combined across these two waves, coding respondents as having a lifetime diagnosis either if they met criteria in the baseline interview or in the follow-up interview, the differences between the ECA and NCS prevalence estimates virtually disappear. That is, the NCS appears to have obtained in a single interview very similar prevalence estimates to those obtained in two ECA interviews.

The most plausible interpretation of this result is that the methodological innovations in the NCS led to more complete recall than in the baseline ECA but that the second chance provided by the ECA reinterview made up for this difference. Several observations are consistent with this interpretation. First, there was evidence of substantial recall failure in the ECA. Focusing on major depression as an example, the estimated lifetime prevalence in the ECA increased by 78% over the 1-year reinterview period and the vast majority of this increase came from respondents in the reinterview reporting episodes of depression that they said occurred before the baseline interview but that were not reported in the baseline interview. In comparison, a community survey in Canada that used the NCS interview approach and a 1-year follow-up interview found an increased lifetime prevalence estimate of depression only about one fourth as large as this, suggesting that a much larger proportion of all potentially reportable episodes are captured in the baseline interview when the NCS procedures are used (R. J. Turner, personal communication, November 1998).

Second, if the two-wave ECA data are comparable to the cross-sectional NCS data, we would expect to find not only that the prevalence estimates are similar but also that more subtle aspects of the data, such as symptom profiles, are similar. This is, in fact, what was found in the comparative analysis. The rank-order correlations of relative symptom prevalences among cases in the two surveys were in the range between .6 and .8 for all diagnoses considered. And critical marker symptoms were quite similar as well. For example, the conditional lifetime prevalences of reported suicide attempts among NCS and ECA lifetime depressives were very similar, indicating that the diagnostic classifications tapped into the same level of syndrome severity.

Third, data from the ECA and NCS validity studies show that despite the much higher prevalences in the NCS than the baseline ECA, the NCS respondents classified as cases were equally as likely as baseline ECA cases to be confirmed as true cases in blind clinical reinterviews. There is some slippage in this comparison because the methods and procedures in the ECA (Helzer, Robins, McEvoy, & Spitznagel, 1985) and NCS (Wittchen, Kessler, Zhao & Abelson, 1995; Wittchen et al., 1996) validity studies differ in several important ways. Nonetheless, if the much higher lifetime prevalence estimates in the NCS are due to false positives, we would expect that a much lower proportion of NCS cases than ECA cases would be confirmed as true cases by clinicians. This is not what we found. The positive predictive value of diagnoses was as high or higher in the NCS as the reported ECA validity study for every diagnosis.

FUTURE DIRECTIONS

Although the modifications described previously appear to have been successful in improving the CIDI, considerable work remains to be done. As noted previously, the WHO CIDI Field Trials (Wittchen, 1994) and the NCS clinical reappraisal studies (Blazer et al., 1994; Kessler, Crum, et al., 1997; Wittchen et al., 1995; Wittchen et al., 1996) both found that the correspondence between CIDI diagnoses and independent clinician-based diagnoses of most disorders is far from perfect. The CIDI validities are unacceptably low for mania (Kessler, Rubinow, et al., in press) and nonaffective psychosis (Kendler et al., 1996).

More detailed analysis of criterion-level correspondence between the CIDI and clinician-based interviews shows that the validity problem can be traced to only one or two criteria in most diagnoses. For example, the NCS clinical reappraisal study of *DSM–III–R* generalized anxiety disorder (GAD; Wittchen et al., 1995) found that the only criterion with serious disagreements between the CIDI and the clinical interviews was A2, which stipulates that the worries must be "excessive or unrealistic" (APA, 1987, p. 251). Most of these discrepancies occurred when respondents reported worries that they considered not to be either excessive or unrealistic associated with two or more objectively serious life problems, but the clinical interviewers judged that the worries were excessive or unrealistic.

When the source of invalidity is isolated in this way, it is likely that an improvement in just one criterion would have a dramatic impact on overall diagnostic validity. In the case of GAD, for example, the Kappa coefficient describing the diagnostic consistency between the CIDI and the clinical interviews increases from .47 to .66 when we delete the stipulation in Criterion A2 that the worries must be excessive or unrealistic, a deletion consistent with ICD–10 (WHO, 1993).

Pinpointing the source of invalidity in this way can also focus thinking about corrective possibilities. It might be that a simple change in question wording will be enough. Or perhaps a series of questions need to be used instead of only one question to operationalize an especially complex criterion. In still other cases, there might be a confusion in the diagnostic system itself. This last possibility is what underlies the problem with the CIDI operationalization of GAD Criterion A2, as *DSM–III–R* gives little guidance on how to make this evaluation. Fortunately, this criterion was clarified in *DSM–IV* (APA, 1994), where it is stated that although patients with GAD may deny that their worries are excessive, this can be inferred from the existence of subjective distress due to constant worry, difficulty controlling the worry, or role impairment due to the worry. It is likely that this clarification will lead to greater consistency between a revised series of CIDI questions and a more focused evaluation of this criterion in future validation studies.

Another challenging issue for future investigation concerns the difficult question of whether respondents are honest either with the interviewer or with themselves in discussing their mental health. The issue of honesty is a problematic one. The methodological literature on the accuracy of respondent reports shows clearly that the perceived social desirability of responses is as important as understanding or memory in determining the accuracy of reports (Kessler & Wethington, 1991; Sudman & Bradburn, 1974). We have no way of assessing the magnitude of this problem with available data, but it clearly needs to be taken into consideration as research in this area moves forward.

ACKNOWLEDGMENTS

The National Comorbidity Survey (NCS) is a collaborative epidemiologic investigation of the prevalences, causes, and consequences of psychiatric morbidity and comorbidity in the United States supported by the National Institute of Mental Health (R01 MH46376, R01 MH49098, and RO1 MH52861) with supplemental support from the National Institute of Drug Abuse (through a supplement to MH46376) and the W. T. Grant Foundation (90135190), Ronald C. Kessler, Principal Investigator. Preparation for this report was also supported by a Research Scientist Award to Kessler (K05 MH00507). Collaborating NCS sites and investigators are: The Addiction Research Foundation (Robin Room), Duke University Medical Center (Dan Blazer, Marvin Swartz), Harvard Medical School (Richard Frank, Ronald Kessler), Johns Hopkins University (James Anthony, William Eaton, Philip Leaf), the Max Planck Institute of Psychiatry Clinical Institute (Hans-Ulrich Wittchen), the Medical College of Virginia (Kenneth Kendler), the University of Miami (R. Jay Turner), the University of Michigan (Lloyd Johnston, Roderick Little), New York University (Patrick Shrout), SUNY Stony Brook (Evelyn Bromet), and Washington University School of Medicine (Linda Cottler, Andrew Heath). Portions of this chapter previously appeared in *Assessment in Child and Adolescent Psychopathology* (eds. D. Shaffer and J. Richters), New York: Guilford Press; and *Sociology of Mental Health and Illness* (eds. V. Horwitz and T. L. Scheid), New York: Cambridge University Press.

A complete list of all NCS publications along with abstracts, study documentation, interview schedules, and the raw NCS public use data files can be obtained directly from the NCS Homepage by using the URL: http://www.hcp.med.harvard.edu/ncs

REFERENCES

American Psychiatric Association. (1980). *Diagnostic and statistical manual of mental disorders* (3rd ed.). Washington, DC: Author.
American Psychiatric Association. (1987). *Diagnostic and statistical manual of mental disorders* (Rev. 3rd ed.). Washington, DC: Author.

American Psychiatric Association. (1994). *Diagnostic and statistical manual of mental disorders* (Rev. 4th ed.). Washington, DC: Author.

Belli, R. F. (1988). Color blend retrievals: Compromise memories or deliberate compromise responses? *Memory and Cognition, 16,* 314–326.

Belson, W. A. (1981). *The design and understanding of survey questions.* Aldershot, England: Gower.

Biderman, A. (1980). *Report of a workshop on applying cognitive psychology to recall problems of the national crime survey.* Washington, DC: Bureau of Social Science Research.

Blazer, D. G., Kessler, R. C., McGonagle, K. A., & Swartz, M. S. (1994). The prevalence and distribution of major depression in a national community sample: The National Comorbidity Survey. *American Journal of Psychiatry, 151,* 979–986.

Bradburn, N., & Sudman, S. (1979). *Improving interview method and questionnaire design: Response effects to threatening questions in survey research.* San Francisco: Jossey-Bass.

Brewer, W. F. (1986). What is autobiographical memory? In D. C. Rubin (Ed.), *Autobiographical memory* (pp. 25–49). New York: Cambridge University Press.

Brown, G. W. (1989). Life events and measurement. In G. W. Brown & T. O. Harris (Eds.), *Life events and illness* (pp. 3–45). New York: Guilford.

Cannell, C. F., Fowler, F. J., & Marquis, K. H. (1968). The influence of interviewer and respondent psychological and behavioral variables on the reporting in household interviews. *Vital and Health Statistics, 26*(2), 1–65.

Cannell, C. F., Miller, P. V., & Oksenberg, L. (1981). Research on interviewing techniques. In S. Leinhardt (Ed.), *Sociological methodology 1981* (pp. 389–437). San Francisco: Jossey-Bass.

Centers, R. (1964). A laboratory adaptation of the conversational procedure for the conditioning of verbal operants. *Journal of Abnormal and Social Psychology, 67,* 334–339.

Clark, H. H., & Schober, M. F. (1992). Asking questions and influencing answers. In J. M. Tanur (Ed.), *Questions about questions: Inquiries into the cognitive bases of surveys* (pp. 15–48). New York: Russell Sage Foundation.

Dohrenwend, B. P., & Dohrenwend, B. S. (1965). The problem of validity in field studies of psychological disorder. *Journal of Abnormal Psychology, 70,* 52–69.

Dohrenwend, B. P., Yager, T. J., Egri, G., & Mendelsohn, F. S. (1978). The psychiatric status schedule (PSS) as a measure of dimensions of psychopathology in the general population. *Archives of General Psychiatry, 35,* 731–739.

Endicott, J., & Spitzer, R. (1978). A diagnostic interview: The schedule for affective disorders and schizophrenia. *Archives of General Psychiatry, 137,* 837–844.

Faris, R. E. L., & Dunham, H. W. (1939). *Mental disorders in urban areas.* Chicago: University of Chicago Press.

Feighner, J. P., Robins, E., & Guze, S. B. (1972). Diagnostic criteria for use in psychiatric research. *Archives of General Psychiatry, 26,* 57–63.

Gilman, S. (1988). *Disease and representation: Images of illness from madness to AIDS.* Ithaca, NY: Cornell University Press.

Gurin, G., Veroff, J., & Feld, S. (1960). *Americans view their mental health.* New York: Basic Books.

Helzer, J. E., Robins, L. N., McEvoy, L. T., & Spitznagel, E. (1985). A comparison of clinical and diagnostic interview schedule diagnoses. *Archives of General Psychiatry, 42* 657–666.

Hollingshead, A. B., & Redlich, F. C. (1958). *Social class and mental illness: A community study.* New York: Wiley.

Hunter, R., & Macalpine, I. (Eds.). (1963). *Three hundred years of psychiatry.* New York: Oxford University Press.

Illich, I. (1975). *Medical nemesis: The expropriation of health.* London: Calder and Boyars.

Jabine, T., Straf, M., Tanur, J. M., & Tourangeau, R. (Eds.). (1984). *Cognitive aspects of survey methodology: Building a bridge between disciplines.* Report of the Advanced Research Seminar on Cognitive Aspects of Survey Methodology. Washington, DC: National Academy Press.

Jobe, J. B., White, A. A., Kelley, C. L., Mingay, D. L., Sanchez, M. J., & Loftus, E. F. (1990). Recall strategies and memory for health care visits. *The Milbank Quarterly, 68,* 171–189.

Keller, M. B., Lavori, P. W., Nielsen, E. (1987). *SCALUP (SCID Plus SADS-L)*. Providence, RI: Department of Psychiatry, Butler Hospital.

Kendler, K. S., Gallagher, T. J., Abelson, J. M., & Kessler, R. C. (1996). Lifetime prevalence, demographic risk factors, and diagnostic validity of nonaffective psychosis as assessed in a U.S. community sample: The National Comorbidity Survey. *Archives of General Psychiatry, 53,* 1022–1031.

Kessler, R. C., Crum, R. M., Warner, L. A., Nelson, C. B., Schulenberg, J., & Anthony, J. C. (1997). The lifetime co-occurrence of DSM–III–R alcohol abuse and dependence with other psychiatric disorders in the National Comorbidity Survey. *Archives of General Psychiatry, 54,* 313–321.

Kessler, R. C., McGonagle, K. A., Zhao, S., Nelson, C. B., Hughes, M., Eshleman, S., Wittchen, H.-U., & Kendler, K. S. (1994). Lifetime and 12-month prevalence of DSM–III–R psychiatric disorders in the United States: Results from the National Comorbidity Survey. *Archives of General Psychiatry, 51,* 8–19.

Kessler, R. C., & Mroczek, D. K. (1995). Measuring the effects of medical interventions. *Medical Care, 33,* AS109–AS119.

Kessler, R. C., Mroczek, D. K., & Belli, R. F. (in press). Retrospective adult assessment of childhood psychopathology. In D. Shaffer & J. Richters (Eds.), *Assessment in child and adolescent psychopathology*. New York: Guilford.

Kessler, R. C., Rubinow, D. R., Holmes, C., Abelson, J. M., & Zhao, S. (1997). The epidemiology of DSM–III–R bipolar I disorder in a general population survey. *Psychological Medicine, 27,* 1079–1089.

Kessler, R. C., & Wethington, E. (1991). The reliability of life event reports in a community survey. *Psychological Medicine, 21,* 723–738.

Kessler, R. C., Wittchen, H-U., Abelson, J. M., McGonagle, K. A., Schwarz, N., Kendler, K. S., Knäuper, B., & Zhao, S. (1998). Methodological studies of the Composite International Diagnostic Interview (CIDI) in the U.S. National Comorbidity Survey. *International Journal of Methods in Psychiatric Research, 7,* 33–55.

Kessler, R. C., & Zhao, S. (in press). The prevalence of mental illness. In A. V. Horwitz & T. L. Scheid (Eds.), *Sociology of mental health and illness*. New York: Cambridge University Press.

Knäuper, B., Cannell, C. F., Schwarz, N., Bruce, M. L., & Kessler, R. C. (in press). Improving accuracy of major depression age of onset reports in the U.S. National Comorbidity Survey. *International Journal of Methods in Psychiatric Research*.

Leighton, A. H. (1959). *My Name is Legion. Vol. I of the Stirling County Study*. New York: Basic Books.

Leventhal, H., Nerenz, D., & Steele, D. J. (1984). Illness representations and coping with health threats. In A. Baum, S. E. Taylor, & J. E. Singer (Eds.), *Handbook of Psychology & Health* (Vol. 4, pp. 219–252). Hillsdale, NJ: Lawrence Erlbaum Associates.

Loftus, E. F., & Palmer, J. C. (1974). Reconstruction of automobile destructions: An example of the integration between language and memory. *Journal of Verbal Language and Verbal Behavior, 13,* 585–589.

Markus, H., & Zajonc, R. B. (1985). The cognitive perspective in social psychology. In G. Lindzey & E. Aronson (Eds.), *The handbook of social psychology* (3rd ed., pp. 137–230). New York: Random House.

Marlatt, G. A. (1972). Task structure and the experimental modification of verbal behavior. *Psychological Bulletin, 78,* 335–350.

Marquis, K. H., & Cannell, C. F. (1969). *A study of interviewer-respondent interaction in the urban employment*. Ann Arbor: University of Michigan.

Means, B., & Loftus, E. F. (1991). When personal history repeats itself: Decomposing memories for recurring events. *Applied Cognitive Psychology, 5,* 297–318.

Menon, A. (1994). Judgements of behavioral frequencies: Memory search and retrieval strategies. In N. Schwartz & S. Sudman (Eds.), *Autobiographical memory and the validity of retrospective reports* (pp. 161–172). New York: Springer-Verlag.

Miller, P. V., & Cannell, C. F. (1977). Communicating measurement objectives in the survey interview. In P. M. Hirsch, P. V. Miller, & F. G. Kline (Eds.), *Strategies for communication research* (Vol. 6, pp. 127–151). Beverly Hills, CA: Sage.

Moss, C., & Goldstein, H. (Eds.). (1979). *The recall method in social surveys*. London: NFER Publishing.

Newman, S. C., Shrout, P. E., & Bland, R. C. (1990). The efficiency of two-phase designs in prevalence surveys of mental disorders. *Psychological Medicine, 20,* 183–193.

Oksenberg, L., Cannell, C. F., & Kanton, G. (1991). New strategies for pretesting survey questions. *Journal of Official Statistics, 7,* 349–365.

Oksenberg, L., Vinokur, A., & Cannell, C. F. (1979a). Effects of commitment to being a good respondent on interview performance. In C. F. Cannell, L. Oksenberg, & J. M. Converse (Eds.), *Experiments in interviewing techniques* (DHEW Publication No. (HRA) 78-3204, pp. 74–108). Washington, DC: Department of Health, Education, and Welfare.

Oksenberg, L., Vinokur, A., & Cannell, C. F. (1979b). The effects of instructions, commitment and feedback on reporting in personal interviews. In C. F. Cannell, L. Oksenberg, & J. M. Converse (Eds.), *Experiments in interviewing techniques* (DHEW Publication No. (HRA) 78-3204, pp. 133–199). Washington, DC: Department of Health, Education, and Welfare.

Pearson, R. W., Ross, M., & Dawes, R. M. (1992). Personal recall and the limits of retrospective questions in surveys. In J. M. Tanur (Ed.), *Questions about questions: Inquiries into the cognitive bases of surveys* (pp. 65–94). New York: Russell Sage Foundation.

Radloff, L. S. (1977). The CES-D Scale: A self-report depression scale for research in the general population. *Applied Psychology Measurement, 1,* 385–401.

Regier, D. A., Farmer, M. E., Rae, D. A., Locke, B. Z., Keith, B. J., Judd, L. L., & Goodwin, F. K. (1990). Comorbidity of mental health disorders with alcohol and other drug abuse. *Journal of the American Medical Association, 264,* 2511–2518.

Regier, D. A., Kaelber, C. T., Rae, D. S., Farmer, M. E., Knäuper, B., Kessler, R. C., & Norquist, G. S. (1998). Limitations of diagnostic criteria and assessment instruments for mental disorders: Implications for research and policy. *Archives of General Psychiatry, 55,* 109–115.

Regier, D. A., Narrow, W. E., Rae, D. S., Manderscheid, R. W., Locke, B. Z., & Goodwin, F. K. (1993). The de Facto U.S. Mental and Addictive Disorders Service System: Epidemiologic catchment area prospective 1-year prevalence rates of disorders and services. *Archives of General Psychiatry, 50,* 85–94.

Robins, L. N., Helzer, J. E., Croughan, J. L., & Ratcliff, K. S. (1981). National Institute of Mental Health Diagnostic Interview Schedule: Its history, characteristics and validity. *Archives of General Psychiatry, 38,* 381–389.

Robins, L. N., & Regier, D. A. (1991). *Psychiatric disorders in America: The Epidemiologic Catchment Area Study.* New York: The Free Press.

Seiler, L. H. (1973). The 22-item scale used in field studies of mental illness: A question of method, a question of substance, and a question of theory. *Journal of Health and Social Behavior, 14,* 252–264.

Simon, G. E., & Von Korff, M. (1995). Recall of psychiatric history in cross-sectional surveys: Implications for epidemiologic research. *Epidemiologic Reviews, 17,* 221–227.

Skelton, J. A., & Croyle, R. T. (Eds.). (1991). *Mental representation in health and illness.* New York: Springer-Verlag.

Spitzer, R. L., Williams, J. B. W., Gibbon, M., & First, M. B. (1992). The structured clinical interview for DSM-III-R. I: History, rationale and description. *Archives of General Psychiatry, 49,* 624–629.

Srole, L, Langer, T. S., Michael, S. T., Opler, M. K., & Rennie, T. A. C. (1962). *Mental health in the metropolis. The Midtown Manhattan Study.* New York: McGraw-Hill.

Sudman, S., & Bradburn, N. M. (1974). *Response effects in surveys: A review & synthesis.* Chicago: Aldine.

Tanur, J. M. (Ed.). (1992). *Questions about questions: Inquiries into the cognitive bases of surveys.* New York: Russell Sage Foundation.

Thase, M. E., Buysse, D. J., Frank, E., Cherry, C. R., Cornes, C. L., Mallinger, A. G., & Kupfer, D. J. (1997). Which depressed patients will respond to interpersonal psychotherapy? The role of abnormal EEG sleep profiles. *American Journal of Psychiatry, 154*, 502–509.

Vinokur, A., Oksenberg, L., & Cannell, C. F. (1979). Effects of feedback and reinforcement on the report of health information. In C. F. Cannell, L. Oksenberg, & J. M. Converse (Eds.), *Experiments in interviewing techniques.* Ann Arbor: University of Michigan.

Weissman, M. M., Bruce, M. L., Leaf, P. J., Florio, L. P., Holzer, C., Ill. (1991). Affective disorders. In L. N. Robins & D. A. Regier (Eds.), *Psychiatric disorders in America. The Epidemiologic Catchment Area Study* (pp. 53–80). New York: The Free Press.

Weissman, M. M., & Myers, J. K. (1978). Affective disorders in a U.S. urban community. *Archives of General Psychiatry, 35*, 1304–1311.

Wittchen, H. U. (1994). Reliability and validity studies of the WHO-Composite International Diagnostic Interview (CIDI): A critical review. *Journal of Psychiatric Research, 28*, 57–84.

Wittchen, H.-U., Kessler, R. C., Zhao, S., & Abelson, J. (1995). Reliability and clinical validity of UM–CIDI DSM–III–R generalized anxiety disorder. *Journal of Psychiatric Research, 29*, 95–110.

Wittchen, H.-U., Zhao, S., Abelson, J. M., Abelson, J. L., & Kessler, R. C. (1996). Reliability and procedural validity of UM-CIDI DSM–III–R phobic disorders. *Psychological Medicine, 26*, 1169–1177.

World Health Organization. (1977). *International classification of diseases—9th Revision.* Geneva, Switzerland: Author.

World Health Organization. (1990). *Composite international diagnostic interview (CIDI, Version 1.0).* Geneva, Switzerland: Author.

World Health Organization. (1993). *International classification of diseases—10 classification of mental and behavioral disorders: Diagnostic criteria for research.* Geneva, Switzerland: Author.

World Health Organization. (1997). *Composite international diagnostic interview (CIDI). Core Version 2.1.* Geneva, Switzerland: Author.

15

"I Took the Medicine Like You Told Me, Doctor": Self-Report of Adherence With Medical Regimens

Cynthia S. Rand
Johns Hopkins University

> *[The physician]* should keep aware of the fact that patients often lie when they state that they have taken certain medicines.
>
> —Hippocrates

Patient adherence with medical regimens is often inadequate (Gordis, 1976; Jay, Litt, & Durant, 1984; Kasl, 1975; Masur, 1981; Melnikow & Kiefe, 1994; Varni & Wallander, 1984) and is associated with poor clinical outcomes (The Coronary Drug Research Project Group, 1980; Korsch, Fine, & Negrete, 1978; Richardson, Shelton, Krailo, & Levine, 1990; Wall et al., 1995). Nonadherence with health care provider recommendations can take many forms including not taking all prescribed doses of medication, neglecting preventive measures, such as immunizations or breast cancer screening, as well as failing to change damaging behaviors, such as smoking or a high-fat diet. Nonadherence with therapy can be costly and risky to an individual's health as well as expensive to society in terms of unnecessary health care costs (Smith, 1985).

Considerable research has examined not only the extent of nonadherence but also the possible predictors of poor adherence and potential intervention strategies for improving patient adherence with therapy. Identifying nonadherent behavior in patients or research participants is the necessary prerequisite to accurately measuring the impact of nonadherence and evaluating the efficacy of adherence-promotion interventions. The most commonly used clinical and research strategy for assessing patient adherence is self-report (Rand, 1990). However, the reliability and validity of self-reports of adherence with therapy have been found to be highly variable across a wide range of diseases and medical regimens. This chapter reviews the importance of accurate assessments of adherence as well as the research findings on the accuracy of self-reported adherence in clinical and research settings. Those factors that can influence the reliability and validity of self-report are discussed as well as the relationship between measurement strategy and the predictors of adherence. Finally, a rationale and a strategy for improving the usefulness and the validity of self-reported adherence in both a research and a clinical setting are offered.

THE CONSEQUENCES OF ADHERENCE MISCLASSIFICATION

In Clinical Care

The indigent, minority patient with unstable diabetes and the White college professor with uncontrolled diabetes may share a disease diagnosis. However, they are unlikely to share an adherence classification. Physicians' reliance on clinical judgment to determine patient adherence can lead to misjudgments about patient behaviors based on personal characteristics such as education and social class (Sackett & Haynes, 1976). Physicians often fail to directly question patients about their adherence with therapy, or, if they do ask, they may employ an interviewing style that discourages candor about nonadherence (e.g., you didn't stop taking your medicine did you?; Steele, Jackson, & Gutmann, 1990). When patients fail in treatment, misclassifications of adherence can result in unnecessary changes in prescribed therapy. Patients may have stronger medications prescribed, with greater risk of side-effects, or they may have additional drugs added to their regimen. The physician, puzzled by an apparently adherent patient's lack of response to treatment, may order costly diagnostic procedures. Unnecessary referrals for specialist care may follow from such adherence misclassifications. Because determinations about patient's adherence can influence the distribution of scarce or costly resources, such as organ donations (Olbrisch & Levenson, 1995; Surman & Cosimi, 1996; Swanson et al., 1991) for transplant or protease inhibitor therapy for AIDS (Ickovics & Meisler, 1997), inaccurate evaluations can have life-or-death consequences (Vanhove, Schapiro, Winters, Merigan, & Blaschke, 1996).

In Clinical Research

Clinical trials of new therapies are predicated on an expected rate of subject adherence with the study treatment. The power of a study—that is, the probability of making a Type II error (i.e., incorrectly accepting the null hypothesis)—is calculated, in part, on the assumption that a defined number of subjects in the treatment group will be adequately exposed to the experimental treatment (Goldsmith, 1979). Inaccurate assessment of subject adherence can complicate the interpretation of clinical trial outcomes. Research has consistently shown that adherence measures tend to overestimate adherence and that self-report is particularly biased toward overestimation of adherence (Mawhinney, Spector, Kinsman et al., 1991; Rand, Nides, Cowles, Wise, & Connett, 1995; Rand, Wise, Nides et al., 1992; Rudd, Ahmed, Zachary, Barton, & Bonduelle, 1990). When a trial shows no treatment effect, post hoc analysis based on biased self-report measures will be unable to distinguish between a treatment's lack of efficacy or the failure of participants to adhere to an effective treatment. In studies that do yield a significant treatment effect, the general bias present in most studies toward overestimation of subject adherence can lead to underestimation of a treatment's efficacy and potentially inaccurate and dangerous dose-response calculations (Feinstein, 1977; Marston, 1970; Stone, 1979).

MEASURING ADHERENCE BY SELF-REPORT

Overview of Self-Report Measures

Patient self-report is the most widely used measure of adherence in both clinical care and research (Dunbar, 1980). In a patient care setting, self-report is usually collected by interview (DeGeest, Borgermans, Gemoets et al., 1995), whereas in a research setting, interview may be replaced or supplemented by self-monitoring adherence diaries (Matsui et al., 1994; Rodewald & Pichichero, 1993) or questionnaires (Kruse, Nikolaus, Rampmaier, Weber, & Schlierf, 1993; Moriskey, Green, & Levine, 1986). Self-report is an inexpensive, simple measurement strategy that is applicable to different medical regimens, is generally brief, and has face validity (Table 15.1). In addition, self-report is the best strategy for evaluating those unique patient factors that may influence adherence with therapy. Although many studies have developed measures of patient adherence with treatment, most of these instruments have not been evaluated for reliability and validity (Rand, 1990). No cross-disease adherence questionnaire has been developed and vali-

TABLE 15.1
Advantages of Self-Report Measures of Adherence

• Fast	• Face validity
• Flexible	• Potentially rich source of data on adherence patterns and barriers
• Inexpensive	• High specificity for nonadherence
• Easy	

dated, in part because most self-report questionnaires of adherence have been designed for specific diseases and studies, and because adherence self-report measures are often no more than one or two questions embedded within general disease self-management measures.

Strengths of Self-Report Adherence Measures

Self-report measures of adherence are used by clinicians in patient management because of their ease and appropriateness to the clinical interaction. Self-report of adherence is a flexible strategy that can be matched to the characteristics of the regimens being evaluated. Querying patients about their patterns of use and experience with medications or other forms of therapy can provide the health care provider with valuable and rich information about the feasibility of the selected regimen, its side-effects, and any patients' concerns. Asking patients directly about their adherence with a prescribed treatment is intuitively appropriate and generally simple to implement. For most medication regimens and behavioral treatments (e.g., dietary or exercise), there are few or no objective measures available to measure adherence. Biochemical analysis of blood, urine, or other bodily excretions to objectively measure medication or by-product levels is available for only a few drugs and the cost and practicality of applying this strategy in a clinical setting is usually prohibitive.

Self-report (particularly in the clinical setting) is generally the only measure that will capture information about patient beliefs, attitudes, and experiences with medication regimens and how these beliefs may affect adherence with therapy. Although pill counts or biochemical assays may be ideal, and perhaps even superior for identifying the nonadherent patient, only self-report measures can reveal that the reason for the nonadherence is that the patient misunderstands the dosing regimen or that she has altered her regimen because of a fear of side-effects (Britten, 1994; Donovan & Blake, 1992). Personal, financial, social, or physical barriers to adherence can be uncovered by sensitive measurement of patient self-reports. Self-report is also the most appropriate measure for evaluating important cultural and ethnic differences that may affect adherence behaviors. Patients may alter therapy because their cultural beliefs about health and therapy are not congruent with those of the prescribing health care provider. Morgan (1995) interviewed Afro-Caribbean patients from inner-city London who were using anti-hypertensive medications, and found that traditional cultural beliefs among these patients about the long-term harmful effects led to reduced adherence with prescribed therapies and increased use of herbal remedies. Among Puerto Rican families, Pachter and Weller (1993) found that a lower level of acculturation to Western culture was associated with poorer medication adherence. These investigators suggested that incorporating nonjudgmental questions about cultural preference for mode of therapy or concerns about Western medical practices into self-report adherence measures might yield more accurate and useful adherence information.

An additional strength of self-report that is often neglected is the generally high specificity of this measurement strategy for identifying nonadherence. Although many personal and social factors may influence patients and research participants to overreport adherence, there is evidence to suggest that when patients tell a health care provider that they are not adhering with therapy, this information can be considered reliable and valid (Gordis, 1976; Hasford, 1991; Rand, Nides, Cowles, Wise, & Connett, 1995). Thus, regular clinical and research application of this measurement technique would allow the simple identification of many candid nonadherers.

Weaknesses of Self-Report Adherence Measures

Despite the potential strengths and advantages of self-report measures of adherence, this measurement strategy is vulnerable to several sources of bias (Table 15.2). When patients are asked to recall medication use over a several-month period, they may be able to report correctly their usage over the past week; however, their ability to accurately recall their medication use 4 months prior to their physician visit may be poor. This recency effect in memory recall will bias adherence self-reports toward the most proximal patterns of use (Neath, 1993). Patients with any level of memory impairment (related to illness, age, concurrent medications, or stress), will also have difficulty reporting their usage pattern of any one medication. The desire to please the health care provider or researcher may also encourage patients to exaggerate reports of medication adherence. The extent that this social desirability effect (Carnrike, McCracken, & Aikens, 1996; Raghubir & Menon, 1996) occurs may be influenced by the setting where assessment occurs, as well as the relationship to the interviewer. If the consequences of candor are perceived as negative (e.g., being judged a neglectful parent, not receiving research payments, etc.), patients may be discouraged from admitting problems with adherence. Physicians' and investigators' sensitivity and skill in eliciting adherence self-reports may influence the patient's willingness to

TABLE 15.2
Disadvantages of Self-Report Measures of Adherence

Highly Variable Degree of Validity Based on the Following Factors:	
• Social desirability	• Patient factors, including: memory,
• Recency effect	language, health beliefs, culture, mental
• Perceived consequences of candor	health, substance abuse
• Interviewer skill	

be candid about problems with following the prescribed regimen (Steele, Jackson, & Gutmann, 1990).

Additional problems may face the pediatric health care provider in assessing adherence in children and adolescents. Responsibility for following prescribed therapy may be shared among parents, relatives, daycare providers, and the child. As children grow, they typically assume a growing level of responsibility for adherence with treatment. As a result of this shifting responsibility, physicians may collect inaccurate self-report information if they do not query all involved parties.

Research on the Reliability and Validity of Self-Report as a Measure of Adherence

When validated against an objective criterion of patient adherence, such as pill counts or biochemical measures, self-report has been found to have a highly variable degree of accuracy (Francis, Korsch, & Morris, 1969). This discrepancy between self-report and objective measures has been observed across a wide-range of therapies including anti-hypertensive medications, (Rudd, Byyny, Zachery et al., 1989) anti-epileptics (Cramer, Mattson, Prevey, Scheyer, & Oullette, 1989), and arthritis medications (Dunbar-Jacob, 1993; Kraag, Gordon, Menard, Russell, & Kalish, 1989).

Stewart (1987) evaluated the validity of self-reported adherence measured by clinical interview against pill-count adherence in a sample of 98 adult medical patients visiting their family doctor. Patients were asked very specific medication-use questions (e.g., What was it [the medication] for? How many times a day were you to take it? Have you done this every day or might you have missed some doses? How many doses might you have missed in the past ten days?) by a research assistant and pill counts were conducted at the end of a home interview. This interview-based self-report assessment was found to have an overall accuracy of 75%, with a sensitivity of 80%, and a specificity of 70%. Positive predictive value (i.e., percent of interviewer-identified adherers were similarly categorized by pill count) was 69% and negative predictive value (i.e., what percent of interviewer-identified nonadherers were similarly categorized by pill count) was 80%. These findings contrast with five other studies of the accuracy of self-reported adherence that were reviewed by Stewart (Table 15.3). In general, these studies had similar overall accuracy, much lower sensitivity, and, for the majority, higher positive predictive value. Stewart also found that the accuracy of self-report was significantly influenced by patient characteristics such as age and prescribed regimen, with self-report a less accurate measure for younger patients and those on more complicated regimens. These calculations of agreement may be an overestimation because of the limitations of pill count as an objective measure (Rand, Wise, et al., 1992). Burney,

TABLE 15.3

Review of Papers That Have Compared Subjective Assessments of Compliance to an Objective Measure

	Park and Lipman	Gordis	Sackett	Gilbert	Inui
Subjective measure quote	Asked whether they had taken prescribed pills. If so, asked to estimate number of pills missed.	"In general how often does your child take his pills?" "In the last two months was there anytime he missed taking his pills for more than one day?"	"People often have difficulty taking their pills for one reason or another . . . have you had any difficulty taking your pills?"	"Many people have difficulty taking medications. Did you ever miss your digoxin? How many pills per week?"	"Many patients find it difficult to take their medication or stick to their diets as their doctors say they should. Over the past two months . . . do you think you have taken your medicine as you should, on schedule and regularly?"
Objective measure	Pill count (all pills = compliant)	Urine test for penicillin (75% tests positive = compliant)	Pill count (80% pills = compliant)	Pill count (80% pills = compliant)	Pill count (75% pills = compliant)
Percentage noncompliant on the objective measure	51.3	42.2	41.5	29.6	62.2
Setting	Psychiatric clinic of a hospital	Pediatric clinic	84 primary care practices	10 family practices	General medical clinic
n	42 outpatients	45 child outpatients	123 men discovered by a hypertension screening program	71 patients on digoxin for more than 3 months	241 hypertensives under treatment, predominantly female
Accuracy (%)	59.8	68.9	78.1	70.4	67.6
Sensitivity (%)	25.0	46.2	53.0	19.1	55.3
Positive predictive value (%)	88.2	100.0	90.0	50.0	88.3

Note. Reprinted by permission of Elsevier Science from "The validity of an interview to assess a patient's drug taking," by M. Stewart, 1987, *American Journal Preventive Medicine, 3*, pp. 95–100. Copyright © 1987 by American Journal of Preventive Medicine.

Krishnan, Ruffin, Zhang, and Brenner (1996) used an electronic pill monitor to measure adherence to a single dose of aspirin in a chemoprevention trial and found that adherence rates by self-report were 73%, but by electronic monitoring, only 44% were classified as adherent.

Coutts, Gibson, and Paton's (1992) medication monitor (Nebulizer Chronolog) in a pilot study examined adherence with inhaled steroid therapy in 14 children ages 9 to 16. Children were monitored for 1 to 3 months and asked to maintain asthma diaries as well as use the monitored inhaler (Table 15.4). The investigators noted significant discrepancies between asthma diary notations of adherence and the Chronolog record of inhaler use, with children's diaries always reporting better compliance than electronically recorded, even though they were aware that the adherence was being monitored. This discrepancy appeared to increase the more complex the regimen.

Spector, Kinsman, Mawhinney, et al. (1986) were one of the first investigative teams to use an electronic medication monitor (the Nebulizer Chronolog) to measure adherence to inhaled asthma medications. Nineteen adult asthmatic patients were studied for 12 weeks with a cromolyn-like drug. Patients' adherence with the four times a day therapy was poor, with a mean of 47% adherent days. Underuse of this preventive medication was much more common than overuse, with all subjects underusing the medication at times. Patients were also asked to maintain asthma diaries as a part of this study, and comparative analysis of Nebulizer Chronolog data and diary found that whereas all subjects self-reported using the inhaler on more than half of the study days, the measured medication usage indicated that only 52.6% of the subjects actually did so.

In a series of small (9–11 patients) studies using an electronic monitor, Yeung, O'Connor, Parry, and Cochrane (1994) examined inhaled corticosteroid use over a period of 2 to 3 weeks. When patients were aware of monitoring, 60% of the patients were fully compliant, 20% were partially

TABLE 15.4
Compliance of Children With Inhaled Corticosteroids

Prescribed Frequency (No. of Times per Day)	No. of Children	No. of Study Days	Reported Compliance in Days (%)*	No. (%) of Days of Recorded Compliance	No. (%) of Days Recorded Underuse	No. (%) of Days Recorded Overuse
2	5	233	96	166 (71)	63 (27)	5 (2)
3	3	80	90	27 (34)	49 (61)	4 (5)
4	6	224	69	41 (18)	181 (81)	2 (1)

Note. From "Measuring compliance with inhaled medication in asthma," by J. A. P. Coutts, N. A. Gibson, and J. Y. Paton, 1992, *Archives of Disease in Childhood, 67,* pp. 332–333. Copyright © 1992 by BMJ Publishing Group. Reprinted with permission.

*Expressed as a percentage of completed diary card days.

compliant (taking just 70% of the prescribed dose), and 20% were nonadherent. When patients were unaware of the monitoring, 6 out of 11 took between 30% and 51% of the prescribed doses. In both of these studies, patients tended to overreport inhaled steroid use. In a separate study of as-needed inhaled bronchodilator use, the investigators found that patients tended to underreport use of this rescue medication.

Rand, Wise, Nides et al. (1992) examined the validity of self-reported adherence with inhaled medications in the Lung Health Study. Adherence was measured by three different adherence measures: self-report, change in canister weight, and the Nebulizer Chronolog™ electronic record of adherence. When adherence classifications by canister weight and self-report were compared, participants were found to consistently overestimate their adherence (Table 15.5). The most accurate self-reports were for those participants who admitted to being poor adherers. In the subset of participants who were electronically monitored, 73% of the participants self-reported using their inhaler an average of three times daily. However, electronic monitoring showed that only 15% of the people used the inhaler an average of 2.5 or more times per day and that only 42% of the people used the inhaler an average of 1.5 to 2.4 times per day. Within this monitored group, 13.7% of participants showed a pattern of sporadic heavy actuation of their inhalers with more than 100 actuations within a 3-hour interval. Figure 15.1 shows the pattern of inhaler use of one individual in this study identified as a medication dumper. The investigators labeled this behavior canister dumping. By self-report and canister weight, these participants were classified as highly adherent; however, by appropriate use, they were found to be poor to very poor adherers. Rand et al. interpreted this usage pattern to reflect deliberate emptying of inhalers to appear to be in good adherence with the prescribed study regimen. The phenomenon of medication dumping is

TABLE 15.5

Self-Reported Inhaler Use Compared to Canister Weight Determined Inhaler Use (%) at One Year in the Lung Health Study (n = 2838)

	Canister Weight				
Self-Report	Over	Good	Satisfactory	Poor	Very Poor
Over	16.7	25.0	50.0	8.3	0.0
Good	13.4	39.7	38.8	5.7	2.4
Satisfactory	6.6	11.9	54.6	20.5	6.4
Poor	3.0	2.2	26.1	38.1	30.6
Very Poor	0.7	1.6	10.7	17.5	69.4

Note. From "Long-term metered-dose inhaler adherence in a clinical trial," by C. S. Rand, M. Nides, M. K. Cowles, R. A. Wise, and J. Connett, 1995, *American Journal of Respiratory & Critical Care Medicine, 152*, pp. 580–588. Copyright © 1995 by American Lung Association. Reprinted with permission.

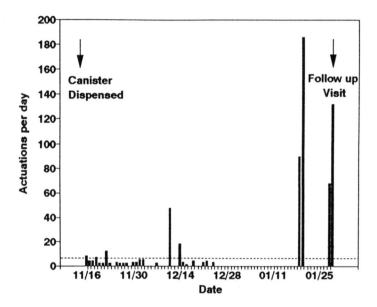

FIG. 15.1. Nebulizer Chronolog (NC) usage by a participant who shows a dumping pattern. The arrows indicate the date that the NC was dispensed, and the date of the follow-up visit. The horizontal dotted line indicates the prescribed number of inhalations. The usage pattern suggests that there is initially satisfactory compliance. After periods of underuse, there is frequent actuation of the MDI. Particularly heavy use is present in the days prior to the scheduled follow-up visit. This participant's self-report indicated inhaler usage at three times a day and canister weight change at 100% of prescribed MDI adherence. The expected change in canister weight for the 628 actuations was 42.5 g compared with the measured change in canister weight of 42.6 g. (From "Metered-dose inhaler adherence in a clinical trial," by C. S. Rand et al., 1992, *American Journal of Respiratory & Critical Care Medicine, 146*, pp. 1559–1564. Copyright © 1992 by American Lung Association. Reprinted with permission.)

nearly impossible to detect by traditional methods of adherence assessment, and inclusion of dumping data into a dose-response analysis can yield counterintuitive results; highly adherent subjects may show a poorer response than moderately adherent subjects. This phenomenon of medication discarding has been documented in several studies that have collected both self-report and objective measures of adherence (Braunstein, Trinquet, & Harper, 1996; Rudd, Byyny, Zachary, et al., 1989; Spilker, 1991).

The discrepancy between self-report and objective measures of adherence may in part be attributable to forgetting or a recency effect; however, both Yeung, O'Connor, Parry, and Cochrane (1994) and Nides et al. (1993) have reported that subjects' self-reports are more concordant with electronic adherence measures when subjects are aware that they are being monitored than when they are kept masked to the monitoring. This suggests that a desire to be perceived as adherent is influencing subjects to self-report more adherent use of medication.

IMPROVING THE ACCURACY AND USEFULNESS OF SELF-REPORT MEASURES OF ADHERENCE

Matching the Tool to the Purpose: Selecting the Right Adherence Measure

Like any measurement instrument, self-report measures should be carefully matched to the requirements and goals of the assessment. Determining when and how to use self-report measures of adherence, and when to incorporate more objective adherence measures (such as pill counts, biochemical assays, or electronic monitoring) requires the clinician or investigator to define the dimensions of adherence that are important. How good adherence is defined should determine how best to measure adherence. The parameters of good adherence should be explicitly delineated and appropriate for the medication regimen or health behavior under study. In a clinical care setting, a broadly defined, flexible criteria of acceptable adherence may be appropriate and not need precise measurement methodology. However, when detailed and exact adherence data are necessary, the measurement instruments should be comparably precise. In both clinical care and research settings, measuring and classifying patients' patterns of medication use may be as important as assessing overall adherence level. Evaluations of these patterns of use may provide important information about the efficacy of therapy as well as the contribution of nonadherence to disease exacerbation.

Self-Report in a Research Setting

In a clinical trial of medications, measures of adherence are necessary to both confirm that subjects adhered with the study drug as projected (i.e., the power of the study) as well as to determine dose-response relationships. Although it is generally preferable and appropriate for clinical trials to include objective measures of adherence to confirm patient adherence, self-report measures still serve an important function in clinical research. When objective adherence measures that provide cumulative data are used, such as pill counts, self-report can fill in the details of patterns of medication use. When biochemical measures are collected, self-report measures of adherence will provide information about adherence outside the timeframe measured by the biochemical measure. Self-report is the only source for information about side-effects, patient response to the treatment, barriers to adherence, and patient beliefs about the therapy. For some treatments (such as behavioral regimens like diet or exercise), no objective adherence measurement is generally possible. And very often, the practical difficulties in obtaining objective measures of adherence, because of cost, setting, or inappropriateness, necessitate that self-report is the only source of adherence data within a study.

If self-report is to become a truly useful and valid measure within a research setting, criteria for the development and evaluation of such an instrument should be as rigorous as for any standardized, psychometric tool (Table 15.6). Ideally, self-report measures of adherence used for research would meet the following criteria: (a) validation of the self-report measure against objective criteria, such as biochemical measures or medication monitors; (b) demonstration of adequate internal consistency and test–retest reliability as appropriate to the measure; (c) inclusion of questions or items that assess daily patterns of use with each regularly prescribed therapy; and (d) measurement of frequency of use of as-needed medications or therapy and triggering events for use. Additional areas of measurement that would help clarify and interpret patterns of medication use could include: (a) patients' confidence that they will adhere appropriately to their medical regimen; (b) patients' self-report of what they believe their prescribed regimen to be; (c) patients' criteria for adequate or appropriate adherence; and (d) reasons for nonadherence or erratic adherence, including physical, psychological, social, and financial barriers.

Because of the difficulty in identifying nonadherence and the costs and consequences associated with this behavior, many investigators have attempted to ascertain predictors of nonadherence. Efforts to identify a compliant personality type have not been successful, nor has the literature consistently found a relationship between patient characteristics and adherence behavior. Although disruptive psychopathology, some addictive disorders, and chaotic family situations have been implicated as risks for nonadherence, sociodemographic characteristics and health beliefs have yielded

TABLE 15.6
Self-Report Measures of Adherence Can Be Improved to Enhance Accuracy
and Usefulness in Profiling Adherence Behavior by:

- Demonstrating adequate psychometric properties, including: adequate test–retest reliability and validity (using objective adherence criteria—biochemical, medication measurement, pharmacy database, or electronic monitoring)
- Evaluating detailed pattern of medication use (e.g., drug holidays, self-regulation, self-titration, etc.)
- Assessing the patient-perceived prescribed regimen and criteria for adequate adherence
- Evaluating barriers (personal, financial, social, cultural, structural) to appropriate adherence

inconsistent results. This failure to find reliable predictors of adherence has led researchers to focus on the characteristics of the treatment regimen, such as complexity and duration, as the most powerful predictors of adherence. It is clear from these studies that stereotyping of patients' likely adherence by personal characteristics is an unsupported (and potentially dangerous) strategy for determining adherence. Nevertheless, the often contradictory findings about the personal and sociodemographic predictors of adherence may be attributable, in part, to the frequently small sample sizes of these studies that lack sufficient power to detect modest, but significant relationships.

In a large-scale study that monitored adherence with an inhaled bronchodilator, Rand, Nides, Cowles, Wise, and Connett (1995) found that married, older, better-educated, women participants were more likely to have satisfactory self-reported inhaler adherence. However, when a validated measure of adherence (canister weight confirmed self-report) was used in the analyses, both education level and gender dropped out of the model, suggesting that gender and education level were more strongly associated with reporting behavior than with actual medication use behavior. In contrast, no significant relationship was observed between race and adherence for self-reported adherence, however, analysis using confirmed adherence data found that non-Whites were less likely to have satisfactory adherence levels (in this particular study). This suggests that although Whites and non-Whites had similar adherence reporting behavior, in actual use, non-Whites were less likely to have satisfactory adherence levels (in this particular study). Overall, these results suggest a possible explanation for why previous studies examining predictors of adherence have yielded such conflicting and inconsistent results. That is, those variables that are related to reporting adherent medication use may be different from those related to actual medication adherence.

Self-Report in a Clinical Setting

Although physicians may endorse the importance of assessing patient adherence with therapy, all too often patients are never directly asked about their adherence with prescribed treatments. And when a health care provider does query a patient about adherence, it may only be triggered by stereotypes and clinical biases. The ability of a health care provider to effectively gather self-reported adherence information from patients and identify patient nonadherence has been shown to be highly variable and dependent on interviewing skill and style. Further, physicians' self-assessments of their own communication skills have been shown to not be related to observer ratings of their communication skills (Manzella et al., 1989; Marteau, Humphrey, Matoon, Kidd, Lloyd, & Horder, 1991).

Steele, Jackson, and Gutmann (1990) examined audiotaped interactions between patients and providers utilizing a qualitative, sociolinguistic methodology in order to classify the interviewing strategies used by primary care physicians to assess patient adherence with antihypertensive therapies. After seeing each patient, participating physicians were asked to identify which patients were nonadherent. In 38 critical case encounters, these physicians identified only 53% of the adherence problems. Physicians who used indirect approaches to assessment (e.g., "Have you noticed any changes since you started taking your medicines?") were the least successful in identifying adherence problems (0/9). Information-intensive strategies (open-ended queries about patterns of medication use) were the most successful (8/10 correct).

The investigators conclude that a nonaccusatory, open-ended, information-intensive approach can be a sensitive and productive tool for the diagnosis of a patient's adherence status.

Traditionally, communication skills and attention to psychosocial issues are not a focus of medical education and training, which may account for physicians' apparent lack of skill in identifying patients with adherence difficulties. Physician interviewing skills and the qualities of the patient–provider interaction are important in both measuring and facilitating adherence behaviors (Roter & Hall, 1987). Use of an information-intensive and nonjudgmental style of interviewing (Table 15.7) has been suggested as a strategy for improving the accuracy of patient self-reported adherence. In recent years, increasing attention has been directed at incorporating communication skills training into medical curriculums through the use of simulated patients and role-playing. Research suggests that this skills building can improve physician communication concerning sensitive or emotional issues (Dimatteo, Sherbourne, Hays, et al., 1993; Dunbar-Jacob, 1993; Heszen-

TABLE 15.7
Effective Clinical Interview Skills That Improve the Accuracy
and Usefulness of Self-Reported Adherence

- Directly evaluate exact adherence behaviors in an Information-Intensive approach— "Which medications are you taking? What dose? How Often? Have you had any side effects?"
- Probe for nonadherence in a nonjudgmental and nonthreatening manner—"Many people have trouble remembering to take their medication. Do you ever forget to take yours? Do you ever intentionally stop taking your medication?"
- Ask patients about possible barriers (personal, financial, social, cultural, and structural) to adherence—"Do you have any worries or questions about the treatment I've prescribed? Have you been able to follow the plan? Can you afford the medications? Do you have any problems getting refills? Do you have any problems using the inhaler the way I prescribed?"

Note. From "Physicians interviewing styles and medical information obtained from patients," by D. L. Roter and J. A. Hall, 1987, *Journal of General Internal Medicine, 2*, pp. 325–329. Copyright © 1994 by American Medical Association. Reprinted with permission.

TABLE 15.8
Self-Report is the Best Measure for Understanding and
Classifying Patient Adherence and Nonadherence

❖ *Erratic*	❖ *Unwitting*	❖ *Deliberate*
• Forgetful	• Misunderstands regimen	Patient self-regulates
• Changing schedule	• Language–cultural barriers	therapy because therapy
• Too busy	• Mental impairment	is perceived to be/have:
• Running out of medication		• not working
		• not needed
		• wrong dosage
		• too dangerous
		• addicting
		• too costly
		• too many side-effects

Klemens & Lapinska, 1984; Holloway, Rogers, & Gershenhorn, 1992; Sackett & Haynes, 1976).

Thoughtful, nonjudgmental assessment of self-report in the clinical setting presents an opportunity to the clinician to explore and understand the nature of patients' adherence difficulties. Adherence with therapy is not a simple, dichotomous variable with patients following a prescribed regimen in a completely adherent or nonadherent fashion. Instead, adherence can be a mutable behavior, highly dependent on the environment and patient knowledge and beliefs. As shown in Table 15.8, nonadherence may have several sources, and each type of adherence difficulty will require a different intervention strategy.

Erratic nonadherence is the failure to consistently follow a regimen that is understood and endorsed by the patient because of personal, logistical, or organizational barriers. Patients may report that they forget because they get busy, they do fine until the weekend when their schedule changes, or they just cannot quite get to the pharmacy to get refills before it closes. Dolce, Crisp, Manzella, Richard, Hardin, and Bailey (1991) examined adherence with medications for chronic obstructive pulmonary diseases and found that forgetting, and other forms of erratic adherence were most often mentioned by patients as the causes when they were not adherent. Erratic adherence may be attributable to unrealistic dosing regimens that do not match lifestyles (e.g., take two tablets five times a day, do not take within 1 hour of eating). School children may have problems using medications during the school day because of policies that require that all medications be delivered by school nurses. Some patients have difficulty remembering to use their preventive medication when they are asymptomatic (e.g., use of antibiotics for acne); however, they may resume appropriate adherence after symptoms, a disease flare, or even a doctor's appointment. Identifying erratic nonadherence requires that patients be queried about the frequency of forgetting doses, the feasibility of the prescribed regimen, and any barriers to regular, sustained use of the treatment. Interventions to ameliorate erratic nonadherence begin first with modifying the regimen, if possible, to fit the patient's lifestyle. Additional strategies may involve suggesting environmental cues or organizational strategies (e.g., keeping medications beside a toothbrush, using a day-by-day pill box, setting a watch alarm), and addressing structural or organizational barriers (e.g., finding a 24-hour pharmacy for refills, arranging for a school to allow medication self-administration, etc.).

A more insidious form of failure to adhere is unwitting nonadherence. Unwitting nonadherence includes patients who do not understand their prescribed therapy either because they never received sufficient education and instruction from their health care provider to adequately adhere or because they forget or confuse instructions. For some patients, comprehension of the prescribed regimen may be impaired by language and cultural differences, cognitive or emotional impairment, or by physician use of medical jargon. The frequent failure of health care providers to provide explicit written instructions may result in patients being unclear about the correct use of medications when they return home from the doctor's. Patients may not understand the parameters for using medications that are prescribed to be used as needed. Underuse of prophylactic therapies may result from patient confusion about the difference between preventive regimens and symptom-driven treatments. Unwitting nonadherence is frequently not identified because the patient is not aware of their inappropriate adherence with therapy and the physician fails to explicitly ask about the regimen the patient is following. Although this form of adherence problem is often difficult to spot, remediation may be relatively straightforward. Strategies include using language- and culturally appropriate educational interventions and materials (written, audio, or video), demonstrations, where appropriate, (e.g. metered-dose inhalers) by health care providers and the patient, and monitoring to assure that drift in understanding does not occur.

Patients often make personal choices to alter therapies. This deliberate nonadherence is often called *intelligent nonadherence*, reflecting a reasoned choice rather than a necessarily wise choice (Hindi-Alexander & Thromm, 1987) Patients who feel better may decide that they no longer need to take prescribed medications. Fear of side-effects or long-term medication use may cause some patients to reduce or discontinue dosing. Patients may abandon a therapy because taste, complexity, or interference with daily life may convince them that the disadvantages of therapy outweigh the benefits. Patients may find that some variation of the prescribed therapy works better than the doctor-prescribed regimen. This deliberate nonadherence, like all nonadherence, does not necessarily result in a worsening disease. In every clinical practice, there are patients who have knowingly altered their prescribed therapy, yet this modification may never be uncovered by their physician. Good physician–patient communication should identify these patient-initiated changes in therapy, discuss the reasons for the alterations, address any misconceptions that might have contributed to the decision, and explore with the patient the personal costs and/or benefits of different treatment options. Regardless of the source of medication nonadherence, the necessary first step to addressing the problem is identifying the problem through effective, open-ended patient–provider communication.

SUMMARY AND RECOMMENDATIONS

Self-report measures of adherence are common but often unreliable and invalid. Multiple factors in the measurement process may influence the accuracy of this measure, including the setting, the demand characteristics, the interviewer or instrument used, and the skill of the interviewer. Self-report can be a valuable source of data and insight into both the behavior of adherence and the efficacy of therapy, however, current self-report measures and strategies often fail to gather this rich detail. Improved measures to evaluate patient adherence would contribute to both clinical care and research. Research is needed to develop standardized self-report instruments of adherence with therapy that are reliable and have been validated against objective measures of adherence, such as electronic monitoring or pharmacy records. Instruments are needed that can distinguish different types of nonadherence with therapy, as well as structural, personal, cultural, and financial barriers to adherence. Measures that have been validated with patients from different cultures and ethnicities would be of value. Special attention should be given to how best to measure adherence in pediatric populations with consideration given to developing parallel forms of a self-report adherence measure, suitable for both parents and children to complete. Finally, given the central role played by health care providers in measuring self-reported adherence, continuing education and research is warranted to improve medical education programs and training in both communication skills and adherence assessment techniques.

REFERENCES

Braunstein, G. L., Trinquet, G., & Harper, A. E. (1996). Compliance with nedocromil sodium and a nedocromil sodium/salbutamol combination. Compliance Working Group. *European Respiratory Journal, 9*, 893–898.

Britten, N. (1994). Patients' ideas about medicines: A qualitative study in a general practice population. *British Journal of General Practice, 44*, 465–468.

Burney, K. D., Krishnan, K., Ruffin, M. T., Zhang, D., & Brenner, D. E. (1996). Adherence to single daily dose of aspirin in a chemoprevention trial. An evaluation of self-report and microelectronic monitoring. *Archives of Family Medicine, 5*, 297–300.

Carnrike, C. L. M. J., McCracken, L. M., & Aikens, J. E. (1996, March). Social desirability, perceived stress, and PACT ratings in lung transplant candidates: A preliminary investigation. *Journal of Clinical Psychology in Medical Settings, 3*(1), 57–67.

The Coronary Drug Research Project Group. (1980). Influence of adherence to treatment and response of cholesterol on mortality in the coronary drug project. *New England Journal of Medicine, 303*, 1038–1041.

Coutts, J. A. P., Gibson, N. A., & Paton, J. Y. (1992). Measuring compliance with inhaled medication in asthma. *Archives of Disease in Childhood, 67*, 332–333.

Cramer, J. A., Mattson, R. H., Prevey, M. L., Scheyer, R. D., & Oullette, V. L. (1989). How often is medication taken as prescribed? A novel assessment technique. *Journal of the American Medical Association, 261*, 3273–3277.

De Geest, S., Borgermans, L., Gemoets, H., Abraham, I., Vlaminck, H., Evers, G., & Vanrenterghem, Y. (1995). Incidence, determinants, and consequences of sub-clinical noncompliance with immunosuppressive therapy in renal transplant recipients. *Transplantation, 59*, 340–347.

Dimatteo, M. R., Sherbourne, C. D., Hays, R. D., Ordway, L., Kravitz, R. L., McGlynn, E. A., Kaplan, S., & Rogers, W. H. (1993). Physicians' characteristics influence patients' adherence to medical treatment: Results from the medical outcomes study. *Health Psychology, 12*(2), 93–102.

Dolce, J., Crisp, C., Manzella, B., Richard, J. M., Hardin, M., & Bailey, W. C. (1991). Medication adherence patterns in chronic obstructive pulmonary disease. *Chest, 99*, 837–841.

Donovan, J. L., & Blake, D. R. (1992). Patient non-compliance: Deviance or reasoned decision-making? *Social Sciences, 34*(5), 507–513.

Dunbar, J. M. (1980). Assessment of medication compliance: A review. In R. B. Haynes, M. E. Mattson, & T. O. Engebretson, Jr. (Eds.), *Patient compliance to prescribed antihypertensive medication regimens: A report to the National Heart, Lung, and Blood Institute* (NIH Publication No. 81-2102, pp. 59–82). Washington, DC: Government Printing Office.

Dunbar-Jacob, J. (1993). Contributions to patient adherence: Is it time to share the blame? *Health Psychology, 12*(2), 91–92.

Feinstein, A. L. (1977). Hard science, soft data, and the challenges of choosing clinical variables in research. *Clinical Pharmacology & Therapeutics, 22*, 485–498.

Francis, V., Korsch, B. M., & Morris, M. J. (1969). Gaps in doctor-patient communications. *New England Journal of Medicine, 280*, 535–540.

Goldsmith, C. H. (1979). The effect of differing compliance distributions on the planning and statistical analysis of therapeutic trials. In R. B. Haynes, D. W. Taylor, & D. L. Sackett (Eds.), *Compliance in Health Care* (pp. 297–308). Baltimore: Johns Hopkins University Press.

Gordis, L. (1976). Methodologic issues in the measurement of patient compliance. In D. L. Sackett & R. B. Haynes (Eds.), *Compliance with therapeutic regimens* (pp. 51–66). Baltimore: Johns Hopkins University Press.

Hasford, J. (1991). Biometric issues in measurement and analyzing partial compliance in clinical trials. In J. A. Cramer & B. Spilker (Eds.), *Patient compliance in medical practice and clinical trials* (pp. 265–281). New York: Raven.

Heszen-Klemens, I., & Lapinska, E. (1984). Doctor-patient interaction, patients' health behavior and effects of treatment. *Social Science & Medicine, 19*(1), 9–18.

Hindi-Alexander, M. C., & Thromm, J. (1987). Compliance or noncompliance: That's the question! *American Journal of Health Promo, 1*(4), 5–11.

Holloway, R. L., Rogers, J. C., & Gershenhorn, S. L. (1992). Differences between patient and physician perceptions of predicted compliance. *Family Practice, 9*(3), 318–322.

Ickovics, J. R., & Meisler, A. W. (1997, April). Adherence in AIDS clinical trials: A framework for clinical research and clinical care. *Journal of Clinical Epidemiology, 50*, 385–391.

Jay, S., Litt, I. F., & Durant, R. H. (1984). Compliance with therapeutic regimens. *Journal of Adolescent Health Care, 5*, 124–136.

Kasl, S. V. (1975). Issues in patient adherence to health care regimens. *Journal of Human Stress, 1*, 5–17.

Korsch, B. M., Fine, R. N., & Negrete, V. F. (1978). Noncompliance in children with renal transplants. *Pediatrics, 61*, 872–876.

Kraag, G. R., Gordon, D. A., Menard, H.-A., Russell, A. S., & Kalish, G. H. (1994). Patient compliance with tenoxicam in family practice. *Clinical Therapeutics, 16*(3), 581–593.

Kruse, W., Nikolaus, T., Rampmaier, J., Weber, E., & Schlierf, G. (1993). Actual versus prescribed timing of lovastatin doses assessed by electronic compliance monitoring. *European Journal of Clinical Pharmacology, 45*(3), 211–215.

Manzella, B. A., Brooks, C. M., Richards, J. M., Jr., Windsor, R. A., Soong, S., & Bailey, W. C. (1989). Assessing the use of metered dose inhalers by adults with asthma. *Journal of Asthma, 26*, 223–230.

Marston, W. V. (1970). Compliance with medical regimens: A review of the literature. *Nursing Research, 19*, 312–323.

Marteau, T. M., Humphrey, C., Matoon, G., Kidd, J., Lloyd, M., & Horder, J. (1991, March). Factors influencing the communication skills of first-year clinical medical students. *Medical Education, 25*, 127–134.

Masur, F. T. (1981). Adherence to health care regimens. In C. K. Prolop & L. A. Bradley (Eds.), *Medical Psychology* (pp. 441–470). New York: Academic Press.

Matsui, D., Hermann, C., Klein, J., Berkovitch, M., Olivieri, N., & Koren, G. (1994). Critical comparison of novel and existing methods of compliance assessment during a clinical trial of an oral iron chelator. *Journal of Clinical Pharmacology, 34*, 944–949.

Mawhinney, H., Spector, S. L., Kinsman, R. A., Siegel, S. C., Rachelefsky, G. S., Katz, R. M., & Rohr, A. S. (1991). Compliance in clinical trials of two nonbronchodilator, antiasthma medications. *Annals of Allergy, 66*, 294–299.

Melnikow, J., & Kiefe, C. (1994). Patient compliance and medical research: Issues in methodology. *Journal of General Internal Medicine, 9*(2), 96–105.

Morgan, M. (1995). The significance of ethnicity for health promotion: Patients' use of anti-hypertensive drugs in inner London. *International Journal of Epidemiology, 24*, S79–S84.

Moriskey, D., Green, L., & Levine, D. (1986). Concurrent and predictive validity of a self reported measure of medication adherence. *Medical Care, 24*, 67–74.

Neath, I. (1993). Contextual and distinctive processes and the serial position function. *Journal of Memory & Language, 32*(6), 820–840.

Nides, M. A., Tashkin, D. P., Simmons, M. S., Wise, R. A., Li, V. C., & Rand, C. S. (1993). Improving inhaler adherence in a clinical trial through the use of the nebulizer chronolog. *Chest, 104*, 501–507.

Olbrisch, M. E., & Levenson, J. L. (1995, May-June). Psychosocial assessment of organ transplant candidates. Current status of methodological and philosophical issues. *Psychosomatics, 36*, 236–243.

Pachter, L. M., & Weller, S. C. (1993). Acculturation and compliance with medical therapy. *Journal of Developmental & Behavioral Pediatrics, 14*, 163–168.

Raghubir, P., & Menon, G. (1996). Asking sensitive questions: The effects of type of referent and frequency wording in counterbiasing methods. *Psychology & Marketing, 13*(7), 633–652.

Rand, C. S. (1990). Issues in the measurement of adherence. In Shumaker (Ed.), *The handbook of health behavior change* (pp. 102–110).

Rand, C. S., Nides, M., Cowles, M. K., Wise, R. A., & Connett, J. (1995). Long-term metered-dose inhaler adherence in a clinical trial. *American Journal of Respiratory & Critical Care Medicine, 152*, 580–588.

Rand, C. S., Wise, R. A., Nides, M., Simmons, M. S., Bleecker, E. R., Kusek, J. W., Li, V. C., & Tashkin, D. P. (1992). Metered-dose inhaler adherence in a clinical trial. *American Review of Respiratory Disease, 146*, 1559–1564.

Richardson, J. L., Shelton, D. R., Krailo, M., & Levine, A. M. (1990, Feb.). The effect of compliance with treatment on survival among patients with hematologic malignancies. *Journal of Clinical Oncology, 8,* 356–364.

Rodewald, L. E., & Pichichero, M. E. (1993). Compliance with antibiotic therapy: A comparison of deuterium oxide tracer, urine bioassay, bottle weights, and parental reports. *Journal of Pediatrics, 123,* 143–147.

Roter, D. L., & Hall, J. A. (1987, September-October). Physician's interviewing styles and medical information obtained from patients. *Journal of General Internal Medicine, 2,* 325–329.

Rudd, P., Ahmed, S., Zachary, V., Barton, C., & Bonduelle, D. (1990). Improved compliance measures: Applications in an ambulatory hypertensive drug trial. *Clinical Pharmacology and Therapeutics, 48*(6), 676–685.

Rudd, P., Byyny, R. L., Zachary, V. et al. (1989). The natural history of medication compliance in a drug trial: Limitations of pill counts. *Clinical Pharmacology and Therapeutics, 46*(2), 169–176.

Sackett, D. L., & Haynes, R. B. (1976). *Compliance with therapeutic regimens.* Baltimore: Johns Hopkins University Press.

Smith, M. (1985). The cost of noncompliance and the capacity of improved compliance to reduce health care expenditures. In Anonymous (Ed.), *Improving medication compliance: Proceedings of a symposium* (pp. 35–42). Washington, DC: National Pharmaceutical Council.

Spector, S. L., Kinsman, R., Mawhinney, H., Siegel, S. C., Rachelefsky, G. S., Ktaz, R. M., & Rohr, A. S. (1986). Compliance of patients with asthma with an experimental aerosolized medication: Implications for controlled clinical trials. *Journal of Allergy and Clinical Immunology, 77,* 65–70.

Spilker, B. (1991). Methods of assessing and improving patient compliance in clinical trials. In J. A. Cramer & B. Spilker (Eds.), *Patient compliance in medical practice and clinical trials* (pp. 37–56). New York: Raven.

Steele, D. J., Jackson, T. C., & Gutmann, M. C. (1990). Have you been taking your pill? The adherence-monitoring sequence in the medical interview. *The Journal of Family Practice, 30,* 294–299.

Stewart, M. (1987). The validity of an interview to assess a patient's drug taking. *American Journal of Preventive Medicine, 3,* 95–100.

Stone, G. C. (1979). Patient compliance and the role of the expert. *Journal of Social Issues, 35,* 34–59.

Surman, O. S., & Cosimi, A. B. (1996, November). Ethical dichotomies in organ transplantation. A time for bridge building. *General Hospital Psychiatry, 18,* 13S–19S.

Swanson, M. A., Palmeri, D., Vossler, E. D., Bartus, S. A., Hull, D., & Schweizer, R. T. (1991). Noncompliance in organ transplant recipients. *Pharmacotherapy, 11,* 173S–174S.

Vanhove, G. F., Schapiro, J. M., Winters, M. A., Merigan, T. C., & Blaschke, T. F. (1996, December 25). Patient compliance and drug failure in protease inhibitor monotherapy [letter]. *Journal of American Medical Association, 276,* 1955–1956.

Varni, J. W., & Wallander, J. L. (1984). Adherence to health-related regimens in pediatric chronic disorders. *Clinical Psychology Review, 4,* 585–596.

Wall, T. L., Sorensen, J. L., Batki, S. L., Delucchi, K. L., London, J. A., & Chesney, M. A. (1995, March). Adherence to zidovudine (AZT) among HIV-infected methadone patients: A pilot study of supervised therapy and dispensing compared to usual care. *Drug and Alcohol Dependence, 37,* 261–269.

Yeung, M., O'Connor, S. A., Parry, D. T., & Cochrane, G. M. (1994). Compliance with prescribed drug therapy in asthma. *Respiratory Medicine, 88,* 31–35.

16

Real-Time Self-Report of Momentary States in the Natural Environment: Computerized Ecological Momentary Assessment

Saul Shiffman
University of Pittsburgh

The bulk of behavioral research on humans relies on retrospective self-report. We rely on study participants to tell us what they are feeling, how they typically behave, how often they have engaged in particular acts, and so on. This applies to much medical research as well: Patients report their experience of symptoms, their consumption of foodstuffs or medications, their exposure to toxins, and so on. Self-report helps human research to bridge an observational gap: Scientists are often interested in people's real-world behavior but have no convenient way of observing it. Thus, we rely on respondents to bring their behavior into the bright light of scrutiny by telling us about it.

Yet, research on autobiographical memory (Bradburn, Rips, & Shevell, 1987; Eisenhower, Mathiowetz, & Morganstein, 1991) suggests that individuals' abilities to provide an accurate account of their experience is limited by the processes by which respondents formulate answers to researchers' questions. These biasing processes are particularly prominent when individuals are asked to rely on recall of past behavior for their responses because autobiographical memory is frequently inaccurate and biased.

In this chapter, I highlight an approach to collection of self-report data that minimizes reliance on recall from memory by relying on respondents' reports of their experience at the moment of the inquiry; that is, by inquiring how participants feel right now, rather than asking how they felt yesterday or how they generally feel. This approach, called Ecological Momentary Assessment (EMA; Stone & Shiffman, 1994), relies for its insights into human behavior on frequent assessment of respondents' momentary state as they go about their business of daily living. The approach has been described in several other publications (Shiffman & Stone, 1998; Stone & Shiffman, 1994). Here, I present the EMA approach as an alternative to soliciting respondents' general beliefs about their own behavior or their recollection of particular experiences of interest to the investigator. Using data from a study of cigarette smokers engaged in the process of quitting smoking, I evaluate the validity of recall data against parallel EMA data. Finally, I summarize several completed and in-progress EMA studies as a means of conveying the range of EMA methods and their prospects.

AUTOBIOGRAPHICAL MEMORY
AND THE LIMITS OF SELF-REPORT

Despite our reliance on it, self-report is often regarded skeptically in research, but perhaps for the wrong reasons. Researchers tend to emphasize the role of motivated distortion over that of natural memory processes. Self-reports are seen as too vulnerable to deliberate bias and misrepresentation by subjects. People are often motivated to misrepresent in order to look good before strangers, to preserve self-esteem, and so on (Ross, 1989). However, in many instances, there is little or no motivation for respondents to distort their research reports; the behaviors in question may not be socially sensitive, they may be motivated to collaborate in the researchers' search for truth, and so forth. Although it is tempting to give greater credibility to respondents' reports in these instances, this ignores a far more important source of bias: biases introduced by the operation of autobiographical memory.

A naïve model of memory presumes that the original encoding of personal experience is perfect and unbiased and that retrieval is simply a matter of restoring that information from this archive, albeit with some loss of fidelity. However, research on autobiographical memory increasingly demonstrates that autobiographical memory is as much a matter of reconstruction as retrieval. We reconstruct personal narratives from fragmentary information stored in memory, organized and supplemented by what we assume must have happened (Ross, 1989).

Arriving at an account of the past is usually aided by heuristic strategies for recall or reconstruction of the past. Such processes introduce not only random error but systematic bias into recall of past events. For example, highly salient events are much more likely to be recalled because they are more prominent to memory or more available to retrieval. As a result, isolated but salient episodes have an undue influence on the retrospective evaluation of experiences in jobs or relationships (Eisenhower et al., 1991).

The use of heuristics allows the present to color the past, too. For example, Bradburn, Rips, and Shevell (1987) showed that people's evaluations of their honeymoons are colored by their current marital satisfaction. Those whose relationships had taken a subsequent course for the worse recalled the honeymoon more negatively, contrary to ratings made at the time. If such retrospective data were taken at face value, they might seem to suggest that marital dissatisfaction has its roots early in the relationship. But the data only show that we use today's experience as a basis for reconstructing past experience. Ross (1989) reviewed the numerous ways in which we alter the past to make it more reasonable in light of the present.

What makes these biases so important is that they are not a product of motivated distortion but rather a consequence of how autobiographical memory operates fundamentally. Respondents are not being uncooperative when they use memory heuristics to reconstruct autobiographical experience; they are simply being human. The shortcuts respondents use to respond to research questions are not used out of laziness. Often, the information that the researcher seeks is simply not available in memory. When respondents are asked how often they drank alcohol in the past year, it may simply not be possible to recall and enumerate every episode of drinking in order to arrive at an exact estimate; heuristic estimates are the only viable way to answer the question. The same may be true when we are asked how depressed we have been or how generous we are. An exact answer based on detailed recall is not available to us; we have to use heuristic strategies to arrive at a good-faith estimate, which, unfortunately, is likely to be biased.

VARIETIES OF SELF-REPORT

Recall heuristics and other cognitive processes that assist in the reconstruction of the past bridge the gap between what we are asked to recall and what we have actually encoded in memory. An implication is that bias in self-report can vary with the amount of cognitive processing that is demanded by the question. Thus, self-reports are not all equally subject to bias. Bias will tend to be greatest for those kinds of recall that make the greatest cognitive demands on the respondent. It is useful to divide self-report into three categories:

Global Self-Report. The bulk of self-report data ask respondents for global summaries or judgments of their behavior. We ask people whether they are generous or stingy, how often they typically exercise, and so forth. To respond accurately from memory, a respondent would have to access memories of the relevant occasions and then integrate or summarize them for reporting. Respondents do not (cannot) approach the inquiry in this way and so necessarily generate responses on the basis of bias-prone heuristic strategies. Some reports, of course, require not only recall from memory but also the application of a judgment. Even if one could accurately retrieve the past, one must then decide whether the data fit the categories of the inquiry (does the estimated frequency qualify as often?). Because of the amount of processing and the multiple levels of processing required, global reports are likely to be most subject to distortion.

Episodic Recall. Whereas global self-report asks for a general characterization based on past behaviors, episodic recall inquiries ask for information about a single, particular event. Debriefing of an assault or of an initial onset of clinical symptoms would be relevant examples. Retrieval of such data does not require summary or integration of multiple episodes or occasions and is thus somewhat less subject to cognitive distortions. However, such recall still depends on the accurate initial encoding of the relevant data and is still subject to some distortion in retrieval. Retrieval can be selective or distorted. Recall of a specific occasion is often colored by schematic recall in which the retrospective narrative is shaped to conform to a template for the class of occasions (e.g., "if we were out to dinner, we must have had wine, because that's what we usually do.").

Immediate Report. Questions about the respondent's current state—for example, What are you doing now?—do not require retrieval of data from memory but simply access to and accurate reporting of current information. Accurate reporting still requires access to the relevant information (e.g., the ability to discern what one is feeling) and a willingness to report it accurately, but it does not require retrieval from memory or other processing—both of which are also presumed by other forms of self-report. Accordingly, immediate reporting is least subject to bias and distortion due to cognitive processing. Although it is the least subject to distortion, immediate report is the least used form of self-report in behavioral research. The key reason is that we are seldom interested in the subject's state at the time of reporting, which is usually a highly artificial occasion; our focus is not on their state at the time they come into our laboratory but on what they experience or do in general in their natural environment or under particular circumstances.

ECOLOGICAL MOMENTARY ASSESSMENT

Some investigators have used strategies for collecting immediate reports of subjects' state in subjects' natural environments. We have labeled these strategies EMA (Stone & Shiffman, 1994). EMA emphasizes collection of data about respondents' momentary, or current, state so as to avoid biases associated with recall. Because the target of inquiry is often the subject's real-world behavior, EMA focuses on collection of data in the subject's natural environment, hence the ecological emphasis. Although our focus here is on self-report, we should note that EMA assessments are not limited to self-reports but can include, for example, directly measured physiological parameters (e.g., Kamarck et al., 1998).

EMA studies usually consist of repeated assessments of subjects' momentary state as they go about the tasks of daily living in their natural environment. Classical examples come from studies using the Experience Sampling Method (ESM; Csikszentmihalyi & Larsen, 1987). In these studies, subjects carry pagers that are activated to beep at random to prompt subjects to complete a written assessment. Repeated assessments over time are then used to characterize and compare individuals or situations. For example, Johnson and Larson (1982) studied women with and without bulimia and found that bulimic women spent more time alone than normal women. Among the bulimic women, Johnson and Larson found that episodes of binge eating were associated with increased emotional upset.

SAMPLING APPROACHES FOR EMA DATA

The repeated assessments that characterize EMA studies essentially constitute a sample of subjects' momentary states. This sampling task can be approached in several ways, which have been characterized by Wheeler & Reis (1991):

Interval-contingent assessment involves completion of assessment at regular intervals. Common implementations include blood pressure assessments at regular intervals and daily diaries (although these are not truly momentary assessments).

Event-contingent assessments are completed when a particular event occurs. The most common example is self-monitoring, where the subject is supposed to record every episode of eating, hair-pulling, or some other behavior of interest (McFall, 1977). Obviously, this approach leads to a sample of such events and not necessarily to a representative sample of the subject's general state. It also requires a clear definition of the triggering event and consistent detection of and response to the event.

Signal-contingent recording is exemplified by ESM, where an external signal cues recording. Usually the signal is timed to be emitted at random (otherwise, it falls into one of the other two sampling approaches) and requires the use of a signaling device. Beepers, electronic watches, and palmtop computers have been used. This strategy can produce a representative sample of subjects' momentary states.

EMA data can be analyzed in different ways for different purposes. Multiple observations are sometimes aggregated within each subject to characterize the subject's general behavior, as in Johnson and Larson's (1982) comparisons of mood among bulimic and normal women. One might also compare different classes of observations within the same subject in order to understand how situational factors (e.g., social interaction, Guyll & Contrada, 1998; or bulimic episodes, Johnson & Larson, 1982) affect a process. Alternatively, if one is studying a process that varies over time, the observations might be analyzed as a time series or using event history frameworks (Affleck, Tennen, Urrows, & Higgins, 1991; Shiffman, Engberg, et al., 1997) or as correlated time series (Kamarck et al., 1998). Finally, investigators interested in particular events can isolate and analyze examples from the data (e.g., Shiffman, Paty, Gnys, Kassel, & Hickcox, 1996). All of the approaches (except possibly the last) treat assessments as a sample of moments and emphasize the need to ensure that a representative and unbiased sample is obtained. In all cases, the approach relies on momentary reports to avoid the problems introduced by retrospective recall.

COMPUTERIZED EMA: THE ELECTRONIC DIARY

Most EMA studies have collected data using paper-and-pencil diaries. Even when a high-tech device has been used to prompt subjects to complete an assessment, the assessment itself has been completed on paper. This approach has significant limitations, most notably that it is easy to fake compliance by completing the diary after-the-fact. Litt, Cooney, and Morse (1998) recently reported on a study in which alcoholic subjects were studied in a signal-contingent EMA study. The subjects were beeped several times daily by pre-programmed electronic watches, at which time they were to complete an assessment card. The apparent rate of compliance, as assessed by the number of completed cards, seemed high. However, debriefing revealed that the majority of subjects (70%) had faked at least some of their entries every single day by writing in the time when they were first prompted but then completing the diary card at their convenience, thus completely subverting the momentary assessment strategy.[1] Thus, having a method to verify the time data are entered is essential to a valid EMA strategy.

I have approached this issue by collecting data using small palm-top computers. In this chapter, I present my approach and, in particular, my application to a specific research problem as an illustration of computerized EMA methods. Participants in our studies carry a computer, which we call an Electronic Diary, or ED, as they go about their daily lives. ED prompts

---

[1]Indeed, one has to assume that this procedure introduced systematic bias because the moments when subjects chose to complete the diary cards are bound to have differed from the random moments at which they were prompted.

for data and records responses while also recording the time of data entry, thus precluding after-the-fact or bunched entry of data. ED issues randomly scheduled audible prompts to solicit data and will only accept data when the subject is responding to a prompt that has just been issued. ED prompts subjects audibly for 2 minutes, after which the prompt is considered to have been missed and is recorded as such. The number of prompts recorded as missed provides a built-in objective measure of compliance.

Implementing EMA data collection on a palmtop computer also addresses other challenges of EMA research. Diary data are often quite "dirty"—subjects leave gaps in the data, give formally invalid responses (i.e., responding "7" to an item with a 1–6 scale), or violate skip patterns within an assessment. ED incorporates data entry features to minimize or eliminate these problems. Data are entered in fixed multiple-choice format with the user selecting a response from among a set of offered alternatives so it is impossible to enter formally invalid responses. ED also enforces and manages skip patterns and does not permit skipping questions, thus eliminating missing data. ED is programmed to check for and filter some invalid response profiles (e.g., saying "no" to all activities when offered an exhaustive list), thus minimizing them. Subjects have the opportunity to review and correct errors within the current assessment but cannot view or change prior assessments. ED also handles prompting schedules more flexibly than other devices. For example, prompting frequency can be modified on the basis of data recorded by the participant.

Traditionally, EMA studies using signal-contingent data collection (i.e., beeping or otherwise prompting subjects) have limited their data collection to certain hours of the day (e.g., 8 am to 8 pm) in order to avoid beeping subjects while they were sleeping. ED incorporates an alarm clock function that subjects use to eliminate prompting while they are sleeping and to wake them up and reinitiate prompting when they wake up. As a result, prompts can be scheduled randomly throughout the day to more validly capture subjects' entire experience. This is not a trivial matter: In a recent study (reported later this chapter), 26% of assessments fell outside an 8 am to 8 pm time window and assessments outside this window differed significantly from those within the window. Thus, the ability to sample the entire waking day enhances the representativeness of EMA data.

ED can also be used to collect event-contingent data. Subjects can initiate entries for any of several events that are defined in ED software and are administered an appropriate assessment. ED can help solve one problem in applying traditional self-monitoring approaches to frequent behaviors such as cigarette smoking, which typically occurs 20 or more times per day. On the one hand, assessing every instance of smoking is unduly burdensome (and differentially burdensome for heavier smokers). On the other hand, allowing subjects to select which events are assessed introduces substantial bias. Our approach has been to instruct subjects to report every event (e.g., each cigarette) to ED. ED then randomly selects a subset of events for assessment, thus eliminating the potential for bias in selection of events for assessment. However, it should be noted that subjects may not notice all eligible events or report all the events they are aware of; this may introduce bias.

In EMA protocols using the ED, subjects are first trained in the use of the device. (Subjects need not be computer-savvy.) They are then instructed to carry ED with them throughout the day, making event entries as needed and responding to random prompts as they occur. They turn ED off when they go to sleep, setting an alarm for waking up. On periodic lab visits, data from ED are uploaded to a PC for summary, review, and analysis. The instant availability of data provides an opportunity to give subjects reinforcement and–or corrective feedback for their compliance or lack thereof.

EMA methods do have substantial limitations as well. They impose significant burdens on both investigators and research subjects. The methods are costly to implement, they require high levels of technical skill in development, and they are labor intensive. The sheer volume of data and its complexity pose significant logistical and intellectual challenges to investigators. EMA methods also demand a good deal of effort and cooperation from subjects and may not be suitable to certain subject populations. For example, elderly patients may have difficulty hearing prompts or reading small diary cards or computer screens. The demands of EMA protocols may be inconsistent with some occupational demands or personality styles.

THE SMOKING MONITORING STUDY

We used ED to implement an EMA study of cigarette smoking and smoking cessation. The study can be used to illustrate EMA methodology and also to test the validity of EMA data against more traditional self-report methods. By comparing real-time EMA data with other self-reports, data from this study can be used to evaluate the accuracy of global self-reports and recall of specific events.

The study tracked the behavior of cigarette smokers who were recruited for smoking cessation treatment. The approach used a simple naturalistic longitudinal design in which subjects monitored their behavior and subjective state multiple times daily over a 6-week period. For the initial 2 weeks, considered a baseline period, subjects were instructed to smoke ad lib and to record each cigarette. At the end of this period came the Target Quit Date, when subjects were expected to stop smoking. After cessation, subjects continued to track their experience—including the experience of any lapses back to smoking—for up to 4 weeks. After quitting for 24 hours, subjects were instructed to record any episodes of smoking (lapses) or episodes of intense temptation to smoke (tempts). Initial lapses were always assessed. Subjects continued to be prompted at random. Finally, participants were invited to return for follow-up approximately 2 months after the end of the monitoring period. Of the 306 smokers who entered the study, 275 completed baseline monitoring, 215 of these quit smoking for at least a day, 105 of these recorded a lapse during monitoring, and 87 of these completed follow-up. (Findings from this study are reported in Shiffman, Engberg et al., 1997; Shiffman, Hickcox et al., 1996; Shiffman, Hufford et al., 1997; and Shiffman, Paty et al., 1996.)

Compliance

During 2 weeks of baseline monitoring, subjects were instructed to record every cigarette on ED. ED randomly sampled these occasions so as to assess an average of 5 smoking occasions per day. Subjects entered an average of 22 cigarettes per day during the first week of monitoring. Simultaneous with monitoring of smoking, ED prompted subjects at random for assessment.[2] Subjects completed an average of 4.75 (SD = 2.29) random assessments per day. They missed only 9% of all prompts during baseline. This demonstrates that very high rates of compliance can be obtained using these methods and that subjects will engage in very high rates of interaction with an appropriately designed monitoring computer.

Report of Smoking Patterns

There has long been an interest in stimulus control of smoking; that is, in how the local context—who else is present, whether the smoker has been drinking, how the smoker is feeling, and so forth—may prompt or suppress smoking. For example, most leading theories of smoking suggest that smoking is cued by the experience of negative emotions and that smoking in turn relieves negative affect (Brandon, 1994; Hall, Munoz, Reus, & Sees, 1993). Other local conditions, such as consumption of alcohol or coffee, are also thought to promote cigarette smoking (Istvan & Matarazzo, 1984; Shiffman & Balabanis, 1995). These supposed associations are important not only theoretically but also clinically and form the basis for many treatment regimens.

---

[2]Assessments were not completely random but were constrained by design to avoid the period immediately following a smoking episode or a previous random prompt. This provided for better separation between samples of smoking occasions and nonsmoking occasions and also minimized the prospect that subjects would be irritated by repeated assessments one after the other.

These stimulus-associations have typically been assessed by global self-report measures. Several questionnaires—known collectively as "smoking typology" measures—are widely used to assess individual differences in smoking patterns. These measures ask smokers to characterize their smoking patterns, reporting whether they typically smoke when drinking, smoke when upset, and so forth. Although these scales have demonstrated good reliability and a consistent pattern of correlations with some external measures such as smoking rate (Shiffman, 1993), their validity as measures of actual smoking patterns is in question.

To assess the validity of globally reported smoking patterns, we first characterized the smoking patterns of 275 subjects based on their ED records of smoking during a baseline week of ad-lib smoking and then compared these to self-described smoking patterns reported by questionnaire. To facilitate the comparison, we elicited global reports of smoking patterns using a questionnaire modeled directly on the assessment used by ED to characterize smoking episodes. To characterize EMA-reported smoking patterns, we summarized ED data from a week of ad lib smoking during baseline. ED assessed approximately 5 cigarettes per day, selected at random from among these recorded on ED. Thus, a week's data comprised approximately 35 assessments of the situations where the subject smoked cigarettes. We summarized data about these episodes for individual items in the domains of mood (14 items; the mean rating for each item), location (7 options; the percentage of cigarettes smoked in each location), and activity (10 items; the percentage of cigarettes accompanied by each activity). Then, we correlated these summaries with corresponding self-report data from the questionnaire administered at entry into the study.

The results were dramatic. The average correlations were 0.09, 0.09, and 0.08 for mood, location, and activity, respectively. The correlations for individual items were uniformly low and sometimes negative. Essentially, global self-reports are almost completely unrelated to actual smoking patterns as recorded in real time!

One possible explanation could be that self-reports take into account the actual association between smoking and situational factors, not just their co-occurrence, and thus require incorporation of data about control non-smoking situations (Paty, Kassel, & Shiffman, 1992). That is, smokers may report whether they smoke more when they are drinking, which requires estimates of the likelihood of smoking when drinking and when not drinking, or data about drinking when smoking and when not smoking. Accordingly, we summarized data from approximately 35 nonsmoking situations assessed during the same baseline week and recomputed the correlations while controlling for the nonsmoking data. The correlations were essentially unchanged when we controlled for the base rate of each antecedent in nonsmoking situations: Global self-reports still show little correspondence with self-monitoring data.[3]

Although almost all the correlations were very low, a few variables showed modest correspondence between self-reported and self-monitoring data, and examination of these is instructive. The highest correlations achieved were for the frequency of smoking at home (0.38), smoking in the workplace (0.37), and smoking during job-related work activity (0.28).[4] In all likelihood, these aspects of smoking are influenced by what smoking restrictions are enforced in the smoker's workplace. In any case, this pattern of results suggests that smokers can characterize with modest accuracy only the most coarse and dramatic aspects of their smoking patterns, such as where they smoke. Smokers may also be accurate in reporting these aspects of smoking because they can infer their likelihood of smoking just by knowing what smoking regulations apply where.

The low validity of self-report may be due, in part, to the enormous cognitive demand that is implicit in questions about smoking patterns. Many subjects in this study had smoked on almost 10,000 occasions in the preceding year, and perhaps on nearly 200,000 occasions in their lifetime. Considering this, it seems implausible that anyone could accurately recall and summarize this experience in order to accurately answer the questions posed on typology questionnaires. This suggests that global self-reports of smoking may represent a particularly challenging task for respondents. It is possible that global self-reports tapping a less frequent behavior would be more accurate. This remains to be proven.

If smokers' reports of smoking patterns are not accurately based on their actual patterns, what are they related to? An earlier analysis (Shiffman, 1993) suggested that smokers' global reports of smoking patterns are very heavily colored by their perceived addiction: More addicted smokers report a higher frequency of smoking across all situations. It is also likely that subjects' global perceptions of their smoking patterns are heavily colored by a few highly salient experiences. For example, a smoker who has repeatedly experienced smoking relapse in stressful situations may conclude that his or her smoking is strongly linked to mood although this event is unrepresentative and constitutes a trivial fraction of the person's smoking occasions.

It should be noted that this instance exemplifies the aphorism that reliability does not imply validity. Smoking typology have repeatedly demonstrated reliability; that is, repeatable responses (Shiffman, 1993). They also

---

[3]The results using standard smoking typology measures (not shown) yield the same conclusions.

[4]Two out of three of these associations became stronger when we control for nonsmoking data (partial *r*s of .36, .45, and .38, respectively).

demonstrate a reproducible factor structure. Nevertheless, they may not measure what they purport to measure. The suggestions above may explain how this can be so: They may be stable measures of other beliefs or biases.

Obviously, what holds for characterization of smoking may not hold for self-reports in other domains. As noted, smoking is so frequent that it may pose unique challenges to autobiographical memory. By the same token, however, the act of smoking, and the questions typically asked about it, are far more concrete than questions about anxiety or pain. This suggests that the implications of these findings for other domains of research are not to be minimized. The validity and expected relationship between self-reports of behavior and the actual behavior cannot be taken for granted.

Recall of Lapse Episodes

Whereas most research focuses on global characteristics such as those putatively assessed in smoking typology measures, researchers are sometimes interested in the details of particular singular events. In the case of smoking, a good deal of attention has focused on smoking lapses—initial episodes of smoking after a period of abstinence. Unfortunately, most attempts to quit smoking end in relapse—by some estimates, 80% of those who quit smoking relapse within 3 months (Garvey, Bliss, Hitchcock, Heinold, & Rosner, 1992). Of course, all relapses begin with an initial lapse, when the line is first crossed between abstinence and smoking. It has been proposed that such lapses are typically precipitated by situational contexts, such as exposure to smoking cues (e.g., a pack of cigarettes, or someone smoking) or emotional upset (Marlatt & Gordon, 1985), and studies have repeatedly confirmed this (Bliss, Garvey, Heinold, & Hitchcock, 1989; O'Connell & Martin, 1987; Shiffman, Paty et al., 1996). However, these data on initial lapses are usually collected at follow-up visits months after the actual episode and thus rely critically on smokers' recall of a long-distant event. It may be plausible that smokers can recall these details long after the fact because these episodes are highly salient watersheds in their efforts to quit smoking, perhaps making them truly memorable.

To evaluate the accuracy of lapse recall, we solicited recall of initial lapses from the smokers who had participated in ED monitoring of their quit experience (Shiffman, Hufford et al., 1997). Recall was solicited at a scheduled follow-up session that fell an average of 72.44 ($SD = 13.67$) days after the initial lapse. Subjects were asked to report on their first episode of smoking by completing a questionnaire paralleling the situational assessment they completed on ED. We then evaluated the correspondence between their retrospective account and the real-time account, as recorded on ED.

Lapse Dating. We first evaluated the accuracy of participants' dating of the lapse. Few participants could accurately remember the day on which their lapse episode occurred. Only 23% were exactly accurate; on average, participants were off by about 2 weeks. Further, some estimates were wildly inaccurate: 5% of participants placed their first lapse as occurring prior to the day they first quit smoking, and 25% placed the lapse outside the 4-week monitoring period. This is particularly striking because participants were enrolled in a structured cessation program with a fixed quit date and had systematically monitored their behavior. Furthermore, dating errors were asymmetric: Consistent with the literature on recall of events (Thompson, Skowronski, & Lee, 1988), participants tended to "telescope" recall to bring the date about 2 weeks closer to the date of follow-up. Inaccuracy in dating of lapse events is serious, as such data are often used to analyze the outcome of smoking cessation by survival analysis.

Recall of Context. We evaluated the accuracy of recall by comparing recall and recorded data in four domains: Mood (represented by 14 items), Activity (10 items), Triggers (factors thought to have triggered the lapse: 9 items), and Reactions (cognitive and emotional responses to the lapse itself: 5 items). Within each domain, we computed item-by-item correlations between recall and ED data. Correlations averaged around 0.32, suggesting that only about 10% of the variance in recall was due to accurate retrieval of information about the episode. The results were similar when the two sources of data were compared using profile correlations (Cronbach & Gleser, 1953), which compare the pattern of data across the two sources, rather than making the comparison one variable at a time. Recall was poor for the items of most interest to students of relapse; for example, recall of the most important trigger corresponded to ED entries less than one third of the time (32%, kappa = 0.19).[5]

Individual Differences in Recall. We expected that some participants would have better recall of the lapse than others and might be able to

---

[5]When participants misstated the date of their initial lapse, this complicated evaluation of the accuracy of the rest of their recall data. If the recall of the episode details was inaccurate, one has to consider that perhaps it is because they are (accurately?) recalling a different episode or occasion. To address this, we used a two-phase procedure to elicit recall of the first lapse. Participants were first asked to recall the first lapse—including its date—without prompting. When the date of the first lapse was misstated, we then solicited a second round of recall, prompting participants with the recorded lapse date and asking them to recall that episode. This did not improve recall. Indeed, prompting with the date generally produced less accurate recall of the situation. Accordingly, our subsequent analyses focused on the unprompted recall.

recognize and report the strength of their recollections. Unfortunately, participants' confidence in their accuracy was completely unrelated to their actual accuracy. In other words, even for those smokers who were quite certain they could accurately recall their first lapse, recollection of this critical incident bore scant resemblance to the original event, both overall and in critical details.

Discussion. Of course, the study and its interpretation is subject to some limitations: The average recall interval in the study was over 2 months; memory might be better for more recent events. The fact that participants experienced and recorded a number of similar events (i.e., later lapses) may have obscured the memory of the index event. The repeated experience may also have promoted the development of an event schema to summarize the entire class of events rather than specific recall of the index event. We relied on unprompted, spontaneous recall of events; the study also does not address the possibility for improving recall through the use of cognitive interviewing strategies.

Nevertheless, the finding that first lapse episodes are not recalled accurately is particularly striking, for several reasons: First, retrospective data on first lapses has been widely used in research on the cause of addictive lapses (Bliss et al., 1989; O'Connell & Martin, 1987); thus, the finding throws into question much of the existing literature on the topic. Second, the real-time recording on ED should have ensured that the details of the episode were initially encoded, thus enhancing recall. Third, for smokers, the first lapse represents a significant transition from abstinence to smoking and the beginning of failure in a major self-change effort; accordingly, it was expected to be a highly salient, emotionally relevant life event, and thus to be quite memorable. Fourth, whereas the literature on autobiographical memory has largely focused on memory for incidental details (e.g., what one had for lunch), either among cognitive scientists (Wagenaar, 1986) or among undergraduate psychology students (Brewer, 1988), this study focused on community adults dealing with a real-life challenge and recalling a significant life event. Thus, the inability of respondents to accurately recall their initial lapses bodes ill for the use of retrospective recall as a method of collecting data about particular past events.

The Influence of Schematic Recall. Why should recall be so inaccurate? One reason, proposed by students of autobiographical memory, is that memories are often reconstructed based on schema—abstract representations or prototypical scripts of event types, from which accounts of particular instances are derived when recall is solicited (Bradburn et al., 1987). In this case, respondents may have a general concept for what a smoking relapse episode looks like. Respondents' use of schemata—essentially stereotypes of the target situation—to reconstruct an episodic memory can yield reasonable, believable—but inaccurate—accounts of the situation (Holmberg & Holmes, 1994; Neisser, 1981).

The use of schematic recall could help explain an apparent paradox: On the one hand, smokers appear to be inaccurate in recalling lapse episodes; on the other hand, the retrospective descriptions they provide strongly resemble (in the aggregate) those based on real-time data. Given the apparent inaccuracy of retrospective data, the description of lapse characteristics drawn from the aggregate real-time data (Shiffman, Paty et al., 1996) largely matched those obtained from prior studies using retrospective data (Bliss et al., 1989; O'Connell & Martin, 1987; see Sutton, 1992). This may be because participants generated descriptions based on an accurate schema of relapse situations although they could not accurately recall their own particular experience.

To explore whether schematic reconstruction of smoking lapse situations could account for the recall data, we sought to compare their respective accounts of lapse episodes to an account representing the schema for smoking lapses. We could not rely on smokers' reports to establish the characteristics of the schema. Any reports from smokers about smoking lapses might be contaminated by actual experience and thus might not represent the schema. Conversely, we reasoned that nonsmokers, having never smoked, would have available to them only schematic information, based on a socially shared sense of smoking lapse episodes, rather than direct experience. Thus, their impressions of smoking lapses would represent the schema or stereotypic description of smoking lapse episodes, unsullied by actual experience.

Accordingly, we asked 30 people who had never smoked to describe what they thought a typical smoking lapse was like, using the same questionnaire that had been used to elicit the recall data. To compare their schematic accounts with those of the smokers in the study, we computed profile correlations for each of the domains we had used in analyzing the lapse episode (mood, activity, triggers, and after-effects). The profile correlation compared smokers' and nonsmokers' average responses over a range of variables in each domain. The profile correlation is sensitive to the shape of the profile (e.g., the pattern of activities endorsed), but not to the level (e.g., the intensity of affect endorsed); thus, it compares the pattern of responses, rather than requiring a match on any particular variable (Cronbach & Gleser, 1953). As hypothesized, smokers' recall data strongly resembled the hypothetical reports received from nonsmokers. Profile rs relating the never-smokers' mean data and those from smoking subjects' retrospective reports were 0.67, 0.57, 0.74, and 0.77 for Mood, Activities, Triggers, and AVE, respectively. In other words, never-smokers, who had no experience with smoking lapses, were able to reproduce the pattern of the retrospective data. This was not true for the data recorded on ED; $rs = 0.01$, 0.59, 0.61, and 0.16, respectively. Thus, the typical pattern of relapse data can be produced without any experiential base at all, consistent with the idea that participants' recall was influenced by general beliefs about smoking relapse episodes and accounting for the plausibility of participants' inaccurate retrospective accounts.

Moderators of Recall Accuracy. In our analyses, we found few moderators of recall accuracy; few subject characteristics or episode characteristics affected accuracy. One of the most striking, however, was that participants who had been smoking in the 2 weeks preceding recall were less accurate in recalling some aspects of the lapse, perhaps because the recent smoking episodes interfere with recall of the distant lapse. It may also be that those who were abstinent at the time of recall may more easily recall the lapse because their abstinent state at the time of recall matches their state at the time of the first lapse. However, we were surprised to find that factors such as participant's emotional state at the time of the lapse (presumably an index of its salience and memorability) were not related to recall accuracy.

Bias in Recall. Analyses of accuracy deal with errors that are presumed to be random (although note the systematic telescoping bias in recall of dates). Autobiographical memory processes can also introduce bias—systematic differences between the actual event and its recollection. The fact that recall data were collected on written forms, whereas real-time recordings were made on a computer, introduced differences in response distributions that made evaluation of bias difficult. Nevertheless, we were able to assess several forms of bias. For example, we found that respondents systematically overstated their negative affect during the lapse. This may reflect an attempt to justify their behavior ("I was feeling so badly that I just *had to* smoke") or to bring the episode into conformity with the schematic stereotype that lapses occur when people are feeling upset. Interestingly, respondents who had been smoking more steadily during the 2 weeks preceding recall exaggerated in retrospect how much the lapse made them feel like giving up their effort to quit, as though they sought to adjust their past experience to better explain their current smoking behavior. Biases such as these are particularly pernicious in a research context because they introduce into the data associations that might be misinterpreted as real causal relationships. For example, the finding in retrospective data that those who most felt like giving up subsequently engaged in more smoking could be interpreted to mean—indeed has been interpreted to mean (Curry, Marlatt, & Gordon, 1987; O'Connell & Martin, 1987; cf. Shiffman, Hickcox et al., 1996)—that the demoralizing impact of the lapse accelerates the resumption of smoking. Thus, retrospective recall of particular events can introduce not only error but systematic bias into data, which may lead to erroneous conclusions.

Summary. In sum, data on lapse recall suggests that retrospective self-report of past events is unreliable, inaccurate, and systematically biased. Although the generalizability of these findings to recall for other events has yet to be demonstrated, the findings counsel against accepting at face value even compelling recollection of singular life events. This has profound and troubling implications both for research and for clinical practice, where a respondent's recall of a past event is typically the only source of information about the event. Obviously, real-time monitoring is not always, or even typically, a viable alternative to retrospective recall. This suggests an urgent need to develop methods to improve recall of past events (e.g., Means, Habina, Swan, & Jack, 1992). Even where recall cannot be enhanced, it should at least be treated with appropriate skepticism.

Prospects for EMA

There has been a recent explosion of interest in EMA approaches to data collection. These methods have been of particular interest in behavioral medicine and health psychology (Shiffman & Stone, 1998), where researchers are often interested in understanding the antecedents of transient symptom-states or physiological states. Thus, for example, EMA methods have been used to study the correlates of neuromyalgic and arthritic pain (Affleck, Urrows, Tennen, Higgins, & Abeles, 1996; Stone, Broderick, Porter, & Kaell, 1997), and ongoing studies are examining correlates of migraine headache and episodes of Reynaud's syndrome. EMA methods have also long been used to study environmental and psychological influences on heart rate and blood pressure (Goldstein, Jamner, & Shapiro, 1992; Jamner, Shapiro, Goldstein, & Hug, 1991; Kamarck et al., 1998) as well as stress hormones (van Eck & Nicolson, 1994; Ockenfels et al., 1995; Smyth et al., 1997). For similar reasons, EMA methods have proved attractive to students of psychopathology, who have used it to study eating disorders (Johnson & Larson, 1982; Schlundt, 1989), anxiety disorders (Dijkman & deVries, 1987; Dijkman-Caes & deVries, 1991), chronic mental patients (Delespaul, 1995; Delespaul & deVries, 1987), and addictive disorders (Kaplan, 1992). Social and personality psychologists have used EMA methods to characterize normal functioning, focusing on topics such as the experience of emotion, personality, and minor daily illness (Larsen & Kasimatis, 1991), social interaction (Reis & Wheeler, 1991), and descriptions of fundamental psychological states (Csikszentmihalyi & Csikszentmihalyi, 1988). In short, EMA methods have been applied to most domains where investigators seek accurate knowledge of respondents' experience and behavior.

Given the importance of self-report to scientific inquiry into human behavior and the inherent limitations of retrospective self-report, EMA methods hold significant promise for such research. Besides overcoming problems of recall, the ecological validity of EMA data and their ability to analyze environmental and subject-state influences on behavior will allow for more realistic and more subtle models of behavior. Finally, the expanding power of computer technology to facilitate field data collection makes these methods increasingly powerful as well as practical. Together, these factors are likely to make EMA methods the wave of the future in the study of human behavior.

REFERENCES

Affleck, G., Tennen, H., Urrows, S., & Higgins, P. (1991). Individual differences in the day-to-day experience of chronic pain: A prospective daily study of Rheumatoid arthritis patients. *Health Psychology, 10*, 419–426.

Affleck, G., Urrows, S., Tennen, H., Higgins, P., & Abeles, M. (1996). Sequential daily relations of sleep, pain intensity, and attention to pain among women with fibromyalgia. *Pain, 68*, 363–368.

Bliss, R. E., Garvey, A. J., Heinold, J. W., & Hitchcock, J. L. (1989). The influence of situation and coping on relapse crisis outcomes after smoking cessation. *Journal of Consulting and Clinical Psychology, 57*, 443–449.

Bradburn, N. M., Rips, L. J., & Shevell, S. K. (1987). Answering autobiographical questions: The impact of memory and inference on surveys. *Science, 236*, 157–161.

Brandon, T. H. (1994). Negative affect as motivation to smoke. *Current Directions in Psychological Science, 3*, 33–37.

Brewer, W. F. (1988). Memory for randomly sampled autobiographical events. In U. Neisser & E. Winograd (Eds.), *Remembering reconsidered: Ecological and traditional approaches to the study of memory* (pp. 21–90). Cambridge, England: Cambridge University Press.

Cronbach, L. J., & Gleser, G. C. (1953). Assessing similarity between profiles. *Psychological Bulletin, 50*, 456–473.

Csikszentmihalyi, M., & Csikszentmihalyi, I. S. (1988). *Optimal experience—Psychological studies of flow in consciousness.* New York: Cambridge University Press.

Csikszentmihalyi, M., & Larsen, R. (1987). Validity and reliability of the Experience-Sampling method. *Journal of Nervous and Mental Disease, 175*, 509–513.

Curry, S., Marlatt, G. A., & Gordon, J. R. (1987). Abstinence violation effect: Validation of an attributional construct with smoking cessation. *Journal of Consulting and Clinical Psychology, 55*, 145–149.

Delespaul, P. A. E. G. (1995). *Assessing schizophrenia in daily life—The Experience Sampling Method.* Maastricht, The Netherlands: Maastricht University Press.

Delespaul, P. A. E. G., & deVries, M. W. (1987). The daily life of ambulatory chronic mental patients. *Journal of Nervous and Mental Disease, 175*, 537–544.

Dijkman, C. I. M., & deVries, M. W. (1987). The social ecology of anxiety—Theoretical and quantitative perspectives. *Journal of Nervous & Mental Disease, 175*, 550–557.

Dijkman-Caes, C. I. M., & deVries, M. W. (1991). Daily life situations and anxiety in panic disorder and agoraphobia. *Journal of Anxiety Disorders, 5*, 343–357.

Eisenhower, D., Mathiowetz, N. A., & Morganstein, D. (1991). Recall error: Sources and bias reduction techniques. In P. P. Biemer, R. M. Groves, L. E. Lyberg, N. A. Mathiowetz, & S. Sudman (Eds.), *Measurement errors in surveys* (pp. 127–144). New York: Wiley.

Garvey, A. J., Bliss, R. E., Hitchcock, J. L., Heinold, J. W., & Rosner, B. (1992). Predictors of smoking relapse among self-quitters: A report from the normative aging study. *Addictive Behaviors, 17*, 367–377.

Goldstein, I. B., Jamner, L. D., & Shapiro, D. (1992). Ambulatory blood pressure and heart rate in healthy male paramedics during a workday and a nonwork day. *Health Psychology, 11*, 48–54.

Guyll, M., & Contrada, R. J. (1998). Trait hostility and ambulatory cardiovascular activity: Responses to social interaction. *Health Psychology, 17*, 30–39.

Hall, S. M., Munoz, R. F., Reus, V. I., & Sees, K. L. (1993). Nicotine, negative affect, and depression. *Journal of Consulting and Clinical Psychology, 61*, 761–767.

Holmberg, D., & Holmes, J. G. (1994). Reconstruction of relationship memories: A mental models approach. In N. Schwarz & S. Sudman (Eds.), *Autobiographical memory and the validity of retrospective reports* (pp. 267–288). New York: Springer-Verlag.

Istvan, J., & Matarazzo, J. D. (1984). Tobacco, alcohol and caffeine use: A review of their interrelationships. *Psychological Bulletin, 95*, 301–326.

Jamner, L. D., Shapiro, D., Goldstein, I. B., & Hug, R. (1991). Ambulatory blood pressure and heart rate in paramedics: Effects of synical hostility and defensivness. *Psychosomatic Medicine, 53*, 393–406.

Johnson, C. L., & Larson, R. (1982). Bulimia: An analysis of moods and behavior. *Psychosomatic Medicine, 44*, 341–351.

Kamarck, T. W., Shiffman, S., Smithline, L., Goodie, J., Paty, J. A., Gnys, M., & Jong, J. (1998). Effects of task strain, social conflict, and emotional activation on ambulatory cardiovascular activity: Daily life consequences of "recurring stress" in a multiethnic adult sample. *Health Psychology, 17,* 17–29.

Kaplan, C. D. (1992). Drug craving and drug use in the daily life of heroin addicts. In M. W. deVries (Ed.), *The experience of psychopathology: Investigating mental disorders in their natural settings* (pp. 193–218). Cambridge, England: Cambridge University Press.

Larsen, R. J., & Kasimatis, M. (1991). Day-to-day physical symptoms: Individual differences in the occurrence, duration, and emotional concomitants of minor daily illnesses. *Journal of Personality, 59*, 387–421.

Litt, M. D., Cooney, N. L., & Morse, P. (1998). Ecological Momentary Assessment (EMA) with treated alcoholics: Methodological problems and potential solutions. *Health Psychology, 17*, 48–52.

Marlatt, G. A., & Gordon, J. R. (1985). *Relapse prevention.* New York: Guilford.

McFall, R. M. (1977). Parameters of self-monitoring. In R. B. Stuart (Ed.), *Behavioral self-management: Strategies, techniques, and outcome* (pp. 196–214). New York: Brunner/Mazel.

Means, B., Habina, K., Swan, G. E., & Jack, L. (1992). *Cognitive research on response error in survey questions on smoking.* (Publication No. PHS 92-1080). Hyattsville, MD: U.S. Department of Health and Human Services.

Neisser, U. (1981). John Dean's memory. *Cognition, 9*, 1–22.

Ockenfels, M. C., Porter, L. S., Smyth, J. M., Kirschbaum, C., Hellhammer, D. H., & Stone, A. A. (1995). The effect of chronic stress associated with unemployment on salivary cortisol: Overall cortisol levels, diurnal rhythm, and acute stress reactivity. *Psychosomatic Medicine, 57*, 460–467.

O'Connell, K. A., & Martin, E. J. (1987). Highly tempting situations associated with abstinence, temporary lapse, and relapse among participants in smoking cessation programs. *Journal of Consulting and Clinical Psychology, 55*, 367–371.

Paty, J. A., Kassel, J. D., & Shiffman, S. (1992). The importance of assessing base rates for clinical studies: An example of stimulus control of smoking. In M. W. deVries (Ed.), *The experience of psychopathology: Investigating mental disorders in their natural settings* (pp. 347–352). Cambridge, England: Cambridge University Press.

Reis, H. T., & Wheeler, L. (1991). Studying social interaction with the Rochester Interaction Record. *Advances in Experimental Social Psychology, 24,* 269–317.

Ross, M. (1989). Relation of implicit theories to the construction of personal histories. *Psychological Review, 96,* 341–357.

Schlundt, D. G. (1989). Computerized behavioral assessment of eating behavior in bulimia: The self-monitoring analysis system. In W. G. Johnson (Ed.), *Advances in eating disorders: Vol. 2. Bulimia* (pp. 1–32). New York: JAI.

Shiffman, S. (1993). Assessing smoking patterns and motives. *Journal of Consulting and Clinical Psychology, 61,* 732–742.

Shiffman, S., & Balabanis, M. (1995). Associations between alcohol and tobacco. In J. B. Fertig & J. P. Allen (Eds.), *Alcohol and tobacco: From basic science to clinical practice.* (Research Monograph No. 30, pp. 17–36). Bethesda, MD: National Institutes of Health.

Shiffman, S., Engberg, J., Paty, J. A., Perz, W., Gnys, M., Kassel, J. D., & Hickcox, M. (1997). A day at a time: Predicting smoking lapse from daily urge. *Journal of Abnormal Psychology, 106,* 104–116.

Shiffman, S., Hickcox, M., Paty, J. A., Gnys, M., Kassel, J. D., & Richards, T. (1996). Progression from a smoking lapse to relapse: Prediction from Abstinence Violation Effects, nicotine dependence, and lapse characteristics. *Journal of Consulting and Clinical Psychology, 64,* 993–1002.

Shiffman, S., Hufford, M., Hickcox, M., Paty, J. A., Gnys, M., & Kassel, J. D. (1997). Remember that? A comparison of real-time versus retrospective recall of smoking lapses. *Journal of Consulting and Clinical Psychology, 65,* 292–300.

Shiffman, S., Paty, J. A., Gnys, M., Kassel, J. D., & Hickcox, M. (1996). First lapses to smoking: Within subjects analysis of real time reports. *Journal of Consulting and Clinical Psychology, 64,* 366–379.

Shiffman, S., & Stone, A. (Eds.). (1998). Assessment of health-relevant variables in natural environments [Special Section]. *Health Psychology, 17,* 3–52.

Smyth, J. M., Ockenfels, M. C., Gorin, A. A., Catley, D., Porter, L. S., Kirschbaum, C., Hellhammer, D. H., & Stone, A. A. (1997). Individual differences in the diurnal cycle of cortisol. *Psychoneuroendocrinology, 22,* 89–102.

Stone, A. A., Broderick, J. E., Porter, L., & Kaell, A. T. (1997). The experience of rheumatoid arthritis pain and fatigue: Examining momentary reports and correlates over one week. *Arthritis Care and Research, 10,* 185–193.

Stone, A. A., & Shiffman, S. (1994). Ecological momentary assessment (EMA) in behavioral medicine. *Annals of Behavioral Medicine, 16,* 199–202.

Sutton, S. R. (1992). Are "risky" situations really risky? Review and critique of the situational approach to smoking relapse. *Journal of Smoking-Related Disorders, 3,* 79–84.

Thompson, C. P., Skowronski, J. J., & Lee, D. J. (1988). Telescoping in dating naturally occurring events. *Memory and Cognition, 16,* 461–468.

van Eck, M. M., & Nicolson, N. A. (1994). Perceived stress and salivary cortisol in daily life. *Annals of Behavioral Medicine, 16,* 221–227.

Wagenaar, W. A. (1986). My memory: A study of autobiographical memory over six years. *Cognitive Psychology, 18,* 225–252.

Wheeler, L., & Reis, H. T. (1991). Self-recording of everyday life events: Origins, types, and uses. *Journal of Personality, 59,* 339–354.

SELF-REPORTING OF PHYSICAL SYMPTOMS

Arthur A. Stone
State University of New York at Stony Brook

In both clinical practice and in research, the primary method of obtaining information about physical symptomatology is through self-reports. Every day, thousand upon thousands of health care providers ask their patients to describe how they are generally feeling and to discuss specific symptoms. Patients present their doctors with panoply of global states ("I feel lousy," "I am fatigued," "I don't feel right") to very concrete descriptions ("I have a sharp pain in my right knee that is worse on awakening"). Information from these interviews, along with various medical tests, provide the basis for treatment and for the evaluation of its efficacy. In medical research, information of the same sort is obtained with questionnaires and structured interviews. These data-collection methods may provide a more systematic way of gathering physical symptom information, but regardless of the mode of data collection, the information is self-reported. Thus, self-reports of physical symptoms may be considered the mainstay of medical practice and research.

Consistent with the theme of the previous chapters of this volume, caution must be taken in blithely accepting self-reported symptomatology. Several factors have the potential to diminish the validity of these data. Because patients typically see their doctors infrequently, even for those with chronic conditions, they are asked to recall their physical symptoms over substantial time intervals, allowing various retrospecting reporting biases to contaminate the reports. Current psychological states (e.g., mood level) may have influence on reports of past and current physical symptoms. Other factors may also influence the validity of self-reports, including patients' motivation to achieve certain outcomes from the medical visit (e.g., increased medication). These and other factors all need to be considered by both the clinician and researcher with an interest in physical symptomatology.

The three chapters comprising this section of the volume detail some of the most salient influences on self-reports of physical symptomatology. Dr. Pennebaker's chapter shows how certain psychological processes influence people's ability to detect physical states and how a mood state, anxiety, can affect the level of symptoms reported. Dr. Keefe's chapter discusses a fundamental physical symptom, pain, and describes current methods of assessing pain and factors that affect the self-report of pain. Dr. Barsky details the relationship between self-reported symptoms and verified disease states and shows how a number of factors influence that relationship.

Overall, these chapters present information that is essential to understanding and interpreting patients' reports of their physical symptoms. Although we are far from having an exact science concerning the self-report of physical symptoms, the research discussed in the chapters demonstrates substantial progress toward that goal.

17

Psychological Factors Influencing the Reporting of Physical Symptoms

James W. Pennebaker
The University of Texas at Austin

Researchers and practitioners routinely ask individuals about their health. We ask people to what degree they are experiencing a variety of physical symptoms from headache and upset stomach to dizziness and pain. Often, these symptom reports are thought to serve as proxies for underlying physiological activity. Not surprisingly, however, we find that although people may report, for example, a headache, no clear biological referent exists to confirm whether or not the person truly is feeling pain in his or her head. Even when biological measures are available, researchers find that the correspondence between physiological activity and self-reports of physiological activity are modest at best.

The purpose of this chapter is to explore how symptoms in general are perceived and reported. For example, there is little doubt that the physical symptoms of both well-understood disorders, such as influenza, and less-understood problems, such as chronic fatigue syndrome (CFS), are subjectively distressing. Despite their possible physiological bases, the symptoms of both influenza and CFS indicate that psychological and perceptual factors are related to both the etiology and possibly the treatment of their symptoms. Virtually all diseases—whether biologically validated or not—have physical symptoms that are influenced by psychological and individual difference processes.

THE PERCEPTUAL PROCESS: THE ACTIVE
VERSUS PASSIVE PERCEIVER

In most western cultures, the majority of common health problems are associated with a variety of subjective physical symptoms, including fatigue, difficulty concentrating, racing heart, shortness of breath, anxiety, headache, upset stomach, dizziness, and muscle tension. Indeed, these sensations are also among the most common among healthy samples of normal individuals (Pennebaker, 1982), those diagnosed with somatization disorders (e.g., Robbins & Kirmayer, 1991), and even those diagnosed with hypertension (Pennebaker & Watson, 1988) and diabetes (Cox et al., 1985; Pennebaker, Gonder-Frederick, Cox, & Hoover, 1985). Similarly, most of these physical symptoms are also typically associated with diagnoses of clinical depression (APA, 1995). Within the personality literature, these constellations of symptoms are the basis of Negative Affectivity, or NA (Watson & Pennebaker, 1989).

Although many illnesses are associated with a variety of symptoms that do not have clear biological bases, the prevailing opinion is that their reports are subjectively real. That is, when individuals report symptoms and sensations, they subjectively experience significant bodily activity. The question that immediately comes to mind, then, concerns the perceptual information that influences how individuals attend to and interpret their body's ambiguous signals. Research that has addressed this issue has evolved considerably over the last century.

The laboratories of Wundt and Fechner yielded the first scientific investigations relevant to symptom perception. In developing the science of psychophysics, Wundt and others demonstrated a one-to-one correspondence between external stimuli and the perception of stimuli (Boring, 1950). When all extraneous variables were held constant, perceptions of light, sound, touch, and other sensory dimensions were mathematically related to the sources of the percepts.

Gibson (1966, 1979) was one of the first researchers to question the psychophysics tradition within perceptual psychology. The crux of his argument was that organisms relied on information from a variety of sources in order to perceive even the simplest stimulus arrays. Further, this information was processed by virtually all of the senses simultaneously in order to create a stable percept. Accordingly, organisms were not passive recipients of information. Rather, they actively searched the environment in order to understand it better and, consequently, to behave appropriately and efficiently.

Consider how individuals perceive the brightness of the moon at night. Of course, they rely heavily on their eyes and their visual systems in general. But the perception of the brightness of an object depends on much more than the stimulation of a portion of rods and cones within the retina. Visually, perception of brightness will also vary depending on the background of the sky, other visible objects, and the degree of adaptation to darkness. Beyond the visual system, the perception of brightness will also be affected by our beliefs about or needs concerning the object. For example, if we live in a primitive culture and believe that moonlight exerts an evil influence, we may over- or underestimate its brightness. Similarly, an adolescent couple trying to walk undetected in their neighborhood at night may overestimate the moon's brightness. Conversely, their curious neighbors may underestimate its brightness.

More relevant to the present discussion concerns the role of nonvisual information that can affect visual perception. The apparent brightness of an object can be altered if the perceiver experiences intense pain, loses vestibular cues (and a corresponding sense of balance), becomes paralyzed, or even hears a loud noise. The point that modern-day perceptual researchers emphasize is that we simultaneously rely on all of our perceptual systems in making sense of any visual arrays.

The Role of Attention

How do individuals first notice and attend to internal physical sensations as opposed to external visual, auditory, or other cues? Given that individuals can process only a finite amount of information at any given time, we have proposed that internal sensory and external environmental cues compete for attention (Pennebaker, 1982). As the number and salience of external cues increases, attention to internal stimuli will necessarily decrease, and vice versa. When the environment lacks meaningful external information (such as when people engage in boring or tedious tasks), attention will tend to focus more internally, thereby causing an increase in symptom reporting. Thus, people should perceive and report more symptoms in unstimulating environments than in interesting ones.

A great deal of research now supports this competition of cues model. Various experiments demonstrate that people report higher levels of fatigue (Fillingham & Fine, 1986; Padgett & Hill, 1989), increased heart palpitations, and even cough more in boring situations than in stimulating ones (Pennebaker, 1982). Manipulations that heighten self-attention also increase physical symptom reporting (e.g., Schmidt, Wolfs-Takens, Oosterlaan, & van den Hout, 1994). Indeed, symptom reports are elevated when individuals live alone (Mahon, Yarcheski, & Yarcheski, 1993), live in rural environments, or work in undemanding or unstimulating settings (e.g., NCHS, 1980). Conversely, increased focus of attention to the body heightens symptom reports, particularly during times of stress (e.g., Goldman, Kraemer, & Salovey, 1996). It is noteworthy, however, that these increased symptom reports are unrelated to accuracy of perceiving physiological change (e.g., Pennebaker & Watson, 1988).

The competition of cues idea helps to explain when and why distraction can serve as a useful short-term coping method. In a naturally occurring setting where distractions are available, symptoms can be temporarily reduced when attention is diverted elsewhere. During brief periods—such as during sports competitions or when patients are receiving relatively fast injections—distraction can also be beneficial. However, directly training people to distract themselves from bodily stimulation over extended periods of time does not appear to be effective. For example, Yardley (1994) reported that distraction techniques were ineffective in reducing symptoms of vertigo. Similarly, Nolan and Wielgosz (1991) found that distraction was one of the least effective ways for individuals to cope with symptoms following a heart attack. Attempting to directly manipulate focus of attention—even in the short run—may not be effective (cf. Fillingim, Roth, & Haley, 1989). The failure of the direct manipulation of attention may stem from the same processes of failed thought suppression (see Wegner, 1992). When individuals attempt to manipulate their attention away from a forbidden topic, they must still monitor the topic at a low level to be certain that they are not, in fact, attending to it.

The Selective Search for Information

Another line of research is based on the assumption that organisms actively search their environment for information that will enable them to behave more adaptively (e.g., Neisser, 1976). This scanning is not random but, rather, is guided by beliefs or mental sets that direct the ways in which information is sought and ultimately found. This principle is also relevant to the formation of health complaints. Health-related beliefs influence how people attend to and interpret bodily sensations (e.g., Skelton & Croyle, 1991).

Dramatic examples of the power of health beliefs, or schemas, can be seen in cases of medical students' disease and mass psychogenic illness. Regarding the former, approximately 70% of first-year medical students report symptoms of the diseases that they are studying (Woods, Natterson, & Silverman, 1978). The students, who are undoubtedly under stress from sleep deprivation, exams, or other reasons, can detect a number of subtle bodily sensations that probably reflect heightened autonomic activity. When they read about various obscure illnesses associated with ambiguous symptoms, the students now scrutinize their bodies particularly closely. Their disease beliefs or schemas direct the ways they attend to their bodies and interpret their symptoms (see Gijsbers van Wijk & Kolk, 1996, for a nice empirical demonstration of the relative effects of differing perceptual processes on symptom reporting).

Schemas and selective search also play an important role in cases of mass psychogenic illness, or MPI (Pennebaker, 1982). In MPI, large groups of individuals who typically work together report a related set of physical symptoms that have no clear organic basis. MPI usually develops when one person in a setting becomes overtly sick and displays observable symptoms such as vomiting or fainting. These symptoms affect the belief processes of others in the setting—especially friends—who consequently experience similar but less dramatic symptoms such as feelings of nausea or dizziness. It is also important to appreciate that cases of MPI are most likely to occur in settings where people are anxious or tense. Many of the most famous cases have occurred during the height of the production season, in companies with poor worker-management relations, loud and unpredictable noise, and jobs that restrict people from talking to one another (Colligan, Pennebaker, & Murphy, 1982).

Perceptual Learning

Where and how individuals pay attention to their bodies can also be strongly influenced by the rewards and punishments inherent in the environment. In a fascinating analysis of symptom reporting, for example, Whitehead and his colleagues (1994) argued that symptomatic disorders—such as irritable bowel syndrome (IBS)—follow very different reporting patterns than asymptomatic problems—such a hypertension. The authors found that IBS patients with the greatest reporting of symptoms as adults reported being systematically rewarded by their parents in childhood. Symptom reporting, then, contributed to secondary gain. Secondary gain, according to Mechanic (1978), results from the added attention, freedom of everyday responsibilities, and so forth that are inherent in the sick role. Symptom reporting, then, serves as a powerful social signal: If I say that I am feeling numerous symptoms, you should treat me with greater kindness.

Just as symptoms can be reinforced via instrumental conditioning, symptom awareness and reporting can be the result of association or classical conditioning. Individuals who have experienced salient symptoms in a particular setting will be particularly sensitive to their bodies whenever they are in the same situations. A striking example can be seen in cases of anticipatory nausea. Cancer patients who have undergone chemotherapy and have gotten sick at a hospital or treatment center subsequently feel sick and often vomit or gag even on seeing the setting in later weeks, months, or even years (cf. Challis & Stam, 1992).

The perceptual approach is important in clarifying how normal individuals typically detect and report symptoms in the real world. From consideration of these perceptual, learning, and motivational factors, it is apparent that self-reports of symptoms reflect far more than biological state. A report of a racing heart, then, may be based on heart sensations but also reflects the person's situational context, beliefs, emotions, and needs (for an in-depth discussion of these phenomena, see Leventhal & Leventhal, 1993).

GENDER, PERSONALITY, AND LIFE EXPERIENCES
THAT PREDISPOSE PEOPLE TO SYMPTOM
REPORTING

There are large individual differences in both the ways people report symptoms as well as the overall rates of reports. As will be discussed later in this chapter, there is evidence to suggest that gender, Negative Affectivity, and traumatic life events are linked to symptom reporting processes.

Gender Differences in Symptom Reporting
and Information Processing

In most surveys among healthy populations, males and females report comparable levels of most physical symptoms. That is, no strong or consistent sex differences emerge when samples are asked to report the degree to which they are experiencing common symptoms and sensations such as headaches, upset stomachs, dizziness, or racing hearts. Although the baseline levels of symptom reports are comparable, a number of studies now indicate that there are clear sex differences in how individuals notice, define, and react to symptoms. Specifically, women are particularly sensitive to external environmental cues and men to internal physiological cues in defining their symptoms. This conclusion is based on laboratory and field studies that have attempted to learn how accurate individuals are at perceiving specific physiological activity (Roberts & Pennebaker, 1995).

Across a large number of controlled laboratory studies using psychophysics paradigms, men are consistently better able than women to detect heart rate, stomach activity, blood pressure, and blood glucose levels. Recall that psychophysics paradigms eliminate or control for virtually all situational cues—thus requiring participants to make judgments about internal physiological activity using only bodily sensations as information sources. In naturalistic field studies, however, both women and men are equally good at estimating blood pressure, blood glucose, and various autonomic channels (for general review, see Roberts & Pennebaker, 1995). These naturalistic studies, unlike in psychophysics paradigms, allow participants to use extraneous situational cues (e.g., time of day, emotional state, tangential thoughts and perceptions) in helping to define internal state.

In a particularly strong test of this, Cox et al. (1985) asked 19 diabetics who had had experience monitoring their blood glucose levels to participate in a two-phase study in the hospital and, later, at home. In the hospital phase, participants' glucose levels were directly manipulated over the course of a day. A machine that simulated the activity of the pancreas took each diabetic on a blood glucose roller coaster ride over the 8-hour experiment. Once every 10 minutes, subjects estimated their glucose levels. Overall, the correlation between actual and estimated blood glucose was .42 for men and .13 for women. Either in the months before or after the hospital study, the same participants estimated and measured their glucose levels several times each day for 2 weeks at home during their normal days. At home, where a variety of situational cues were present, the correlation between actual and estimated glucose levels were .58 for men and .69 for women.

As discussed elsewhere (Pennebaker & Roberts, 1992), situational cues—such as time of day, room temperature, and so forth—are usually redundant with internal physiological cues. In other words, we can make fairly accurate, educated guesses about people's physiological activity if we know the settings they are in. What is interesting, however, is that men and women differentially rely on internal versus external cues in defining the symptoms that they are feeling.

The use of differential perceptual strategies by men versus women may explain some puzzling gender differences in symptom-reporting patterns. Although the base rates of symptom reports are comparable between women and men in relatively benign settings, certain types of stressful environments indicate differential symptom patterns. Given that women are especially sensitive to situational cues, it would be predicted that their symptom-reporting patterns would reflect the settings that they are perceiving as stressful. Men, however, should often ignore the settings and focus on their physiological cues. Symptom reporting, then, would mirror situational fluctuations in women and physiological changes in men.

Interestingly, these predictions are consistent with cases of mass psychogenic illness (Colligan et al., 1982), sick building syndrome (Bachmann & Myers, 1995; Sternberg & Wall, 1995), video display symptom complaints (Aronsson, Dallner, & Aborg, 1994), and cases of multiple chemical sensitivity (Bell, 1994). In each of these phenomena, women consistently report greater symptom levels than men. In mass psychogenic illness, for example, women have been found to be more prone to episodes than men across cultures (e.g., Phoon, 1982) and over the centuries (e.g., Sirios, 1982). It could be argued that MPI—not unlike sick building syndrome, video display complaints, or multiple chemical sensitivity—is a phenomenon wherein a salient smell or label emerges to help explain the existence of naturally occurring symptoms of stress or illness. The more prominent the situational label, then, the more likely that females may use it to help define their internal state (see also Pennebaker & Memon, 1996).

Interestingly, these sex differences could be both adaptive and maladaptive. If, in fact, low levels of environmental or dietary toxins are directly causing subtle adverse biological activity, females would be more likely to detect it than males. On the other hand, if the situational cues are benign and detectable biological changes are resulting from toxin exposure, males may be slightly more likely to detect them. Note that the gender differences in the perceptual bases of symptom reporting has been found in generally healthy individuals. Further, the effects are moderately strong but not overwhelming. At this point, the findings and explanations are intriguing and worthy of future study.

Negative Affectivity and Physical Symptoms

Within the last few years, researchers have begun to examine the role that personality variables play in the formation and reporting of physical symptoms. Much of this research has been based on a mood-related disposition called Negative Affectivity or trait NA (Watson & Clark, 1984). Trait NA is essentially identical to several other dispositional constructs such as neuroticism (Costa & McCrae, 1987), trait anxiety (Taylor, 1953), pessimism versus optimism (Scheier & Carver, 1993), and so on. Trait NA reflects pervasive individual differences in negative mood and self-concept. High NA individuals experience consistently higher levels of distress and dissatisfaction over time and across different situations. High NA subjects are also more introspective and tend to dwell differentially on their failures and shortcomings. They tend to be negativistic, focusing on the negative aspects of themselves and others.

Virtually any questionnaire scale that taps self-reports of anxiety, worry, stress-proneness, or negative emotions can be considered a measure of NA (see Watson, Clark, & Tellegen, 1988). A growing number of studies indicate that trait NA is highly correlated with virtually all measures of symptom reporting. Across several samples, using different NA scales and various measures of symptom reporting, NA markers typically correlate in the .30 to .50 range with symptom reports, with a mean coefficient of approximately $r = .40$. Interestingly, high NA individuals consistently report all types of sensations and physical symptoms to a greater degree than do low NA individuals—even though high and low NA subjects do not differ noticeably on various objective health markers (Costa & McCrae, 1987; Watson & Pennebaker, 1989).

The reliable link between NA and symptom reporting, in the absence of any NA-related differences in objective health status, indicates that symptom reports are strongly affected by the NA trait. High NA individuals appear to be hypervigilant about their bodies and have a lower threshold for noticing and reporting subtle bodily sensations. Because of their generally pessimistic view of the world, they are also likely to worry about the implications of their perceived symptoms. Indeed, these high NA individuals would also be the ones to worry more about chemicals, pollens, physicians, and the environment.

Any studies using self-reports of physical symptoms as outcome measures must consider the issue of NA. First, consistent with other aspects of the trait, high NA individuals will be more likely than others to report symptoms across all situations and over long time intervals. Because of this, excessive symptom reporting is not only influenced by transient situational stressors but also reflects a stable personality trait. Second, reliance on symptom reports without a concurrent measure of NA can lead to a distorted view of the meaning and significance of these symptoms. Third, researchers and clinicians should be alert to the role of NA as a nuisance factor that must be assessed when trying to evaluate and treat reports of symptoms.

As discussed previously, symptom reports are influenced both by situational cues and by broad dispositional differences in distress and complaining. Closely allied with this evidence is work suggesting that the tendency to report symptoms and negative affect is strongly heritable (e.g., Bouchard, 1994). The genetic argument reflects common assumptions about the phenotypic bases of physiological functioning as well as recent findings concerning the inheritance of perceptual and emotional styles.

The awareness and reporting of physical symptoms depends, to a large degree, on the way information is processed in different parts of the brain. The somatosensory cortex, for example, fundamentally affects how individuals perceive sensations in their bodies. Beyond basic perception, the ability to report symptoms is dependent on the proper functioning of the language centers in the temporal and parietal lobes (e.g., Luria, 1980). Further, it is well documented that central nervous system structure and function are, in turn, strongly genetically determined. Monozygotic twins, for example, have remarkably similar—albeit not identical—cortical structures, neurotransmitter activity, EEG, and autonomic nervous system activation compared with fraternal twins (Young, Waldo, Rutledge, & Freedman, 1996). In short, the brain's biological hardware that underlies symptom perception clearly has a heritable basis.

Of particular relevance are a series of discoveries pointing to the genetic bases of personality dispositions and their associated cognitive-perceptual-behavioral styles. Of greatest relevance are the findings of Tellegen et al. (1988) who conducted a large-scale examination of the heritability of trait NA. The Minnesota researchers investigated over 400 pairs of identical and fraternal twins who were reared either together or apart. Overall, an estimated 55% of the variance on trait NA could be attributed to genetic factors, whereas only 2% was due to the shared familial environment. The remaining 43% of the variance is presumably attributable to measurement error and idiosyncratic situational influences that were not assessed by the researchers. A number of other large-scale studies have now reported similar findings in regard to the heritability of trait NA (cf. Bouchard, 1994).

Unfortunately, the Minnesota project did not directly examine the heritability of symptom reporting. Nevertheless, the heritability of the NA trait strongly suggests that individuals' proclivity to report symptoms and sensations has a similar genetic basis. Given the currently available data, however, it is impossible to point with any certainty to the biological and/or psychological mechanisms underlying the genetics of symptom reporting or, more broadly, the psychiatric diagnosis of somatization disorder—wherein individuals chronically report high levels of physical symptoms. Perhaps the most promising hypothesis links attentional vigilance with specific physiological substrates.

Gray (1982) pointed to the importance of inhibitory centers within the brain (such as those in the septum and hippocampus) as influencing—both directly and indirectly—individual differences in trait NA. When these inhibitory centers are activated, individuals become hypervigilant about the presence of novel stimuli in the environment. Gray believed that high NA subjects, who he called trait anxious, have overactive inhibitory centers that result in their being characterologically hypervigilant. This hypervigilance probably affects symptom reporting in two ways. First, high NA subjects should be more attentive to subtle sensations in their bodies. Second, because their scanning is fraught with anxiety and uncertainty, high NAs may be more likely to interpret minor symptoms and sensations as painful or pathological. Interestingly, Barsky and Klerman (1983) also argued that hypervigilance, selective attention, and the tendency to view somatic sensations as ominous are all important elements in the amplification of symptoms. Thus, the perceptual style of high NAs may be largely responsible for their enhanced somatic complaining.

Traumatic Experiences and Symptom Reporting

Although situational and inherited dispositional factors can be powerful predictors of symptom reporting, certain broad life experiences also appear to influence symptom awareness—often in pathological ways. Symptom reports both with and without underlying objective disease markers increase after traumatic experiences. This is seen in studies where large groups of traumatized individuals are followed for weeks, months, or years after such traumas as rape, death of spouse, or other trauma (e.g., Lehman, Ellard, & Wortman, 1986; Pennebaker, 1989, 1997). Similarly, studies that have focused on large groups of individuals diagnosed with various somatoform disorders typically report trauma rates significantly above those of individuals either without somatoform disorders or other problems. What is it about a trauma that appears to exacerbate symptom reports?

For the last few years, my students and I have been examining this question from several perspectives. One important feature of traumas that is linked to self-reports of health and illness (and even health-related behaviors) is that those traumas that are not openly discussed with others are more problematic than those that are talked about. Across various large-scale surveys, for example, we have consistently found that individuals who report having one or more traumas at any point in their lives about which they did not talk reported having significantly higher rates of reported minor health problems (headaches, upset stomach, racing heart) and well as serious diagnoses (high blood pressure, cancer, ulcers)—see Pennebaker and Susman (1988). Indeed, these symptom and illness rates were significantly higher than for subjects who had experienced the same types of traumas but who did talk about the events.

Why, then, would undisclosed traumas maximally elevate symptom reports? At least four overlapping hypotheses exist:

Long-Term Stress Responses Resulting From the Trauma. One possibility is that these traumas are simply biologically stressful and, in some way, result in adverse autonomic and immune function changes that are accurately detected by the perceivers. This is probably true with many cases. However, closer inspection of people suffering from various somatoform disorders indicates that the majority are simply reporting more physical symptoms in the absence of heightened autonomic activity.

Symptom Reporting as a Distraction. People who have had traumas in their lives and who have not been able to resolve them may adopt certain cognitive strategies that allow them to avoid thinking about these events; they are always in search of distracters. Of all types of information, bodily cues are always available. By focusing on symptoms and sensations, individuals may be able to avoid addressing the overwhelming thoughts of emotional upheavals.

Traumatic Thought Suppression. A related hypothesis assumes that individuals who actively avoid trying to think about their traumas consistently work to block out trauma-relevant thoughts and emotions. In reality, aspects of the trauma are continuously processed on both a conscious and nonconscious level. When a dimension of the trauma pops into the individual's thoughts, he or she can suppress the thought fairly quickly. Of prime importance, the brief appearance of the thought together with the work of trying to suppress it results in an emotional and autonomic response. From the individual's perspective, however, the bodily changes associated with the emotional response are not immediately interpretable because trauma-relevant thoughts continue to be suppressed. In other words, the person experiences an emotion without a perceptible eliciting event. Unable to truly define the bodily state as an emotion, the person's only recourse is to label the emotional changes as their components: physical symptoms (cf. Wegner, 1992; Wegner, Shortt, Blake, & Page, 1990).

Secondary Gain. The reporting of symptoms is ultimately a social act. By telling others of one's symptoms, the person is seeking help in reducing the symptoms, seeking more information about the causes or consequences of the symptoms, and, in some cases, searching for acknowledgment, attention, or other forms of reward from others. Reporting of symptoms following a stressful event has previously been found to bring stressed families closer together (e.g., Minuchin et al., 1975) and allow the symptom reporters a way by which to escape from other stressful situations such as school or work (e.g., Mechanic, 1978).

In many ways, it is beyond the goals of this chapter to explore the many links between stressful life experiences and symptom reporting. Suffice it to say that in cases where ambiguous symptoms are reported at a high rate without a clear environmental or biological correlate, it would behoove the clinician or researcher to explore the patient's earlier traumatic life experiences.

IMPLICATIONS: INTERPRETING PHYSICAL SYMPTOM REPORTING IN THE REAL WORLD

The awareness and reporting of physical symptoms results from natural perceptual processes. As such, it can be misleading to assume that people's perceptions of symptoms reflect their presumed physiological referents. This dilemma is particularly relevant in situations where individuals are reporting symptoms in the absence of objective biological measures that could confirm their symptoms.

Over the last 20 years, we have witnessed the growth and popularization of several disorders that have helped people label and understand their ambiguous symptoms: iron-poor blood, hypoglycemia, chronic fatigue, mitral valve prolapse, Epstein-Barr, Seasonal Affective Disorder, depression, repressed childhood memories, and others. Similarly, a multitude of environmental factors have also been blamed for a comparable group of ambiguous symptoms: ionization of the air, video display terminals, refined sugar, animal fat, food additives, and so forth. Are these disorders and environmental toxins real? Yes, sometimes.

Based on our research on symptom reporting, we would predict that among a group of 100 people who experience the standard symptoms of fatigue, anxiety, racing heart, dizziness, upset stomach, and headache, a small percentage probably have iron-poor blood, low blood glucose, or spend too much time in front of a video display terminal. Similarly, some of these 100 people will be hyper-responsive to low dosages of chemicals. In fact, a few are probably being poisoned to death by the chemicals they fear while their physicians dismiss their symptoms as psychogenic.

But here is the dilemma. Although virtually all of our 100 people will be subjectively feeling the sensations they report, perhaps only a minority will exhibit biological activity that can explain the symptoms. Further, the presence of biological markers will typically be secondary to the power of perceptual and emotional factors in the symptom-reporting process. Unfortunately, it can be quite difficult to disentangle truly dangerous low-level toxic exposure from psychological factors in explaining the elevated symptoms. Using single-session survey or experimental designs, this is an almost impossible task—something akin to proving the null hypothesis. On a case-by-case basis, however, where individuals are repeatedly exposed to potential toxins and placebos in a double-blind fashion, we may be able to distinguish the individual symptom-reporting patterns in responses to substances. Note that this strategy may help to determine the dose-response gradient of toxins to symptoms for a particular individual in a controlled laboratory setting. The degree to which this knowledge generalizes to symptom reports in the real world may still be unknown because, after all, symptoms are subject to the various distortions inherent in the perceptual process.

A useful strategy for clinicians and researchers would be to acknowledge that symptoms are based on a multitude of factors. Certain psychological variables may be particularly potent in driving the symptom reporting process. The following checklist may be helpful in identifying the degree to which cases of elevated symptom reporting are being influenced by perceptual, emotional, or other psychological factors:

Perceptual Factors

1. Boring or tedious environment. People are more likely to pay attention to and to amplify bodily sensations in situations lacking in stimulation.

2. Situations fraught with tension or anxiety. Poor worker–management relations, interpersonal conflict at home, and other forms of stress or pressure can exacerbate physical symptoms. People in settings where they are unable to directly address the causes of their tension may be forced to look elsewhere to define their symptoms. For example, a person who has a specialized job with an abusive boss may not be able to acknowledge the tremendous tension brought about by his or her boss. An alternative label for this tension might be illness.

3. Isolation at work or home. Cases of MPI, for example, are likely to occur in places where individuals are unable or not allowed to talk with others. This can occur in settings with high levels of ambient noise (e.g., factories) or in places where talking is discouraged (e.g., libraries). Lack of interpersonal communication allows people more time to ponder their bodily sensations, may exacerbate tension or anxiety, and may fail to allow for

the normal social comparison that occurs when people try to understand their sensations.

4. An appropriate trigger or causal attribution. A new or unique smell, knowledge of chemical use, or recent exposure in the media of a medical problem or disaster (e.g., sick building, a celebrity diagnosed with cancer or AIDS) can help people organize their symptoms into a coherent explanation. A particularly powerful trigger can be the overt and unexplained sickness or death of a coworker or family member.

5. The social spread of the disorder. Within the workforce, psychogenic diseases have been found to spread along friendship lines rather than by proximity.

6. Secondary gain. Symptoms of all disorders are much more likely to be reported if the person receives some kind of reward from others. The reward could be attention or alleviation of responsibilities at work or in the home. Research within a family systems framework suggests that somatization disorders can help to control the dynamics within the family.

Individual Differences

1. Gender. Females are more likely to suffer from episodes of MPI, sick building syndrome, video display fatigue symptoms, and multiple chemical sensitivity brought about by presumed toxins in the environment. This may be partially due to the fact that males and females rely on different sources of information to interpret bodily state.

2. Negative Affectivity. Individuals with a history of reporting negative moods, thoughts, and symptoms may be especially prone to elevated symptom reporting.

3. Traumatic experiences in childhood. People report far more physical symptoms if they have had a traumatic experience in childhood. Further, those who have not disclosed this trauma to others are more likely to report a variety of health and symptom problems throughout the life cycle.

4. Recent traumatic experiences. Psychological upheavals (death of family member, divorce) in the preceding months may also contribute to elevated symptom reporting.

ACKNOWLEDGMENTS

I am indebted to David Watson for his input in several sections of the paper. Parts of this chapter were reported in Pennebaker (1994). Preparation of this manuscript was made possible by a grant from the National Institute of Mental Health (MH52391).

REFERENCES

American Psychiatric Association. (1995). *Diagnostic and statistical manual of mental disorders* (4th ed., rev.). Washington, DC: Author.

Aronsson, G., Dallner, M., & Aborg, C. (1994). Winners and losers from computerization: A study of the psychosocial work conditions and health of Swedish state employees. *International Journal of Human-Computer Interaction, 6*, 17–35.

Bachmann, M. O., & Myers, J. E. (1995). Influences on sick building syndrome symptoms in three buildings. *Social Science and Medicine, 40*, 245–251.

Barsky, A. J., & Klerman, G. L. (1983). Overview: Hypochondriasis, bodily complaints, and somatic styles. *American Journal of Psychiatry, 140*, 273–283.

Bell, I. R. (1994). Neuropsychiatric aspects of sensitivity to low level chemicals: A neural sensitization model. *Toxicology and Industrial Health, 10*, 277–312.

Boring, E. G. (1950). *A history of experimental psychology.* New York: Appleton-Century-Crofts.

Bouchard, T. J. (1994). Genes, environment, and personality. *Science, 264*, 200–201.

Challis, G. B., & Stam, H. J. (1992). A longitudinal study of the development of anticipatory nausea and vomiting in cancer chemotherapy patients: The role of absorption and autonomic perception. *Health Psychology, 11*, 181–189.

Colligan, M. J., Pennebaker, J. W., & Murphy, L. R. (Eds.). (1982). *Mass psychogenic illness: A social psychological analysis.* Hillsdale, NJ: Lawrence Erlbaum Associates.

Costa, P. T., Jr., & McCrae, R. R. (1987). Neuroticism, somatic complaints, and disease: Is the bark worse than the bite? *Journal of Personality, 55*, 299–316.

Cox, D. J., Clarke, W. L., Gonder-Frederick, L. A., Pohl, S., Hoover, C., Snyder, A., Zimbelman, L., Carter, W. R., Bobbitt, S., & Pennebaker, J. W. (1985). Accuracy of perceiving blood glucose in IDDM. *Diabetes Care, 8*, 529–535.

Fillingim, R. B., & Fine, M. A. (1986). The effects of internal versus external information processing on symptom perception in an exercise setting. *Health Psychology, 5*, 115–123.

Fillingim, R. B., Roth, D. L., & Haley, W. E. (1989). The effects of distraction on the perception of exercise-induced symptoms. *Journal of Psychosomatic Research, 33*, 241–248.

Gibson, J. J. (1966). *The senses considered as perceptual systems.* Boston: Houghton-Mifflin.

Gibson, J. J. (1979). *The ecological approach to visual perception.* Boston: Houghton-Mifflin.

Gijsbers van Wijk, C. M. T., & Kolk, A. M. (1996). Psychometric evaluation of symptom perception related measures. *Personality & Individual Differences, 20*, 55–70.

Goldman, S. L., Kraemer, D. T., & Salovey, P. (1996). Beliefs about mood moderate the relationship of stress to illness and symptom reporting. *Journal of Psychosomatic Research, 41*, 115–128.

Gray, J. A. (1982). *The neuropsychology of anxiety: An enquiry into the functions of the septo-hippocampal system.* New York: Oxford University Press.

Lehman, D. R., Ellard, J. H., & Wortman, C. B. (1986). Social support for the bereaved: Recipients' and providers' perspectives on what is helpful. *Journal of Consulting and Clinical Psychology, 54*, 438–446.

Leventhal, H., & Leventhal, E. A. (1993). Affect, cognition, and symptom perception. In C. R. Chapman & K. M. Foley (Eds.), *Current and emerging issues in cancer pain: Research and practice* (pp. 153–173). New York: Raven.

Luria, A. R. (1980). *Higher cortical functions in man.* New York: Basic Books.

Mahon, N. E., Yarcheski, A., & Yarcheski, T. J. (1993). Health consequences of loneliness in adolescents. *Research in Nursing & Health, 16*, 23–31.

Mechanic, D. (1978). *Medical sociology* (2nd ed.). New York: Freeman.

Minuchin, S., Baker, L., Rosman, B. L., Liebman, R., Milman, L., & Todd, T. C. (1975). A conceptual model of psychosomatic illness in children. *Archives of General Psychiatry, 32*, 1031–1038.

National Center for Health Statistics (1980). *Basic data on depressive symptomatology.* Washington, DC: U.S. Government Printing Office.

Neisser, U. (1976). *Cognition and reality.* New York: Freeman.

Nolan, R. P., & Wielgosz, A. T. (1991). Assessing adaptive and maladaptive coping in the early phase of acute myocardial infarction. *Journal of Behavioral Medicine, 14,* 111–124.

Padgett, V. R., & Hill, A. K. (1989). Maximizing athletic performance in endurance events: A comparison of cognitive strategies. *Journal of Applied Social Psychology, 19,* 331–340.

Pennebaker, J. W. (1982). *The psychology of physical symptoms.* New York: Springer-Verlag.

Pennebaker, J. W. (1989). Confession, inhibition and disease. In L. Berkowitz (Ed.), *Advances in experimental social psychology* (Vol. 22, pp. 211–244). New York: Academic Press.

Pennebaker, J. W. (1994). Psychological bases of symptom reporting: Perceptual and emotional aspects of chemical sensitivity. *Toxicology and Industrial Health, 10,* 497–511.

Pennebaker, J. W. (1997). *Opening up: The healing power of expressing emotions* (2nd ed.). New York: Guilford.

Pennebaker, J. W., Gonder-Frederick, L., Cox, D. J., & Hoover, C. W. (1985). The perception of general vs. specific visceral activity and the regulation of health-related behavior. In E. S. Katkin & S. B. Manuck (Eds.), *Advances in behavioral medicine* (Vol. 1, pp. 165–198). San Francisco: JAI Press.

Pennebaker, J. W., & Memon, A. (1996). Recovered memories in context: Thoughts and elaborations on Bowers and Farvolden. *Psychological Bulletin, 119,* 381–385.

Pennebaker, J. W., & Roberts, T. A. (1992). Toward a his and hers theory of emotion: Gender differences in visceral perception. *Journal of Social and Clinical Psychology, 11,* 199–212.

Pennebaker, J. W., & Susman, J. R. (1988). Disclosure of traumas and psychosomatic processes. *Social Science and Medicine, 26,* 327–332.

Pennebaker, J. W., & Watson, D. (1988). Blood pressure estimation and beliefs among normotensives and hypertensives. *Health Psychology, 7,* 309–328.

Phoon, W. H. (1982). Outbreaks of mass hysteria at workplaces in Singapore: Some patterns and modes of presentation. In M. Colligan, J. W. Pennebaker, & L. Murphy (Eds.), *Mass psychogenic illness* (pp. 21–32). Hillsdale, NJ: Lawrence Erlbaum Associates.

Robbins, J. M., & Kirmayer, L. J. (1991). Cognitive and social factors in somatization. In L. J. Kirmayer & J. M. Robbins (Eds.), *Current concepts of somatization* (pp. 107–142). Washington, DC: American Psychiatric Press.

Roberts, T. A., & Pennebaker, J. W. (1995). Women's and men's strategies in perceiving internal state. In M. Zanna (Ed.), *Advances in experimental social psychology* (Vol. 28, pp. 143–176). New York: Academic Press.

Scheier, M. F., & Carver, C. S. (1993). On the power of positive thinking: The benefits of being optimistic. *Current Directions in Psychological Science, 2,* 26–30.

Schmidt, A. J. M., Wolfs-Takens, D. J., Oosterlaan, J., & van den Hout, M. A. (1994). Psychological mechanisms in hypochandriasis: Attention-induced physical symptoms without sensory stimulation. *Psychotherapy & Psychosomatics, 61,* 117–120.

Sirios, F. (1982). Perspectives on epidemic hysteria. In M. Colligan, J. W. Pennebaker, & L. Murphy (Eds.), *Mass psychogenic illness* (pp. 217–236). Hillsdale, NJ: Lawrence Erlbaum Associates.

Skelton, J. A., & Croyle, R. T. (Eds.). (1991). *Mental representation in health and illness.* New York: Springer-Verlag.

Sternberg, B., & Wall, S. (1995). Why do women report "sick building symptoms" more often than men? *Social Science and Medicine, 40,* 491–502.

Taylor, J. A. (1953). A personality scale of manifest anxiety. *Journal of Abnormal and Social Psychology, 48,* 285–290.

Tellegen, A., Lykken, D. T., Bouchard, T. J., Jr., Wilcox, K. J., Segal, N. L., & Rich, S. (1988). Personality similarity in twins reared apart and together. *Journal of Personality and Social Psychology, 54,* 1031–1039.

Watson, D., & Clark, L. A. (1984). Negative Affectivity: The disposition to experience aversive emotional states. *Psychological Bulletin, 96,* 465–490.

Watson, D., Clark, L. A., & Tellegen, A. (1988). Development and validation of brief measures of Positive and Negative Affect: The PANAS Scales. *Journal of Personality and Social Psychology, 54*, 1063–1070.

Watson, D., & Pennebaker, J. W. (1989). Health complaints, stress, and distress: Exploring the central role of Negative Affectivity. *Psychological Review, 96*, 234–254.

Wegner, D. M. (1992). You can't always think what you want: Problems in the suppression of unwanted thoughts. In M. Zanna (Ed.), *Advances in experimental social psychology* (Vol. 25, pp. 193–225). San Diego: Academic Press.

Wegner, D. M., Shortt, J. W., Blake, A. W., & Page, M. S. (1990). The suppression of exciting thoughts. *Journal of Personality and Social Psychology, 58*, 409–418.

Whitehead, W. E., Crowell, M. D., Heller, B. R., & Robinson, J. C. (1994). Modeling and reinforcement of the sick role during childhood predicts adult illness behavior. *Psychosomatic Medicine, 56*, 541–550.

Woods, S., Natterson, J., & Silverman, J. (1978). Medical students' disease: Hypochondriasis in medical education. *Journal of Medical Education, 41*, 785–790.

Yardley, L. (1994). Prediction of handicap and emotional distress in patients with recurrent vertigo: Symptoms, coping strategies, control beliefs and reciprocal causation. *Social Science & Medicine, 39*, 573–581.

Young, D. A., Waldo, M., Rutledge, J. H., & Freedman, R. (1996). Heritability of inhibitory gating of the P50 auditory-evoked potential in monozygotic and dizygotic twins. *Neuropsychobiology, 33*, 113–117.

18

Self-Report of Pain: Issues and Opportunities

Francis J. Keefe
Duke University Medical Center

Pain is a private experience with complex sensory, affective, and evaluative quali-
ties that must be measured if people in distress are to be helped. The sensations,
thoughts, and feelings are salient for the sufferer, but incomprehensible to an
observer unless there are observable manifestations.
—Craig, Prkachin, and Grunau (1992, p. 257)

What is the most common manifestation of pain? Verbal descriptions of pain
are among the most frequent and important pain-related behaviors. In the
clinical setting, self-reports of pain are considered to be one of the primary
means of understanding another's pain experience. In this context, self-reports of pain can have very important consequences. Individuals who can
reliably and accurately describe their pain experience are much more likely
to obtain rapid and effective treatment. Those who, because of language or
physical limitations, are unable to report on their pain, in contrast, may
have great difficulty in obtaining pain relief. Consider, for example, a young
American woman who, during a recent visit to Brazil, had a fish bone caught
in her throat and was unable to communicate her pain and distress verbally.
Her gestures and attempts to talk were incomprehensible to both friends
and health professionals and the resulting delay in treatment left her with
scar tissue and persistent swallowing difficulties.

In the clinical setting, the report of pain also has important social and
occupational consequences. Individuals who complain of persistent pain
may be deemed to be disabled, relieved of their job responsibilities, and be

given financial compensation for pain-related disabilities. Finally, reports of pain can have important legal consequences. Individuals who report persistent pain following an accident may sue for monetary payments to compensate them for their pain and suffering.

The purpose of this chapter is to provide an introduction to methods and issues involved in the self-report of pain. The chapter is divided into three sections. The first section provides a brief overview of the evolution of concepts of pain. The second section describes and critiques several of the most common methods used in assessing pain self-reports. The final section highlights several critical clinical and research issues in this field.

CONCEPTS OF PAIN

To understand current approaches to assessing the self-report of pain, it is important to be aware of the evolution of current conceptualizations of pain. Historically, persistent pain was viewed as mystical or religious in nature (Melzack & Wall, 1996). The ancients believed that individuals afflicted by chronic pain were possessed by evil spirits or suffering retribution for sins they may have committed. The more modern concept of pain as primarily a sensory event can be traced back to the writings of Descartes in the 17th century (Melzack & Wall, 1996). Descartes maintained that pain signals were transmitted from a peripheral site of injury or disease through the spinal cord and to the brain. This concept of a pain pathway received considerable support from subsequent neuroanatomical and physiological studies conducted in the 18th, 19th, and 20th centuries (Melzack & Wall, 1996). These studies supported the specificity theory of pain in that they clearly demonstrated the existence of specific pain receptors, neural pain pathways, and a sensory center in the brain involved in pain perception. By the mid 1950s, the specificity theory was the predominant model of pain.

In the late 1950s and early 1960s, clinical observations began to raise questions about the validity of the specificity theory of pain (Melzack & Wall, 1962, 1965). An important assumption of this theory, for example, is that the level of pain will be proportional to the degree of underlying tissue damage. Thus, individuals having more tissue damage can be expected to have more pain. However, clinical studies had shown that individuals having evidence of tissue damage often fail to report pain. Beecher, a neurosurgeon working on the Anzio beachhead during World War II, found that many of the soldiers wounded in battle reported little or no pain despite having major injuries (Beecher, 1959). More recent research carried out in emergency room settings demonstrated that up to 40% of patients having injuries that should be painful reported little or no pain at all (Melzack & Wall, 1982). Clinical studies also revealed that individuals may report pain in the absence of obvious input from the periphery. The classic clinical example of this phenomenon is phantom limb pain in which a person reports experiencing persistent pain in a limb that has been amputated (Melzack, 1995).

The specificity model of pain also failed to account for the role that psychological factors can play in the pain experience. There is substantial evidence from experimental laboratory studies that psychological factors such as attention, mood, and expectations can influence the perception of carefully controlled pain stimuli (e.g., painful heat, cold, or pressure stimulation; Price & Harkins, 1992). Research has also shown that social and cultural factors can have a major effect on the experience and report of pain (Sternbach & Tursky, 1965).

Problems with the specificity theory of pain stirred interest in the development of new, alternative theories of pain. The gate control theory developed by Melzack and Wall (1965) is the most influential and important of these theories. The gate control theory maintains that in the spinal cord there is a gating mechanism with the function of controlling the flow of impulses from the periphery to the brain. The gate is influenced not only by peripheral input from pain and touch fibers but also by activity in brain areas responsible for cognition and emotion. Thus the gate control theory recognizes the influence that cognitive processes (e.g., attention, memory, and expectations) and emotional reactions (e.g., depression, anxiety, or anger) can have on the transmission of pain signals from the periphery to the brain.

The gate control theory is important for pain measurement because it emphasizes that pain is not a simple sensory experience but rather a multidimensional experience that has emotional and cognitive components (Keefe, Lefebvre, & Starr, 1996). Over the past two decades, a number of studies have attempted to identify the key dimensions underlying the pain experience (Jensen & Karoly, 1992). There appears to be growing agreement that there are at least two basic dimensions of pain that can be assessed in individuals having persistent pain (Jensen & Karoly, 1992; Price & Harkins, 1992). The first dimension, pain intensity, reflects the severity of pain; that is, how much it hurts. The second dimension, pain affect, reflects the emotional arousal related to pain; that is, how unpleasant and distressing the pain is. Pain affect appears to be especially important in understanding the chronic pain experience (Jensen & Karoly, 1992).

PAIN ASSESSMENT METHODS

Traditionally, the main focus of pain assessment has been on pain intensity. How is pain intensity assessed? Two of the most commonly used methods are verbal rating scales and numeric rating scales.

None

Slight

Moderate

Intense

Extremely Intense

FIG. 18.1. Example of a verbal pain rating scale.

A verbal rating scale consists of a series of pain adjective descriptors. Figure 18.1 displays a typical five-word verbal rating scale. As can be seen, the adjective descriptors are arranged in a set ranging from those describing the least to the most intense pain. To score verbal rating scales, each adjective is typically given a numeric value (e.g., from 1 to 5), which is then used in data analysis. The instructions for these scales are quite simple. An individual, for example, might be asked to select the descriptor that best describes the current intensity of their pain (current pain measure). To understand variations in pain, the individual might also be asked to indicate which of the descriptors best describes their worst pain, least pain, and average pain over the past week.

Verbal descriptor scales have several strengths and limitations (Jensen & Karoly, 1992). Their major strength is ease of use. Individuals readily understand these scales. In addition, verbal rating scales take very little time and as a result can be administered quite frequently (e.g., daily or at key points over the course of a laboratory study or treatment program). One limitation of five- to seven-word verbal rating scales is that respondents have relatively few options with which to rate their pain. Another limitation is that the subjective distance between adjacent steps on a verbal scale (e.g., between moderate and severe pain) may not be equal for different individuals but may be treated so in data analyses.

A numeric rating scale consists of a set of numbers (e.g., 0 to 100) whose endpoints are labeled (e.g., 0 = no pain, 100 = pain as bad as it can be). The respondent is asked to select the number that best describes the intensity of their pain for a given time period (e.g., now, past week, etc.). Numeric rating scales, like verbal rating scales, are easy to use. They have two advantages over verbal scales (Jensen & Karoly, 1992). First, they usually provide more response options. Second, one can treat these scales as ratio scales, thereby meeting the requirements of many parametric statistical tests. The major disadvantage of pain intensity measures is that they focus on only one dimension of a multidimensional experience.

A number of self-report measures have been developed to assess both pain intensity and pain affect. Price and his colleagues, for example, have conducted a series of studies in which they have used visual analogue scales to assess pain intensity and pain unpleasantness (Price, Barrel, & Gracely, 1980; Price & Harkins, 1987; Price, Harkins, & Baker, 1987; Price, Harkins, Rafii, & Price, 1986; Price, McGrath, Rafii, & Buckingham, 1983). A visual analogue scale consists of a line (often 100 mm in length) whose endpoints are labeled with pain descriptors. The individual is instructed to place a mark along the line to indicate their current pain level. In their research, Price and colleagues employed two visual analogue scales: (a) one to assess pain intensity—whose endpoints were no pain sensation and most intense pain sensation imaginable, and (b) one to assess pain unpleasantness—whose endpoints were not at all unpleasant and most unpleasant imaginable. These visual analogue scales have been shown to be highly reliable and sensitive to treatment effects (Price & Harkins, 1992).

Price, Bush, Long, & Harkins (1994) also developed a novel mechanical visual analogue scale that consists of a slide rule algometer designed to assess pain intensity and pain unpleasantness. Figure 18.2 depicts this algometer. The individual is handed the algometer and first asked to rate the intensity of the pain by pulling the slider on the ruler from left to right to indicate the level of pain experienced. The slide ruler is 150 mm long and

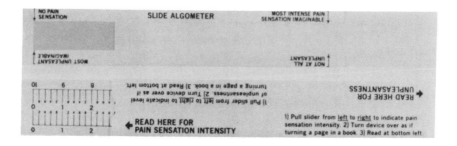

FIG. 18.2. A mechanical, visual anologue slide rule algometer used to rate pain intensity and pain unpleasantness. The view on top displays the front of the algometer as seen by patients. The view on the bottom displays the back of the algometer that shows the numerical rating given by the patient. Reprinted from *Pain*, Vol. 56, Price, Bush, Long, and Harkins, A comparison of pain measurement characteristics of mechanical visual analogue and simple numerical rating scales, pp. 217–226, copyright © 1994, with kind permission from Elsevier Science - NL, Sara Burgerhartstraat 25, 1055 KV Amsterdam, The Netherlands.

uses the same endpoints as previously used by Price and Harkins (1987). As the slider is pulled out, it exposes progressively more of an underlying red bar. Once the rating is made, the slide ruler is turned over and the pain intensity rating can be read off in millimeters. The slide ruler is then turned over to reveal endpoints for pain unpleasantness, and the individual is asked to rate the unpleasantness of the pain in a similar fashion.

This slide rule algometer has several advantages. First, it is easy to use in research or clinical settings. A researcher could easily gather multiple assessments of pain intensity and pain affect over the course of an experiment without having to ask the subject to complete a questionnaire or provide a verbal report of the pain. A clinician could carry the algometer in his or her pocket and, at key time points during the clinical encounter, ask the patient to rate the intensity and unpleasantness of their pain. Second, the algometer is plastic and therefore maintains its shape. Visual analogue scales that are photocopied or printed tend to shrink when they are printed on paper. With repeated copies of an original, the shrinkage can amount to 10% or more, thereby reducing a 100 mm line to 90 mm or less.

Psychophysical scaling techniques have also been used to examine different dimensions of the pain experience, such as pain intensity and pain unpleasantness. Investigators have used cross modality matching to have individuals scale verbal descriptors referring to pain intensity and pain unpleasantness (Fillingim, Keefe, Light, Booker, & Maixner, 1996; Tursky, 1976). The main potential advantage of this procedure in scaling pain intensity, for example, is that respondents are able to indicate their own individual judgments about the intensity value of each pain descriptor. In cross modality matching, the respondent is presented with stimuli (e.g., 12 verbal descriptors of pain intensity) and asked to rate each stimulus using two response modalities (e.g., numerical values, line lengths).

We conducted a study of cross modality matching in pain clinic patients (Urban, Keefe, & France, 1984). Each patient was initially asked to rate a set of 12 words describing the intensity of pain. The patient was first presented with the word "moderate" and instructed that the numeric value assigned to this word was 50 and the line length assigned was 50 mm. The patient was then asked to assign a number proportional to each intensity descriptor as each was presented individually. The patient then was asked to draw a line proportional to the each of intensity descriptors. An identical procedure was then used for scaling of the pain's unpleasantness descriptors.

This experiment was repeated in two groups of pain clinic patients. Patients in Group 1 were given only one opportunity to scale the descriptors. Patients in Group II repeated the scaling procedure three times. Patients were considered to be reliable in their scaling if the correlation between their numeric and line-length estimates exceeded a correlation coefficient of .90.

Figure 18.3 displays a graph of the line production versus numerical estimates for psychophysically scaled pain intensity descriptors. Examination of this figure reveals two important findings. First, when one examines how the pain intensity descriptors are distributed along the best-fitting line between the data points, it is immediately evident that the distance between descriptors is quite variable. For example, there is a large group of descriptors arranged toward the bottom of this line and then a fairly large gap between the words mild and moderate. This finding indicates that the subjective distance between descriptors such as weak and mild is much smaller than that between mild and moderate even though, on conventional verbal rating scales, these distances are usually treated as equal. Second, as can be seen, a total of 16 out of 20 patients in Group I were able to reach the criterion for reliability of scaling these descriptors (a correlation coefficient of greater than .90), and 17 out of 20 patients in Group II met this criterion. Thus, the vast majority of patients were able to reliably scale psychophysical descriptors of pain intensity. Further, there was no notable improvement in reliability when comparing patients who were given one opportunity to do the scaling (Group I) versus those who had three opportunities to do the scaling procedure (Group II).

Figure 18.4 displays a graph of the line production versus numerical estimates for psychophysically scaled pain unpleasantness descriptors for subjects in Group I and Group II. A similar pattern to the pain intensity descriptors is evident if one examines the distribution of unpleasantness descriptors along the best fitting line between the data points; that is, the subjective distance between adjacent descriptors varies considerably with some descriptors being grouped quite close together (e.g., intolerable and unbearable), whereas others are much farther apart (e.g., distressing and miserable). Once again, this finding raises concerns about the usual practice of treating the distance between such descriptors as equal. A second important finding was that relatively few patients were able to reliably scale the pain unpleasantness descriptors. As can be seen, only 4 of 20 patients were able to reliably scale these descriptors when given a single opportunity to do so (Group I), and only 10 of 20 were able to do so after given three opportunities at scaling. Data analyses were conducted to compare those patients who were able to reliably scale the unpleasantness descriptors versus those who were not. There were no differences between these groups in demographic variables (education level, employment), medical or pain history variables (duration of pain, number of operations, narcotic use, disability–compensation status), or psychiatric diagnosis. There were differences, however, based on responses on the SCL-90R, a measure of psychological distress. Patients who were able to reliably scale these descriptors tended to have higher scores on almost all of the SCL-90R subscales, with significant elevations noted for the Group II patients on anxiety, paranoid

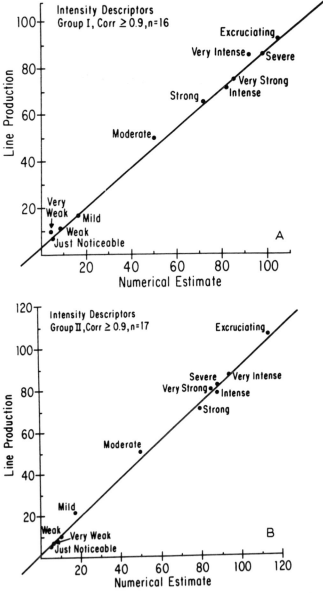

FIG. 18.3. Display of line production versus numerical estimates produced during cross modality matching procedure for pain intensity descriptors. Pain clinic patients in this study were provided either with one opportunity to scale the descriptors (Group 1) or three opportunities to scale the descriptors (Group 2). Reprinted from *Pain*, Vol 20, Urban, Keefe, and France, A study of psychophysical scaling in chronic pain patients, pp. 157–168, copyright © 1984, with kind permission from Elsevier Science - NL, Sara Burgerhartstraat 25, 1055 KV Amsterdam, The Netherlands.

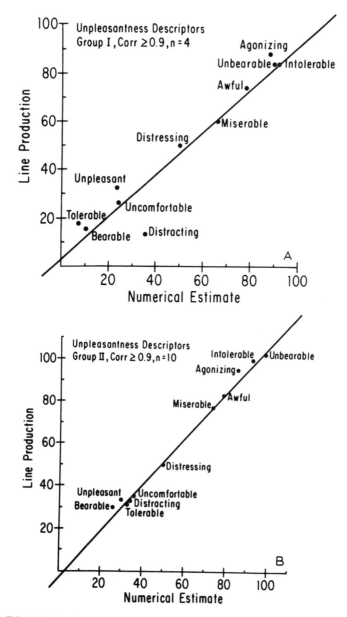

FIG. 18.4. Display of line production versus numerical estimates produced during cross modality matching procedure for pain unpleasantness descriptors. Pain clinic patients in this study were provided either with one opportunity to scale the descriptors (Group 1) or three opportunities to scale the descriptors (Group 2). Reprinted from *Pain*, Vol. 20, Urban, Keefe, and France, A study of psychophysical scaling in chronic pain patients, pp. 157–168, copyright © 1984, with kind permission from Elsevier Science - NL, Sara Burgerhartstraat 25, 1055 KV Amsterdam, The Netherlands.

ideation, and psychoticism. These findings suggest that patients who are more psychologically distressed tend to be more accurate in their scaling of adjectives related to the affective or emotional component of pain. It may be that, because of the distress, this dimension is more salient. In any event, the failure to achieve higher rates of reliability for the unpleasantness descriptors is a concern and raises questions about the use of such cross-modality matching procedures when assessing pain affect in clinical practice.

The adjective checklist of the McGill Pain Questionnaire (MPQ; Melzack, 1975) is probably the most widely used multidimensional pain rating scale. As can be seen in Fig. 18.5, the MPQ adjective checklist consists of a series of 20 groups of pain adjective descriptors. Each set is designed to assess a different aspect of pain (e.g., the seventh set assesses thermal qualities of pain with the adjectives hot, burning, scalding, and searing). Within each set, the adjectives are arranged in order of intensity from least to most severe. The respondent is instructed to select a single adjective in each set that is relevant to the pain. If a set contains no adjectives that are descriptive of the respondent's pain, he or she is asked to skip it. The sets of descriptors are grouped into three major groups, each corresponding to one of the major dimensions of the pain experience elaborated in the Gate Control Theory of pain: (a) sensory, (b) evaluative, and (c) affective. The MPQ has been found to have excellent test–retest reliability (Love, Leboeuf, & Crisp, 1989). Factor analytic studies also support the breakdown of the descriptor sets into three major groups (Melzack & Katz, 1992).

Measures of pain affect can be very helpful in understanding the pain experience and patients' response to pain treatments. Studies have shown that medications can have different effects on pain intensity versus pain affect. Gracely and his colleagues at the National Institutes of Dental Research, for example, conducted several studies in this area. For example, in one study they showed that Fentanyl reduces the intensity, but not the unpleasantness, of painful tooth pulp stimulation (Gracely, McGrath, & Dubner, 1979). In contrast, in another investigation they demonstrated that Diazepam reduces the unpleasantness of pain while having minimal effects on pain intensity (Gracely, McGrath, & Dubner, 1978). Certain psychological variables may have more of an effect on pain affect than on pain intensity. For example, in a recent study, we examined how self-efficacy for arthritis pain (i.e., confidence that one has the capability of controlling arthritis pain) was related to arthritis patients' perceptions of a series of painful heat stimuli (Keefe, Lefebvre, Maixner, Salley, & Caldwell, 1997). Although self-efficacy for arthritis pain was significantly related to judgments of the unpleasantness of the heat stimuli, it was not related to judgments of the intensity of the stimuli. Individuals who scored high on self-efficacy for arthritis pain rated the unpleasantness of the painful stimuli as much lower than those scoring low on self-efficacy. Finally, it is possible that certain psychological

McGill Pain Questionnaire

Patient's Name _____ Date _____ Time_____am/pm

PRI: S_____ A_____ E_____ M_____ PRI(T)_____ PPI____
      (1-10)   (11-15)   (16)   (17-20)   (1-20)

1 FLICKERING	11 TIRING
QUIVERING	EXHAUSTING
PULSING	
THROBBING	12 SICKENING
BEATING	SUFFOCATING
POUNDING	13 FEARFUL
2 JUMPING	FRIGHTFUL
FLASHING	TERRIFYING
SHOOTING	14 PUNISHING
3 PRICKING	GRUELLING
BORING	CRUEL
DRILLING	VICIOUS
STABBING	KILLING
LANCINATING	15 WRETCHED
4 SHARP	BLINDING
CUTTING	16 ANNOYING
LACERATING	TROUBLESOME
5 PINCHING	MISERABLE
PRESSING	INTENSE
GNAWING	UNBEARABLE
CRAMPING	17 SPREADING
CRUSHING	RADIATING
6 TUGGING	PENETRATING
PULLING	PIERCING
WRENCHING	18 TIGHT
7 HOT	NUMB
BURNING	DRAWING
SCALDING	SQUEEZING
SEARING	TEARING
8 TINGLING	19 COOL
ITCHY	COLD
SMARTING	FREEZING
STINGING	20 NAGGING
9 DULL	NAUSEATING
SORE	AGONIZING
HURTING	DREADFUL
ACHING	TORTURING
HEAVY	PPI
10 TENDER	0 NO PAIN
TAUT	1 MILD
RASPING	2 DISCOMFORTING
SPLITTING	3 DISTRESSING
	4 HORRIBLE
	5 EXCRUCIATING

BRIEF	RHYTHMIC	CONTINUOUS
MOMENTARY	PERIODIC	STEADY
TRANSIENT	INTERMITTENT	CONSTANT

E = EXTERNAL
I = INTERNAL

COMMENTS:

FIG. 18.5. The McGill Pain Questionnaire. Copyright © 1975 by Ron Melzack.
Reprinted from Melzack and Katz (1992).

treatments for pain (e.g., relaxation) are effective primarily because they alter pain affect while having minimal effects on pain intensity.

ISSUES IN PAIN SELF-REPORT

Researchers and clinicians who ask individuals to report their pain face a number of important issues. In this section, six important issues are highlighted: (a) the reliability of single versus multiple ratings of pain, (b) the relationship of clinical pain to experimental–laboratory pain measures, (c) the effects of social reinforcement on pain self-reports, (d) the relationship of self-reports of pain to nonverbal pain behavior, (e) the influence of mood on pain self-report, and (f) the utility of diary records in pain assessment.

Reliability of Single Versus Multiple Ratings of Pain

In research and practice settings, individuals having pain are often asked to provide a single rating or small number of ratings of their pain. To achieve reliable data on average pain levels, how often must one take ratings of pain? A recent study by Jensen and McFarland (1993) addressed this issue by systematically analyzing data on pain intensity collected from 200 chronic pain patients. All patients in this study had completed 2 weeks of diary records in which they rated their pain hourly using a 0 to 10 numeric scale on which 0 = no pain and 10 = pain as bad as it can be. Data analyses revealed that only one third of the patients reported similar average pain levels across the days of a week. Thus, for the majority of patients, the average of a day's ratings of pain differed substantially from one day to the next. Would increasing the number of pain intensity ratings heighten the test–retest reliability of composite measures of pain? The test–retest reliability of an average based on 2 days had a stability coefficient of .79. To achieve an adequate level of stability (a stability coefficient of over .90), Jensen and McFarland found that one needed to make at least three assessments of pain per day for 4 days. Estimates of pain based on a single rating of pain were not found to be reliable or valid. Estimates based on the average of 12 ratings taken across 4 different days, however, did show adequate reliability and validity.

Taken together, these findings underscore the importance of obtaining multiple pain ratings over multiple days. Researchers and clinicians should be cautious in interpreting results based on single ratings of pain intensity and should consider incorporating multiple ratings into their data collection protocols. Jensen and McFarland's results are also interesting in suggesting that adequate reliability in an average measure of pain does not have to involve exceptionally burdensome data collection. In this study, three or four daily measures collected over a relatively short time period (4 days) provided an adequate average measure of the patient's pain experience. Further research is needed to replicate these findings in other pain populations and to examine more fully the psychometric properties of composite pain measures based on a smaller versus larger number of pain ratings.

Relationship of Clinical Pain to Experimental–Laboratory Pain Measures

There has been growing interest in the use of experimental pain methods in assessing individuals' responses to pain. The laboratory appears to have several advantages in pain assessment. First, in the laboratory, one can control environmental factors that could potentially influence pain reports (e.g., social situation, noise, visual distractions). Second, the laboratory provides an opportunity to precisely control the timing, duration, and intensity of noxious stimuli. Finally, in the laboratory, one can easily obtain measures of pain threshold and pain tolerance but also judgments of a range of discrete noxious stimuli.

Laboratory pain measures are increasingly being gathered from individuals suffering from clinical pain conditions. An assumption that underlies this approach is that laboratory measurements of pain (e.g., pain threshold or tolerance) can be generalized to clinical pain. Thus, for example, patients who are found in the lab setting to be overly sensitive to pain or to be fairly stoic might be expected to show similar responses to clinical pain experiences. Recently, researchers have begun to examine correlations between laboratory and clinical measures of pain in patients having acute and chronic pain conditions. A good example of this research is a study by Janal, Glusman, Kuhl, and Clark (1994) of patients having angina secondary to coronary artery disease. All patients participated in a laboratory session to assess their pain thresholds for ischemic, electrical, and heat stimuli. As part of their clinical evaluation, these patients had also undergone a treadmill exercise protocol in which exercise demands were gradually increased and patients were asked to report when they first experienced anginal pain. Data analyses compared laboratory pain thresholds for the different noxious stimuli to reports of angina during the treadmill test. The results indicated that the latency to first anginal report during the treadmill exercise test was unrelated to ischemic, electrical, or heat pain thresholds. Interestingly, the three laboratory pain measures were also not found to correlate with each other. These findings suggest that individuals not only can differ substantially in their response to clinical and experimental pain stimuli but that they also can vary in their response to different types of laboratory pain stimuli.

Further research is needed to examine the reliability and validity of laboratory pain measures. At this point, however, one must be cautious about assuming that responses to one laboratory pain stimulus can be useful when making judgments about how an individual will respond to clinical pain.

Effects of Social Reinforcement on Pain Self-Reports

Behavior theorists (Fordyce, 1976) proposed that social factors, such as attention from a solicitous spouse, can affect the report of pain. White and Sanders (1986) conducted an interesting and important study on the effects of social reinforcement on reports of chronic pain. Subjects in this study, four female chronic pain inpatients, were systematically exposed to two different experimental conditions delivered during two randomly selected, 5-minute sessions each day for 7 consecutive days. During the first condition, an experimenter met with the subject, asked them about how they were feeling, and then systematically reinforced verbal complaints about pain with verbal attention, praise, or sympathy. The second condition was identical to the first except that the experimenter verbally reinforced the patient for any comments about feeling better, coping more effectively, or following through with exercise or other treatment recommendations. Immediately after the 5-minute meeting, subjects were asked to rate the intensity of their pain on a 0-to-5 rating scale. Data analyses revealed that there was a significant difference in mean pain intensity across days for the two pain conditions. Subjects consistently reported higher pain ratings following reinforcement for talking about pain topics than following reinforcement for talking about well topics. The magnitude of differences in pain between these two conditions appears to be in the 20% to 25% range.

The results reported by White and Sanders (1986) are interesting in that they were obtained after only a relatively brief (5-minute) manipulation delivered by an experimenter. In naturalistic settings such as the home, patients may receive substantially more reinforcement for discussing pain topics and the individual providing the reinforcement (e.g., a spouse) may be much more salient. Taken together, these results suggest that social reinforcement can have an impact on the pain report of patients having chronic pain. Researchers and clinicians should be alert to the potential influence that their attention to pain complaints may have on subsequent ratings of pain collected from patients. Careful standardization of instructions and the behavior of assessors may be needed to minimize the influence of social reinforcement on pain self-report.

Pain Report and Nonverbal Pain Behavior

Individuals who have pain not only provide self-reports of their experience, they also engage in a variety of nonverbal behaviors that communicate to others the fact that pain is being experienced. These behaviors may include a decrease in activity level, an inability to carry out simple daily tasks (e.g., walking, sitting), moving in a slow or guarded fashion, and the display of facial expressions (e.g., grimacing).

In gauging the significance of an individual's report of pain, clinicians often observe nonverbal pain behaviors. Consider, for example, two people with persistent low back pain, both of whom rate their pain at 8 on a 0-to-10 numerical rating scale. The first person appears to be in obvious discomfort, is unable to work, and reports that his pain wakes him nightly from sleep. The second person reports an identical pain level, but jokes during the physical examination, seems to be walking comfortably, and, although not working, remains relatively active around the house. The behavior of these two people will likely influence the clinician's response. The first person, for example, may be sent for additional medical tests (e.g., diagnostic EMG, myelogram) and may receive careful consideration for medical or surgical intervention. The complaints of the second person, however, are not likely to be taken as seriously. Because of his behavior, this individual may receive much more limited pain assessment and treatment. This is unfortunate because the basis for making this judgment is only a brief sample of behavior exhibited during a clinical encounter that the individual may find stressful. The person's behavior in this setting may not be representative of his or her usual behavior.

Nonverbal pain behaviors are overt and can be carefully and systematically measured by trained observers. Standardized observation protocols have been developed for assessing pain behaviors in laboratories (Keefe & Block, 1982) and in more naturalistic, clinical settings (Keefe, Wilkins, & Cook, 1984). There is considerable support for the reliability and validity of such observation methods in recording pain behaviors (Keefe & Dunsmore, 1992).

What do studies that use such standardized observation methods tell us about the correlation between pain self-report and nonverbal pain behavior? A number of studies have been carried out to address this issue (Jensen, 1997) and the observed correlations have varied considerably. For example, in our own research (Keefe & Block, 1982) we found that the correlation between self-reports of pain on a 0-to-10 scale and nonverbal pain behaviors was high ($r = .71$, $p < .01$). Richards, Nepomuceno, Riles, and Suer (1982), however, found that pain behavior correlated very poorly with ratings of pain given at the time of admission to a comprehensive ($r = .17$, n. s.). In general, the highest correlations between pain ratings and pain behavior have been obtained in studies in which the conditions of observation are more standardized and the observers are very carefully trained in observation methods (Keefe & Dunsmore, 1992).

Why do discrepancies between pain reports and nonverbal pain behavior occur? First, individuals may be motivated to report higher levels of pain because it can affect their treatment (Jensen, 1997). A person having persistent pain, for example, may realize that unless her pain report is high, she will not receive a newly developed neurosurgical procedure that promises to significantly reduce or eliminate her pain. Second, social and cultural factors may play a role. Sternbach and Tursky (1965), in a classic study, found that women of Italian descent had much lower tolerance for electric shock stimulation than women of Old American or Jewish descent. Finally, people may simply be reluctant to report their pain. Cleeland (personal communication, November 7, 1988) found that cancer patients are often reluctant to report their pain to their physicians. He suggested that educational initiatives be undertaken to coach patients how to more accurately report pain and display appropriate pain behaviors. Cleeland suggested that such coaching may significantly improve the management of pain in many persons having cancer pain.

If pain report and pain behavior are discrepant, should one simply focus on pain report and ignore pain behavior? Or should pain behavior be considered to be the most important index of pain? Fordyce (1985), a leading behavioral pain theorist, addressed this issue when he wrote:

> Peripheral stimulation will have, in the normal course of events, elicited a sensation that people, when asked, are likely to identify as "pain" ... that "pain," whether measured in intensity or reactive terms, constitutes another set of events different from, though potentially linkable to, pain behavior. (p. 59)

Fordyce suggested that pain report and nonverbal pain behavior are both important constructs in understanding the pain experience. These constructs focus on different aspects of the pain experience. In some instances, measures of these different constructs may be highly intercorrelated, whereas in other instances, they may not be. Clinicians and researchers need to recognize that both of these constructs are important in pain assessment and need to ensure that they use reliable and valid measures to assess both pain and pain behavior.

Mood and the Self-Report of Pain

Individuals suffering from persistent pain often experience substantial changes in mood and heightened psychological distress. Is there evidence that changes in mood can influence the self-report of pain?

Several studies have examined whether a person's mood at the time of a painful experience can affect their later recall of that experience. Kent (1985), for example, conducted a study examining the relationship of dental anxiety to pain recall. Subjects in this study were 58 individuals undergoing a painful dental procedure. All subjects completed a measure of dental anxiety prior to the procedure. Immediately after the procedure, they were asked to rate the pain experienced during the procedure. Three months later, subjects were contacted and asked to recall the level of pain they had experienced during the procedure. Data analyses revealed that subjects who had initially rated their dental anxiety as high recalled having much higher pain levels than they actually experienced at the time.

Can changes in mood influence the pain experience? Zelman, Howland, Nichols, and Cleeland (1991) conducted an experimental study in which they systematically examined the effects of a mood manipulation on pain tolerance. To assess pain tolerance, all subjects were exposed to a cold pressor pain challenge that involved keeping their hands in cold water for as long as they could tolerate. Two measures of cold pressor pain tolerance were taken, one before mood induction and one after. Subjects were randomly assigned one of three mood induction conditions: positive mood, negative mood, or neutral mood. In this mood induction procedure, subjects read a series of depressive, elative, or neutral statements presented on slides and were asked to experience the mood suggested by the statement. The results of this study indicated that the mood induction had a significant effect on pain tolerance. Subjects who had been exposed to the negative mood induction had a significant decrease in their tolerance for cold pressor pain, whereas those exposed to the positive mood induction showed a significant increase in their pain tolerance.

Taken together, the results of these studies suggest that clinicians and researchers need to be more aware of the fact that mood can influence the report of pain. Researchers need to develop methods to help clinicians gauge the impact of mood on an individual's current reports of pain as well as their recall of past pain experiences.

Diary Records and Pain Assessment

There is growing recognition that one needs to take multiple measurements of pain to achieve the most reliable and valid assessment of the pain experience (Jensen, 1997). Daily diaries provide a convenient means of gathering repeated measures of pain.

Diary methods for assessing pain and pain-related behaviors have long been used by pain clinicians (e.g., Fordyce, 1976). A variety of diary formats have been developed. Some ask patients to provide hourly entries on pain intensity, activity, and medication intake. Others ask patients to provide end-of-the-day ratings in which they rate changes in their pain that occurred over the day. Although diary data are graphed and used to document treatment outcome, relatively few research studies have evaluated their reliability and validity. It seems likely that people may have difficulty with some diary recordkeeping tasks (e.g., rating changes in their pain, keeping up with hourly data entries) and that this may reduce their validity.

Recently, there has been growing interest among researchers in the use of daily diary methods to study how processes such as coping are related to day-to-day variations in pain (Affleck, Tennen, Urrows, & Higgins, 1991). These new daily diary measures not only have been shown to be highly reliable (Affleck et al., 1991), they also enable one to capture how dynamic processes, such as the relationship of coping to pain, unfold over time. We recently conducted a study of daily coping and pain in a sample of 53 patients having pain due to rheumatoid arthritis (Keefe, Affleck et al., 1997). Subjects in this study completed a diary each evening for 30 days in which they reported on: (a) the specific pain coping strategies they had used (e.g., relaxation, distraction, venting emotions), (b) the efficacy of their coping, (c) their joint pain, and (d) their positive and negative mood. The data were analyzed in two ways. First, to examine interrelationships among the measures across all subjects, data gathered over the 30 days were averaged and correlational analyses conducted. These analyses showed that daily coping efficacy was unrelated to pain coping or pain intensity. Second, to examine how these repeated measures related at the within-person level, within-subjects analyses were conducted. Interestingly, the within-person analyses revealed that daily coping efficacy was significantly related to decreases in pain and also to decreases in negative mood and increases in positive mood. Time-lagged effects were also evident in the within-subjects analyses with individuals having higher coping efficacy on a given day reporting lower levels of pain on the next day. Taken together, these findings suggest that a careful within-person analysis of diary data can reveal important relationships between pain and coping.

Stewart, Lipton, Simon, Liberman, and Von Korff (1997) used diary measures of pain to examine the validity of a new questionnaire measure of headache pain (the Impact Questionnaire). Subjects in this study, 226 migraine headache sufferers, completed the Impact Questionnaire based on their headache activity and level of disability (i.e., effects of pain on home, work, and social activities) over the previous 3 months. These questionnaire reports of headache activity were then compared to diary records of their headaches kept over the same 3-month period. The data analyses revealed that there was a strong and positive correlation between the questionnaire reports of headache frequency and actual diary records of headaches (correlation coefficient of .67) and between questionnaire reports of headache intensity and diary records of headache intensity (correlation coefficient of .74). Furthermore, there was also a strong relationship between questionnaire reports of lost work time due to headache and diary records of work loss (correlation coefficient of .60). This study demonstrates the utility of diary measures of pain in validating other pain assessment methods; that is, a standard headache questionnaire. In the future, researchers developing questionnaire measures of pain need to consider validating their instruments against daily diary records of pain.

CONCLUSIONS

The self-report of pain is critical to the understanding of another's pain experience. Newly developed self-report measures of pain aim to capture the multidimensional nature of the pain experience. Reliable and valid measures of two of the most important dimensions of pain—that is, pain intensity and pain affect—are available and are being used in many clinical research studies. Many of these measures are new, however, and will need further development before they can be routinely incorporated into clinical practice. As self-report methods are refined, they are likely to significantly improve our abilities to assess and treat acute and persistent pain.

REFERENCES

Affleck, G., Tennen, H., Urrows, S., & Higgins, P. (1991). Individual differences in the day-to-day experience of chronic pain: A prospective daily study of rheumatoid arthritis patients. *Health Psychology, 10*, 419–426.

Beecher, H. K. (1959). *Measurement of subjective responses.* New York: Oxford University Press.

Craig, K. D., Prkachin, K. M., & Grunau, R. V. E. (1992). The facial expression of pain. In D. Turk & R. Melzack (Eds.), *Handbook of pain assessment* (pp. 257–276). New York: Guilford.

Fillingim, R. B., Keefe, F. J., Light, K. C., Booker, D. K., & Maixner, W. (1996). The influence of gender and psychological factors on pain perception. *Journal of Gender, Culture, and Health, 1*, 21–36.

Fordyce, W. E. (1976). *Behavioral methods for chronic pain and illness.* St. Louis, MO: Mosby.

Fordyce, W. E. (1985). On Rachlin's "pain and behavior": A lightening of the burden. *Behavior and Brain Sciences, 81*, 58–59.

Gracely, R. H., McGrath, P., & Dubner, R. (1978). Validity and sensitivity of ratio scales of sensory and affective verbal pain descriptors: Manipulation of affect by diazepam. *Pain, 35*, 279–288.

Gracely, R. H., McGrath, P., & Dubner, R. (1979). Narcotic analgesia: Fentanyl reduces the intensity but not the unpleasantness of painful tooth pulp sensations. *Science, 203*, 1261–1263.

Janal, M. N., Glusman, M., Kuhl, J. P., & Clark, W. C. (1994). On the absence of correlations between responses to noxious heat, cold, electrical, or ischemic stimulation. *Pain, 58*, 403–411.

Jensen, M. P. (1997). Validity of self-report and observation measures. In T. S. Jensen, J. A. Turner, & Z. Wiesenfeld-Hallin (Eds.), *Proceedings of the 8th World Congress on Pain* (pp. 637–661). Seattle, WA: IASP Press.

Jensen, M. P., & Karoly, P. (1992). Self-report scales and procedures for assessing pain in adults. In D. C. Turk & R. Melzack. *Handbook of pain assessment* (pp. 135–151). New York: Guilford.

Jensen, M. P., & McFarland, C. A. (1993). Increasing the reliability and validity of pain intensity measurement in chronic pain patients. *Pain, 55*, 195–203.

Keefe, F. J., Affleck, G., Lefebvre, J. C., Starr, K., Caldwell, D. S., & Tennen, H. (1997). Coping strategies and coping efficacy in rheumatoid arthritis: A daily process analysis. *Pain, 69,* 43–48.

Keefe, F. J., & Block, A. R. (1982). Development of an observation method for assessing pain behavior in chronic low back pain patients. *Behavior Therapy, 13,* 363–375.

Keefe, F. J., & Dunsmore, J. (1992). Pain behavior: Concepts and controversies. *American Pain Society Journal, 1,* 92–100.

Keefe, F. J., Lefebvre, J. C., Maixner, W., Salley, A. N., & Caldwell, D. S. (1997). Self-efficacy for arthritis pain: Relationship to perception of thermal laboratory pain stimuli. *Arthritis Care and Research, 10,* 177–184.

Keefe, F. J., Lefebvre, J., & Starr, K. (1996). From the gate control theory to the neuromatrix: Revolution or evolution. *Pain Forum, 5,* 143–145.

Keefe, F. J., Wilkins, R. H., & Cook, W. A. (1984). Direct observation of pain behavior in low back pain patients during physical examination. *Pain, 20,* 59–68.

Kent, G. (1985). Memory for dental pain. *Pain, 21,* 187–194.

Love, A., Leboeuf, D. C., & Crisp, T. C. (1989). Chiropractic chronic low back pain sufferers and self-report assessment methods. Part 1. A reliability study of the Visual Analogue Scale, the pain drawing, and the McGill Pain Questionnaire. *Journal of Manipulative and Physiological Therapeutics, 12,* 21–25.

Melzack, R. (1975). The McGill Pain Questionnaire: Major properties and scoring methods. *Pain, 1,* 277–299.

Melzack, R. (1995). Phantom limb pain and the brain. In B. Bromm & J. E. Desmeadt (Eds.), *Pain and the brain* (pp. 73–82). New York: Raven.

Melzack, R., & Katz, J. (1992). The McGill Pain Questionnaire: Appraisal and current status. In D. C. Turk & R. Melzack (Eds.), *Handbook of pain assessment* (pp. 152–168). New York: Guilford.

Melzack, R., & Wall, P. D. (1962). On the nature of cutaneous sensory mechanisms. *Brain, 85,* 331–356.

Melzack, R., & Wall, P. D. (1965). Pain mechanisms: A new theory. *Science, 150,* 971–979.

Melzack, R., & Wall, P. D. (1982). Acute pain in an emergency clinic: Latency of onset and descriptor patterns. *Pain, 14,* 33–43.

Melzack, R., & Wall, P. D. (1996). *The challenge of pain.* London: Penguin.

Price, D. D., Barrel, J. J., & Gracely, R. H. (1980). A psychophysical analysis of experiential factors that selectively influence the affective dimension of pain. *Pain, 8,* 137–179.

Price, D. D., Bush, F. M., Long, S., & Harkins, S. W. (1994). A comparison of pain measurement characteristics of mechanical visual analogue and simple numerical rating scales. *Pain, 56,* 217–226.

Price, D. D., & Harkins, S. W. (1987). The combined use of visual analogue scales and experimental pain in improving standardized assessment of clinical pain. *Clinical Journal of Pain, 3,* 1–8.

Price, D. D., & Harkins, S. W. (1992). Psychophysical approaches to pain measurement and assessment. In D. C. Turk & R. Melzack (Eds.), *Handbook of pain assessment* (pp. 111–134). New York: Guilford.

Price, D. D., Harkins, S. W., & Baker, C. (1987). Sensory-affective relationships among different types of clinical and experimental pain. *Pain, 28,* 291–299.

Price, D. D., Harkins, S. W., Rafii, A., & Price, C. (1986). A simultaneous comparison of fentanyl's analgesic effects on experimental and clinical pain. *Pain, 24,* 197–203.

Price, D. D., McGrath, P. A., Rafii, A., & Buckingham, B. (1983). The validation of visual analogue scales as ratio scale measures for chronic and experimental pain. *Pain, 17,* 45–56.

Richards, R., Nepomuceno, C., Riles, M., & Suer, A. (1982). Assessing pain behavior: The UAB Pain Behavior Scale. *Pain, 14,* 393–398.

Sternbach, R. A., & Tursky, B. (1965). Ethnic differences among housewives in psychophysical and skin potential responses to electric shock. *Psychophysiology, 1,* 241–246.

Stewart, W. F., Lipton, R. B., Simon, D., Liberman, J., & Von Korff, M. (1997). *Validity of an illness severity measure for headache in a population sample of migraine sufferers*. Manuscript submitted for publication.

Tursky, B. (1976). The development of pain perception profile: A psychophysical approach. In M. Weisenberg & B. Tursky (Eds.), *Pain: New perspectives in therapy and research* (pp. 171–194). New York: Plenum.

Urban, B. J., Keefe, F. J., & France, R. F. (1984). A study of psychophysical scaling in chronic pain patients. *Pain, 20*, 157–168.

White, B., & Sanders, S. H. (1986). The influence of patients' pain intensity ratings of antecedent reinforcement of pain talk or well talk. *Journal of Behavior Therapy & Experimental Psychiatry, 17*, 155–159.

Zelman, D. C., Howland, E. W., Nichols, S. N., & Cleeland, C. (1991). The effects of induced mood on laboratory pain. *Pain, 46*, 105–111.

19

The Validity of Bodily Symptoms in Medical Outpatients

Arthur J. Barsky
Harvard Medical School, Boston, MA
Brigham and Women's Hospital, Boston, MA

THE RELATIONSHIP BETWEEN SYMPTOMS AND DISEASE

Although history-taking is the key to diagnosis in clinical medicine, and symptom relief is the goal of medical treatment, symptoms are often unreliable and invalid measures of the extent and severity of medical disease. Disease may unfold without causing symptoms, as is seen for example in silent myocardial infarctions and asymptomatic lumbar disk disease. Conversely, it is common to encounter patients with symptoms but no demonstrable disease, as for instance in chronic pain, somatization, and conversion symptoms. Medical treatment may cure disease without relieving symptoms (as has been demonstrated in peptic ulcers; Bodemar & Walan, 1978; Peterson et al., 1977, and rheumatoid arthritis; Dwosh, Giles, Ford, Pater, & Anastassiades, 1983), and ineffective treatment can bring about a symptomatic cure, as is attested to by the powerful and ubiquitous placebo effect (Harrington, 1997).

There are now a number of studies that reveal how widely symptom severity and the extent of tissue pathology may diverge. Asthmatic patients' dyspnea corresponds poorly to measures of airway obstruction (Burdon, Juniper, Killian, Hargreave, & Campbell, 1982; Kikuchi et al., 1994; Rubinfeld & Pain, 1976), and in chronic obstructive pulmonary disease, little relationship is found between subjective dyspnea and forced expiratory volume (Alonso et al., 1992; Burdon et al., 1982; Mahler, Matthay, Snyder, Wells, &

Loke, 1985; Mahler, Weinberg, Wells, & Feinstein, 1984). Similarly, the presence of a peptic ulcer is only weakly associated with its symptoms (Bodemar & Walan, 1978; Peterson et al., 1977), and measures of urodynamic obstruction are not significantly correlated with the urinary obstructive symptoms in patients with benign prostatic hypertrophy (Frimodt-Moller, Jensen, Iversen, Madsen, & Bruskewitz, 1984). Arthritis pain has been extensively studied in this respect: Osteoarthritis patients show a variable and inconsistent relationship between subjective distress and objective disease, and little relationship can be found between radiological abnormalities and pain (Boden, Davis, Dina, Patronas, & Wiesel, 1990; Hussar & Guller, 1956; Keefe et al, 1987; Summers, Haley, Reveille, & Alarcón, 1988; Wiesel, Tsourmas, Feffer, Citris, & Patronas, 1984). Finally, the symptoms of diabetes correlate more closely with depression than with glycosylated hemoglobin levels (Lustman, Clouse, & Carney, 1988), and in moderately anemic patients there is no statistical association between hemoglobin levels and symptoms (Wood & Elwood, 1966).

We have undertaken several studies to explore the nonmedical factors that contribute to somatic symptom reporting in medical patients. The theoretical model guiding this work has been derived from current knowledge about somatization, and we have proposed that the factors that foster somatization also amplify the somatic symptoms resulting from demonstrable organ pathology as well. In effect, we are suggesting that the same forces that promote medically unexplained symptoms also exacerbate the symptoms resulting from demonstrable disease.

Somatization is the experience and reporting of medically unexplained symptoms, the misattribution of these benign symptoms to serious medical disease, and the seeking of medical attention for them. The phenomenon is ubiquitous. It is estimated that in 25% to 50% of all primary care visits, no serious medical cause is found to explain the patient's presenting symptom (Bridges & Goldberg, 1985; Cartwright, 1967; Gough, 1977; Katon, Ries, & Kleinman, 1984; Kleinman, Eisenberg, & Good, 1978; Kroenke, Arrington, & Mangelsdorff, 1990; Mechanic, 1974). Put another way, 38% to 60% of the patients in primary care practice complain of symptoms that have no serious medical basis (Backett, Heady, & Evans, 1954; Cummings & Vanden Bos, 1981; Follette & Cummings, 1968; Garfield et al., 1976; Hilkevitch, 1965; Pilowsky, Smith, & Katsikitis, 1987; van der Gagg & van de Ven, 1978). And if we focus not on patients or visits as the denominator but rather on symptoms, a similar picture emerges; of all the symptoms patients report, 30% to 75% remain medically unexplained after adequate evaluation. Even when restricted to symptoms that have bothered the patient a lot in the past month, 16% to 33% have no medical explanation (Kroenke et al., 1990, 1994; Kroenke & Mangelsdorff, 1989). Although we tend to think of such symptoms as trivial, in fact medically unexplained symptoms are actually as disabling, more chronic, and more refractory to treatment than are organically based symptoms (Craig, Boardman, Mills, Daley-Jones, & Drake, 1993; Escobar, Burnham, Karno, Forsythe, & Golding, 1987; Escobar, Golding et al., 1987; Kroenke & Mangelsdorff, 1989; Kroenke et al., 1994).

What mechanisms account for this widespread and troubling phenomenon? A good deal is known about the forces that predispose to, precipitate, and/or perpetuate somatization (Bass, 1990; Ford, 1983; Kellner, 1986; Pennebaker, 1982). Certain childhood experiences are thought to predispose to somatizing in adulthood, including having had figures of identity (family members who somatized or suffered from a chronic disease); an exaggerated parental interest in, or attention to, symptoms and health; and childhood neglect, trauma, or abuse. Certain personality traits are also thought to make one more prone to somatization. These include negative affectivity (neuroticism) and certain personality disorders (especially those in *DSM–IV* cluster B). In addition to formative childhood experiences and certain personality traits, an amplifying somatic style is thought to foster somatization. Somatic amplifiers have a relatively enduring propensity to experience bodily sensation in general (including normal physiology and trivial, benign dysfunction) as noxious, intense, and unpleasant.

Several factors precipitate somatization. Distressing life events that require adaptation (particularly those involving loss) have been linked to the onset of medically unexplained somatic symptoms; bereavement is the prototypical such event. Anxiety and depressive disorders are accompanied by prominent somatic complaints and often by disease fears and beliefs as well. Finally, cognitive factors may precipitate somatization. These include the activation of latent health schema used to interpret somatic sensation, heightened bodily vigilance, the misattribution of benign bodily sensation to serious disease, and external locus of control.

A number of factors have been identified as reinforcers that perpetuate or maintain somatization once it has occurred. Secondary gains ensue when one becomes a patient and assumes the sick role. These include the power to control and manipulate others, the ability to postpone obligations and challenges and to avoid seemingly insurmountable problems, and the legitimization of a relationship with a physician. It is important to remember that secondary gains do not imply malingering but rather operate unconsciously to reinforce particular coping behaviors.

A MODEL OF SOMATIC SYMPTOM FORMATION

This brief review provides some guidance in identifying factors that explain why somatic symptom reports are only loosely related to underlying tissue pathology. It suggests that bodily amplification, hypochondriacal concerns,

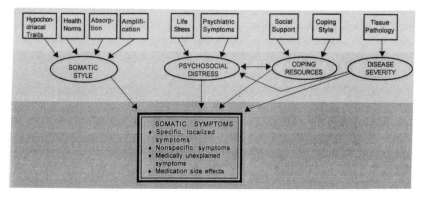

FIG. 19.1. A cognitive–perceptual model of symptom formation.

normative beliefs about health, psychiatric symptoms, and daily life stress
are among the factors that contribute to the inter-individual variation in
somatic symptom reporting among medically ill patients. Based on this, a
conceptual model of somatic symptom formation is presented in Fig. 19.1. I
posit four domains that together determine the degree of symptom distress.
These four domains are termed disease severity, somatic style, psychosocial
distress, and coping resources.

Disease Severity

Medical morbidity, that is, the extent and severity of tissue destruction and
organ pathology, is obviously a key determinant of symptoms. In the case
of pain, the bodily sensation resulting from tissue destruction is referred to
as the nociceptive component of the pain experience. Although most salient
when medical disease is most severe, there are nonetheless occasions when
very severe tissue destruction results in few symptoms (Beecher, 1966).

Somatic Style

Somatic style then filters and embellishes the sensory and nociceptive inputs
that originate in the diseased tissues. It is this cortical and subcortical
processing of sensation that imparts the qualities of discomfort, noxious-
ness, urgency, and alarm. Somatic style is conceptualized as a relatively
stable, enduring characteristic, a propensity to experience bodily sensation
in general (both benign and normal sensations and the symptoms of disease)
as intrusive, noxious, worrisome, and intense. Somatic style is composed of
bodily amplification, hypochondriacal attitudes, normative beliefs about
health, and bodily absorption.

Psychosocial Distress

Psychosocial distress also amplifies bodily symptoms. Recurrent, minor, daily irritations and major stressful life changes requiring adaptation both lead to an increase in bodily distress and somatic symptom reporting. Some portion of this effect may be mediated by the emotional dysphoria that stress engenders. Somatic discomfort is an integral aspect of emotional distress; anxiety and depression, for example, are accompanied by prominent somatic complaints and also cause preexisting symptoms to be intensified.

Coping Resources

Finally, somatic symptoms are modified by the coping behaviors with which patients respond to their illness. Adaptive coping and helpful social supports modulate distress, whereas maladaptive coping responses and social isolation exacerbate symptoms.

The process of symptom formation is, of course, complicated by the reciprocal relationships among these factors, which feed back on and interact with each other. These reciprocal relationships have been omitted from the unidirectional model previously presented in order to simplify it and to emphasize only the fundamental relationships.

THE SYMPTOMS OF UPPER RESPIRATORY TRACT INFECTIONS

We have undertaken several empirical studies of medical outpatients to examine various components of this model of symptom formation, focusing in particular on somatic style. In the first of these, we examined the associations of bodily amplification, psychiatric distress, and tissue pathology with the symptoms resulting from upper respiratory tract infections (URIs; Barsky, Goodson, Lane, & Cleary, 1988; Lane, Barsky, & Goodson, 1988). The study population consisted of consecutive patients presenting to a medical walk-in clinic with a URI. Those with more serious, underlying medical disorders such as pneumonia, asthma, and bronchitis, were excluded. One hundred and fifteen such patients were studied. They completed a series of questionnaires assessing URI symptoms and discomfort, bodily amplification, and psychiatric distress. URI symptoms were measured with a 15-item, self-report questionnaire and subjective self-ratings of global discomfort were also obtained. Amplification (which is defined as the tendency to experience benign, mild, and ambiguous bodily sensation as intense, noxious, and unpleasant) was measured with the Somatosensory Amplification Scale. Anxiety, depression, and hostility were measured with the Hopkins

Symptom Checklist–90. Each patient's physician rated the extent and severity of 11 physical examination findings, including fever, adenopathy, tonsillar exudate, nasal edema, and pharyngeal edema. The sum of these 11 findings was used as a measure of the seriousness of the patient's URI and was termed medical morbidity.

Multiple linear regression analysis was used to examine the contributions of demographic characteristics, medical morbidity, and the psychiatric–perceptual factors to the variability in discomfort and disability. First, we calculated the amount of variance in discomfort explained by sociodemographic characteristics (age, sex, and ethnicity). Next, we calculated the additional variance in discomfort explained when medical morbidity was added to the model. Third, amplification, somatization, hostility, depression, and anxiety scores were added separately to the preceding model. We also tested for an interaction between the psychiatric measures and medical morbidity in order to examine whether or not the effect of the psychiatric characteristics held across all levels of disease.

A wide range in symptoms existed among patients with URIs of comparable severity. This interindividual variability in symptoms was seen even at the extremes, among those patients rated by their physicians as having the mildest infections and those with the most severe infections. Of the 22 patients (19%) rated sickest by the clinicians, eight complained of two or fewer symptoms, whereas nine complained of five or more symptoms. The same broad spectrum was found among the patients with the most benign physical examinations. Of the 18 patients (15.6%) judged least sick, three complained of two or fewer symptoms, whereas six complained of five or more symptoms.

Sociodemographic characteristics explained 17% of the variance of discomfort ($R^2 = 0.17$). When the medical morbidity variables were added, the variance explained increased to 25% ($R^2 = 0.25$). At the next step, each of the individual psychiatric–perceptual variables increased the explanatory power of the model significantly, as shown in Fig. 19.2 and Table 19.1. Somatization was most powerful, raising the variance in discomfort explained to $R^2 = 0.49$. Amplification and somatization together increased the total R^2 to 0.54 ($F = 12.77$). Thus, the best model for predicting discomfort contained the sociodemographic descriptors and medical morbidity together with somatization and amplification. We repeated these regressions, adding an interaction term for each psychiatric–perceptual subscale and medical morbidity. None of the interaction coefficients was significant, indicating that the relationship between discomfort and the psychiatric scales was the same for all levels of physical disease.

Physical examination findings, however, did not significantly contribute to predicting the variance in disability. When the basic model is considered and the emotional–perceptual scales are added in stepwise fashion, only

MODEL: AGE, SEX, ETHNICITY, EXTENT OF PHYSICAL DISEASE

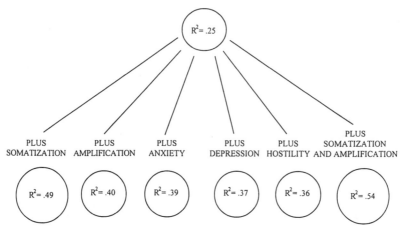

FIG. 19.2. Discomfort in upper respiratory tract infection.

somatization is retained and the overall explanation of the variance remains relatively low. This may, however, have to do with our measure of disability, which had limitations.

We thus found a wide variation in symptom reports among individuals with similar physical findings. Their ratings of subjective discomfort were significantly correlated with measures of affective dysphoria after the extent of the medical disease was taken into account. Somatization and amplification appeared to be the most dominant of these factors. Our results suggest

TABLE 19.1
Predictors of Discomfort in Patients
With Upper Respiratory Tract Infections

	β*	R^2*	F*	p*
Discomfort model:				
Extent of physical disease, adjusted for age, sex, ethnicity				
Plus				
Somatization	0.5998	0.49	46.24	0.0001
or				
Amplification	0.6119	0.40	24.59	0.0001
or				
Anxiety	0.5418	0.39	22.05	0.0001
or				
Depression	0.4062	0.37	18.09	0.0001
or				
Hostility	0.4600	0.36	16.36	0.0001

*β (regression coefficient), F, and p are for each subscale coefficient; R^2 is for the individual regression equations.

that the concept of amplification merits further study. Our measure of amplification increased the prediction of discomfort from 25% to 40% when added to the measures of physical findings and demographic descriptors. It must be remembered, however, that amplification itself was measured with a self-report instrument, not with any objective perceptual test of sensitivity or discriminative ability. This brings up one of the major limitations of this study (and of much research like it): Most of the measures are self-reports and thereby introduce a serious confound. A general tendency or bias toward symptom reporting, such as negative affectivity or neuroticism, could systematically underlie measures of both somatic symptoms and psychiatric symptoms. In addition, because this study was cross-sectional and not longitudinal, no inferences about cause and effect can be drawn. It is just as possible to conclude from these data that particularly intense symptoms lead to anxiety, depression, and bodily amplification as it is to conclude that these psychological characteristics lead to an intensification of bodily sensations.

CARDIAC SYMPTOMS, CARDIAC SENSATIONS, AND CARDIAC DISEASE

Heart disease and cardiac symptoms furnish a particularly interesting set of problems to explore in this regard. Here, the absence of a one-to-one relationship between symptoms and disease has been widely documented and has enormous clinical and public health implications. Angina pectoris is a highly insensitive and nonspecific indicator of ischemic heart disease. Anginal chest pain is often reported by patients in whom extensive medical evaluation reveals no evidence of cardiac disease. Thus, between 10% and 30% of patients with chest pain severe enough to warrant angiography are found to have no significant coronary vessel disease. Conversely, 70% of documented ischemic episodes in patients with coronary artery disease are asymptomatic and 30% of myocardial infarctions are asymptomatic (Deanfield et al., 1983; Epstein, Quyyumi, & Bonow, 1988; Glazier, Chierchia, Brown, & Maseri, 1986; Kannel & Abbott, 1984; Quyyumi, Wright, Mockus, & Fox, 1985).

A similar situation obtains when we turn from ischemic heart disease to disorders of cardiac rhythm. Many patients with palpitations are without arrhythmias and a large proportion of arrhythmias are asymptomatic. When patients complaining of palpitations undergo 24-hour, ambulatory, electrocardiographic monitoring, 39% to 85% manifest some rhythm disturbance (Burckhardt, Luetold, Jost, & Hoffman, 1982; Clark, Glasser, & Spoto, 1980; Goldberg, Raftery, & Cashman, 1975; Grodman, Capone, & Most, 1979; Hasin, David, & Rogel, 1976; Kennedy, Chandra, Sayther, & Caralis, 1978; Lipski et al., 1976; Zeldis, Levine, Michelson, & Morganroth, 1980; the vast majority of these arrhythmias are benign, clinically insignificant, and do not merit treatment). Although as many as 75% of these patients with arrhythmias report their presenting symptom during monitoring (Burckhardt et al., 1982; Clark et al., 1980; Grodman et al., 1979; Hasin et al., 1976; Kunz, Raeder, & Burckhardt, 1977; Morahan, Denes, & Rosen, 1975; Zeldis et al., 1980), in only about 15% of cases do these symptom reports coincide with their arrhythmias (Burckhardt et al., 1982; Clark et al., 1980; Grodman et al., 1979; Kennedy et al., 1978; Kunz et al., 1977; Morahan et al., 1975; Winkle, Derrington, & Schroeder, 1977; Zeldis et al., 1980).

A number of important clinical questions arise from this variable relationship between symptoms and arrhythmias. In part, confusion occurs because physicians and patients alike use the term palpitations imprecisely to refer to changes in rate, rhythm, or force of contraction and to a number of different sensations, including acceleration, irregular rhythm, increased force of contraction, or missing a beat. When treating patients complaining of palpitations, are there characteristic symptom descriptions or clinical histories that are more or less likely to suggest the presence of an arrhythmia? Are there particular symptom descriptions that correspond to particular types of arrhythmias? Are there characteristics of the patients themselves that indicate whose symptom reports are more likely to reflect underlying arrhythmic activity and whose symptom reports are more likely to be medically unexplained? There are also more basic questions that arise as to the sensory pathways that underlie cardiac interoception. Where do sensations of cardiac contraction and awareness or cardiac activity originate and how are they processed in the central nervous system? What is needed here is more exploration and understanding of the neurophysiology and psychophysiology of cardiac interoception. We have undertaken several studies of medical outpatients complaining of palpitations to examine some of these questions. We sought to obtain explicit, precise symptom recordings from patients during daily life to correlate these with concurrent ambulatory ECG recordings and to contrast the clinical characteristics of the patients whose symptoms did and did not coincide with arrhythmias.

The Relationship Between Palpitations and Arrhythmias

We and others have conducted a series of studies of medical outpatients complaining of palpitations to further investigate cardiac symptoms and cardiac perception (Barsky, Ahern, Delamater, Clancy, & Bailey, 1997; Barsky, Cleary, Barnett, Christiansen, & Ruskin, 1994; Macdonald, Sackett, Haynes, & Taylor, 1984; Zeldis et al., 1980). In the first of these, 145 consecutive outpatients referred to an ambulatory electrocardiography (Holter) laboratory for evaluation of palpitations were accrued, along with a comparison sample of 70 nonpatient volunteers who had no cardiac symptoms and no history of cardiac disease. They underwent a research battery consisting of self-report questionnaires, cognitive tests, and structured interviews. Somatization was measured with the Somatic Symptom Inventory. Hypochondriacal attitudes and beliefs were measured with the Whiteley Index, and anxiety was assessed with the Spielberger State–Trait Anxiety Inventory. Psychiatric diagnoses were established with a structured, diagnostic interview (the Diagnostic Interview Schedule). Patients were then given specially designed diaries for recording their symptoms during ambulatory monitoring. They completed an entry for each symptom noted and recorded the exact onset of the symptom with a clock that had previously been synchronized with the monitor. The Holter electrocardiogram was subsequently analyzed in conjunction with the symptom diary to determine cardiac activity preceding each symptom report. A symptom was considered accurate when it followed within 30 seconds after any demonstrated arrhythmia.

To assess the association between symptom reports and cardiac activity, we calculated the average positive predictive value (PPV). This value is equal to the number of reported symptoms that were preceded by an arrhythmia divided by the total number of symptoms reported (true positives / [true positives + false positives]). To estimate the association between patient characteristics and PPV, taking into account the varying number of symptoms reported by the patient, we employed beta-binomial regression models. After estimating the bivariate associations between each characteristic and the PPV, we estimated another model that included all the patient characteristics that had statistically significant bivariate associations with PPV. Because of the statistical association between PPV and the incidence of arrhythmias, we also included the number of arrhythmias occurring during monitoring in the model.

Ninety-nine palpitation patients (68%) reported at least one palpitation during monitoring. Among those patients who were symptomatic, the mean number of diary symptoms reported in 24 hours was 3.7. The mean PPV for all symptom reports among palpitation patients was 0.399, compared with a mean PPV = .118 for the nonpatient volunteer sample (p = .01). In Table 19.2 it can be seen that the palpitation descriptors most likely to be accompanied by electrocardiographic abnormalities are heart stopping, fluttering, and irregular heartbeat. The least predictive descriptive terms used by the patients were racing and pounding. The particular descriptive term chosen by the patient to describe his/her sensation conveyed only a limited amount of diagnostic information. When associated with an arrhythmia, the sensation of the heart stopping always followed a ventricular premature contraction (although there were only 19 such reports). Eighty-five percent of the accurate reports of jumping and pounding followed ventricular premature contractions. In contrast, the complaints of irregular heartbeat and fluttering

TABLE 19.2
Types of Symptoms Reported by Palpitation Patients (n = 145)

Symptom	Number of Symptom Reports	Average Positive Predictive Value*
Stopping	20	.950
Fluttering	111	.811
Irregular heartbeat	156	.782
Jumping	79	.620
Pounding/vigorous heartbeat	125	.392
Racing	105	.210
Faintness	38	.158
Chest pain	49	.143
Shortness of breath	73	.137

Note. Frequency and average positive predictive value by type of symptom reported.
*Number of symptoms accompanied by arrhythmia divided by total number of symptoms reported.

were less predictive: Approximately half of these reports, when accurate, resulted from ventricular premature contractions and approximately half of them followed atrial premature contractions. The descriptor used did not correspond literally to the type of arrhythmia that caused it; stopping never coincided with bradycardia or a prolonged pause, and racing was never associated with tachycardia.

The likelihood that a diary symptom coincided with an arrhythmia was not related to sociodemographic characteristics, the chronicity of the patient's chief complaint or to the presence of diagnosed heart disease (see Table 19.3). Nor was PPV related to the clinical significance of the arrhythmia: Patients with clinically serious arrhythmias did not differ significantly from patients with benign arrhythmias in PPV or in the number of diary symptoms. Accurate awareness of arrhythmias might conceivably be related to medical care use because more contact with doctors and more diagnostic testing could cause patients to scrutinize themselves more and become hypervigilant about bodily sensations. In fact, however, PPV was not significantly associated with physician visits, number of cardiac tests undergone, or emergency room use.

To further examine the accuracy of Holter diary symptoms, subjects whose symptoms corresponded to ECG changes more than two thirds of the time (i.e., PPV > 0.67) were defined as accurate reporters. Defined in this way, accuracy had a bimodal distribution (see Figure 19.3). Thirty four percent of the symptomatic palpitation patients and 11% of the asymptomatic comparison subjects were classified as accurate reporters (p = 0.07). Accurate awareness of arrhythmias was inversely related to somatization, hypochondriasis, the number of psychiatric diagnoses, and the number of

TABLE 19.3
Patient Characteristics and Positive Predictive
Value of Holter Diary Symptoms

	Adjusted Odds Ratio	95% Confidence Interval	
Sociodemographic Characteristics			
Age (years)	1.04	(1.01	1.06)
Gender (female)	1.00	(0.48	2.09)
Socioeconomic position (1–5)	1.08	(0.78	1.49)
Marital status (married)	0.96	(0.47	1.96)
Clinical Characteristics			
Duration of palpitations (months)	1.00	(0.996	1.003)
Percent of patients with known cardiac history	0.94	(0.44	2.02)
Medical Care Utilization			
Previous Holter monitor	1.51	(0.68	3.34)
Previous stress test	1.53	(0.73	3.18)
Number of physician visits, preceding 12 months	1.01	(0.98	1.05)
Number of emergency and walk-in visits, preceding 12 months	0.82	(0.66	1.02)
Number of mental health visits, preceding 12 months	0.21	(0.07	0.61)

Note. Adjusted odds ratios, estimated using beta-binomial regression. These ratios represent the relative likelihood that palpitations are more accurate (i.e., have a higher positive predictive value) in patients with and without each clinical characteristic or in patients with a one-integer increment in the characteristic.

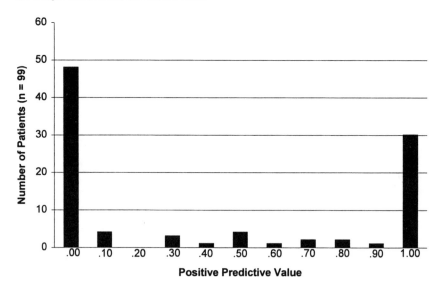

FIG. 19.3. Distribution of positive predictive value of diary symptoms among symptomatic Holter patients.

psychiatric symptoms (see Table 19.4). The accuracy of Holter diary symptoms was also inversely related to self-reported somatosensory amplification. None of the cognitive measures was related to accuracy. When we included all the significant predictors of average PPV in a beta-binomial regression model, the only statistically significant predictor of PPV was the patients' somatization score (OR = 0.41; CI = 0.19; 0.90). Even when the number of cardiac events was added to the model, the somatization score remained significant (OR = 0.41; CI = 0.18; 0.96).

Thus, several significant differences emerge between patients whose symptoms tend to coincide with arrhythmias and patients whose symptoms tend not to. The former somatize less, are less hypochondriacal, and have less psychiatric morbidity. Somatizing and hypochondriacal patients might *a priori* be expected to be more sensitive and more astute interoceptors who notice benign bodily dysfunctions, mild infirmities, and normal physiologic functions that other people are insensitive to or fail to discern. That is, we might expect that somatizers are able to make finer visceral discriminations and detect more subtle cardiac irregularities. However, our findings suggest that this is not the case and instead imply that somatizing and hypochondriacal concerns are better understood as a general response bias toward the expression of bodily distress, a global proclivity to feel uncomfortable. To use a signal detection paradigm, rather than being sensitive

TABLE 19.4
Comparison of Patients With Accurate
and Inaccurate Holter Diary Symptoms

	Patients With PPV > 0.67 (n = 34)	Patients With PPV < 0.67 (n = 65)	p
Perceptual characteristics			
Bodily Amplification (1–5)	2.1	2.5	0.02
Hear pulse throbbing in ear (1–5)	2.2	2.6	0.14
Psychiatric characteristics			
State Anxiety (1–4)	1.7	1.7	0.99
Somatization (1–5)	1.6	2.3	0.000
Hypochondriacal symptoms (1–5)	1.7	2.2	0.003
Patients with ≥ 1 psychiatric diagnosis*	11 (32.3%)	42 (64.6%)	0.004
Mean number of psychiatric symptoms, past year	1.94	3.94	0.000
Mean number of psychiatric symptoms, lifetime	10.9	22.0	0.000
Cognitive characteristics			
Attributional style			
Somatizing (1–4)	1.82	1.82	0.99
Normalizing (1–4)	2.31	2.26	0.65
Psychologizing (1–4)	1.95	2.06	0.34
Health norms (1–24)	18.4	17.1	0.19

*Excluding simple and social phobias.

detectors of weak and infrequent bodily signals, somatizers are less able to discriminate signals from background noise.

The inverse relationship between positive predictive value and psychiatric disorder is not surprising. An extensive body of research indicates that patients with high levels of psychologic distress and psychiatric symptoms report high levels of somatic symptoms as well (Costa & McCrae, 1980, 1985; Pennebaker, 1982, 1991; Watson & Pennebaker, 1989). As Watson and Pennebaker (1989) observed, physical symptoms and negative moods together often reflect a pervasive underlying disposition toward experiencing distress and discomfort in general. Thus, patients who are more psychiatrically disturbed would be expected to report more somatic symptoms in general and more cardiac symptoms (including palpitations) in particular. In many instances then, Holter diary reporting may be viewed as a specific manifestation of a more generalized tendency toward experiencing somatic distress and reporting it.

The tendency to experience and report a wide range of negative emotions—including anxiety, hostility, guilt, and depression—has been termed negative affectivity or neuroticism and has been shown to be a reliable, valid, and stable psychometric construct. Individuals who score high on self-report questionnaires of negative affectivity also report high levels of many somatic symptoms as well. There are several possible explanations for this association between emotional and physical symptoms. It could reflect a true co-occurrence of psychiatric and medical morbidity in the same individuals. Alternatively, because we know that these symptomatic individuals have higher rates of medical utilization, emotionally distressed people may notice preexisting somatic symptoms or verbalize them in order to legitimize their medical help-seeking. Another possible explanation, which may be most relevant to the present study, is that some individuals may have a greater tendency to recognize and report both psychologic and somatic symptoms—that is, to amplify all forms of distress.

From a clinician's perspective, the likelihood that a symptom is indicative of an underlying arrhythmia is the most salient aspect of symptom accuracy. But the converse phenomenon—the sensitivity of symptom reporting (i.e., the likelihood that a given arrhythmia will generate a symptom report) is also of interest. In our study, there was a very low likelihood that any single arrhythmia was noticed and reported as a symptom; palpitations were extremely insensitive indicators of arrhythmias. Of the 137 patients who had arrhythmic activity during Holter monitoring, 87 (64%) detected none of their arrhythmias at all. Only 8 detected more than 10% of the events that occurred, and only 26 detected more than 1%. Even the patients with the highest PPVs were very insensitive and failed to note the vast majority of their arrhythmias. Only 6 of the 30 patients with at least one accurate symptom report had average sensitivities greater than 0.25.

Accurate Awareness of Resting Heartbeat

We also examined the accurate awareness of resting heartbeat as another dimension of the validity of symptom reports of cardiac activity (Barsky, Cleary, Barnett, et al., 1994; Barsky, Cleary, Brener, & Ruskin, 1993; Barsky, Cleary, Sarnie, & Ruskin, 1994). Accurate awareness of resting heartbeat was determined with the Brener-Kluvitse procedure (Brener & Kluvitse, 1988), in which subjects were connected to an electrocardiogram and seated in a dim, sound-attenuated room. They were then presented with six different trains of 20-ms-long auditory tones, each separated from the preceding R-wave by one of six intervals (0, 100, 200, 300, 400, and 500 ms). They were instructed to sample each of the different R-wave to tone intervals and then select the one judged to coincide with heartbeat sensations. Performance on this heartbeat detection (HBD) task was evaluated by analyzing each subject's frequency distribution of preferred intervals over the six R-wave to tone intervals. If this distribution differed significantly from chance (a rectangular distribution) by the chi-square test, that subject was deemed to have detected heartbeat sensations. The distribution was also used to calculate indices of the temporal location of heartbeat sensations (median interval) and the precision of heartbeat detection (interquartile range). The patients in this study also completed many of the same self-report questionnaires described in the earlier study.

The HBD task was completed on 121 palpitation patients and 64 asymptomatic, nonpatient volunteers. Twenty five (20.7%) palpitation patients and 3 (4.7%) comparison patients demonstrated a statistically significant awareness of cardiac contraction ($\chi^2 \geq 11.07$). This intergroup difference is highly significant ($p = 0.01$). Thus, one fifth of the palpitation patients were accurately aware of ventricular systole at rest, a significantly higher proportion than found among the asymptomatic nonpatients. At least two possible explanations for this difference arise. First, it is possible that on innate, preexisting sensitivity to cardiac activity makes those individuals more likely to notice benign ectopy and to label it a palpitation and then to seek medical attention for their symptoms. Alternatively, experiencing a worrisome bodily symptom and consulting a doctor about it may foster bodily hypervigilance, introspection, and self-monitoring. These in turn might improve cardiac awareness, and the individual in effect learns to become a more sensitive heartbeat detector.

We also examined the relationship between HBD ability and a variety of other patient characteristics. These included sociodemographic characteristics, the severity and chronicity of palpitations, the extent of previous medical care, and selected psychiatric and psychological characteristics. The most striking general finding was the lack of association between cardioception and all of these variables. One exception to this pattern of negative findings was that HBD ability was related to normative beliefs about good health. Accurate cardioceptors were significantly more likely to consider ambiguous medical symptoms to be indicative of disease—that is, they had a lower threshold for considering themselves to be sick. It is not immediately apparent why patients who are more aware of cardiac contraction have a lower threshold for deciding that they are sick. Perhaps those who are more aware of their own normal resting heartbeat have a clearer and more explicit picture of normal physiology and good health and are therefore better able to detect deviations from that state and more ready to view these deviations as abnormal and indicative of sickness. This same finding emerged in another, entirely unrelated study (unpublished data), where we again found that among general medical outpatients, accurate awareness of resting heartbeat was significantly and inversely related to normative beliefs about health.

HBD performance was unrelated to the self-reported tendency to amplify bodily sensation; accurate heartbeat detectors did not report they were any more sensitive to benign bodily sensation or find it any more noxious or intense than did inaccurate perceivers. (HBD performance was, however, significantly associated with a single question from the Somatosensory Amplification Scale, the item "I can sometimes hear my heartbeat throbbing in my ear"; $p = 0.03$). Thus the subjective sense that one is exceptionally sensitive to nonpathological bodily discomfort was not corroborated by an objective test of sensitivity to normal cardiac contraction. This is compatible with literature suggesting that subjective and objective measures of interceptive accuracy are not closely related (Katkin, 1985; Pennebaker, 1991; Schandry, 1981; Whitehead, Drescher, Heiman & Blackwell, 1977).

The overall impression, however, is that heartbeat detection was not related to a wide variety of clinical and historical variables studied. This suggests that heartbeat awareness is more like an innate sensory acuity (akin to an accurate musical ear, for example) than a perceptual ability that is developed through practice, the experience of medical illness, or paying more attention to one's body. A large literature exists on the awareness of resting heartbeat (Brener & Kluvitse, 1988; Brener & Ring, 1992, 1995; Jones, 1995; Katkin, 1985; Yates, Jones, Marie, & Hogben, 1985). However most of these studies have been conducted under laboratory conditions, using healthy volunteers rather than ill patients. Several different paradigms have been used, and they have yielded somewhat contradictory results. But they generally suggest that accuracy of heartbeat awareness is greater in males and in subjects who are more anxious and younger. What is largely missing from the literature is work examining heartbeat awareness in symptomatic patients and in patients with cardiac disease. Nor has this research explored the relationship between awareness of normal physiology and awareness of disease and abnormal function.

The Interrelationships Between Measures
of Cardioception

We therefore compared the accuracy of palpitation reports during ambulatory monitoring (i.e., the degree to which patient reports of palpitations coincided with demonstrated cardiac arrhythmias) and the accuracy of resting heartbeat detection (see Fig. 19.4). These two forms of cardioception proved to be unrelated to each other. The average PPV of those who passed and who failed the HBD task was the same (0.40), and the bivariate correlation between the two tests was not significant. In addition, as described previously, these tests had very different patterns of association with the other study variables. Although awareness of arrhythmias was related to several clinical variables, HBD performance was unrelated to any of the sociodemographic, psychiatric, medical, or medical care characteristics

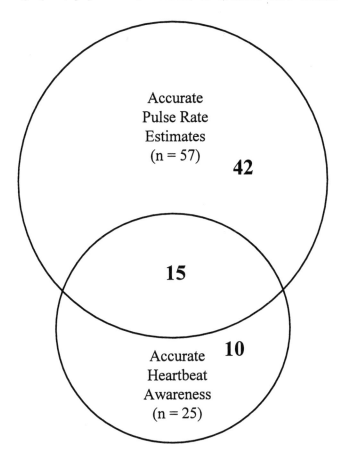

FIG. 19.4. Accurate cardiac perception: two paradigms.

studied. The independence of these two cardioceptive tasks is not surprising because performance on laboratory tests of visceral interoception generally differs from performance in vivo during everyday life (Pennebaker, 1991; Pennebaker, Gonder-Frederick, Cox, & Hoover, 1985; Pennebaker & Watson, 1988; Tyrer, Lee, & Alexander, 1980; Whitehead et al., 1977; an analogous picture emerges in pain research, where the sensitivity to experimental and pathological pain are found to differ; Jamner & Schwartz, 1986; Sternbach, 1974). First, the detection of resting heartbeat is a different psychophysical task from the detection of irregularities in, and departures from, that baseline. In other words, people may be more or less able to perceive the steady state itself than to perceive changes in it (Pennebaker, 1982, 1991). Second, we know that bodily perception is affected by the context in which it occurs (Pennebaker, 1982), and the circumstances and setting of the experimental laboratory differ markedly from those of the natural environment. In daily life, external stimuli compete for attention, different situational feedback occurs, and different cues and external information are available to interpret one's sensory experience. This point has been made by Pennebaker (1991) and Pennebaker and Watson (1988) in studying the awareness of blood pressure and blood sugar. Finally, bodily perception is profoundly influenced by the beliefs, knowledge, and expectations we have about what we perceive. The implications of an arrhythmic sensation, with its alarming and ominous threat to health, are very different from the meaning and significance we attach to sensing one's normal heartbeat.

IMPLICATIONS AND FUTURE RESEARCH

The lack of a fixed, one-to-one relationship between symptoms and disease is enormously important in the practice of medicine. Although the patient's clinical history always remains the cornerstone of the diagnostic process, clinicians must at the same time remember that somatic symptoms are often a manifestation of factors other than disease. Thus the bodily distress that the patients report to their physicians reflects a host of psychosocial and environmental factors such as personality style, life stress, expectations and beliefs about health, anxiety and depression, and the secondary gains of illness.

Symptoms are important not only because they point the way toward underlying disease and guide the diagnostic process but because they cause suffering and their amelioration is an end in itself. And here again, physicians need to understand the psychosocial factors that cause and exacerbate symptoms in order to relieve them. Such knowledge is critical in developing a science of symptom palliation that is as powerful as our science for curing disease. In learning more about the reporting of symptoms and the factors that modulate the symptom experience, it may prove useful to investigate a number of natural experiments such as the placebo effect and the palliative effect of psychosocial therapies such as support groups and hypnosis. The research techniques, strategies, and approaches needed to pursue these studies will come in large measure from psychology and the social sciences rather than from the biomedical sciences.

What is needed is a more comprehensive and more explicit understanding of the entire process of symptom generation, appraisal, experience, and reporting. This would start with an elucidation of the peripheral and central neuroanatomical pathways and of neurophysiological processing of visceral and somatic afferent sensations. Functional brain imaging offers us the exciting prospect of actually visualizing the subcortical and cortical processing of somatic and visceral stimuli. Study of the perceptual process would also encompass rigorous psychophysiological measurement of patients using paradigms in which a quantifiable sensory stimulus is administered and the patient's subjective sensations are then obtained. These studies need to be conducted in such a fashion that the patient's discriminative acuity (his or her ability to accurately detect a stimulus) is distinguished from response bias (the systematic tendency to report that somatic and visceral stimuli in general are bothersome or more intense). Here, signal detection theory and techniques, as have been applied in the study of pain, may be helpful.

ACKNOWLEDGMENT

This chapter was supported by NIMH grant #MH40487 and NIH grant #HL43216.

REFERENCES

Alonso, J., Anto, J. M., Gonzalez, M., Fiz, J. A., Izquierdo, J., & Morera, J. (1992). Measurement of general health status of non-oxygen-dependent chronic obstructive pulmonary disease patients. *Medical Care, 30*, MS125–MS135.

Backett, E. M., Heady, J. A., & Evans, J. C. G. (1954). Studies of a general practice (II): The doctor's job in an urban area. *British Medical Journal, 1*, 109–115.

Barsky, A. J., Ahern, D. K., Delamater, B. A., Clancy, S., & Bailey, E. D. (1997). Differential diagnosis of palpitations: Preliminary development of a screening instrument. *Archives of Family Medicine, 6*, 241–245.

Barsky, A. J., Cleary, P. D., Barnett, M. C., Christiansen, C. L., & Ruskin, J. N. (1994). The accuracy of symptom reporting in patients complaining of palpitations. *American Journal of Medicine, 97*, 214–221.

Barsky, A. J., Cleary, P. D., Brener, J., & Ruskin, J. N. (1993). The perception of cardiac activity in medical outpatients. *Cardiology, 83*, 304–385.

Barsky, A. J., Cleary, P. D., Sarnie, M. K., & Ruskin, J. N. (1994). Panic disorder, palpitations, and the awareness of cardiac activity. *Journal of Nervous & Mental Disease, 182*, 63–71.

Barsky, A. J., Goodson, J. D., Lane, R. S., & Cleary, P. D. (1988). The amplification of somatic symptoms. *Psychosomatic Medicine, 50*, 510–519.

Bass C. (1990). *Somatization: Physical symptoms and psychological illness.* Oxford, England: Blackwell.

Beecher, H. K. (1966). Relationship of significance of wound to pain experience. *Journal of the American Medical Association, 161*, 1609–1613.

Bodemar, G., & Walan, A. (1978). Maintenance treatment of recurrent peptic ulcer by cimetidine. *Lancet, 1*, 403–407.

Boden, S. D., Davis, D. O., Dina, T. S., Patronas, N., & Wiesel, S. W. (1990). Abnormal magnetic-resonance scans of the lumbar spine in asymptomatic subjects. *Journal of Bone & Joint Surgery, 72*, 403–408.

Brener, J., & Kluvitse, C. (1988). Heart beat detection: Judgements of the simultaneity of external stimuli and heart beats. *Psychophysiology, 25*, 554–561.

Brener, J., & Ring, C. (1992). Sensory and perceptual factors in heartbeat detection. In D. Vaitl & R. Scandry (Eds.), *Interoception and cardiovascular processes.* New York: Springer-Verlag.

Brener, J., & Ring, C. (1995). Sensory and perceptual factors in heartbeat detection. In D. Vaitl & R. Scandry (Eds.), *From the heart to the brain* (pp. 193–221). Frankfurt, Germany: Peter Lang.

Bridges, K. W., & Goldberg, D. P. (1985). Somatic presentation of DSM–III psychiatric disorders in primary care. *Journal of Psychosomatic Research, 29*, 563–569.

Burckhardt, D., Luetold, B. E., Jost, M. V., & Hoffman, A. (1982). Holter monitoring in the evaluation of palpitations, dizziness and syncope. In J. Roelandt & P. G. Hugenholtz (Eds.), *Long term ambulatory electrocardiography* (pp. 29–39). The Hague, Netherlands: Martinus Nijhoff.

Burdon, J. G. W., Juniper, E. F., Killian, K. J., Hargreave, F. E., & Campbell, E. J. M. (1982). The perception of breathlessness in asthma. *American Review of Respiratory Diseases, 126*, 825–828.

Cartwright, A. (1967). *Patients and their doctors: A study of general practice.* London: Routledge & Kegan Paul.

Clark, P. I., Glasser, S. P., & Spoto, E., Jr. (1980). Arrhythmias detected by ambulatory monitoring: Lack of correlation with symptoms of dizziness and syncope. *Chest, 77*, 722–725.

Costa, P. T., Jr., & McCrae, R. R. (1980). Somatic complaints in males as a function of age and neuroticism: A longitudinal analysis. *Journal of Behavioral Medicine, 3*, 245–257.

Costa, P. T., Jr., & McCrae, R. R. (1985). Hypochondriasis, neuroticism, and aging. When are somatic complaints unfounded? *American Psychologist, 40*, 19–28.

Craig, T. K. J., Boardman, A. P., Mills, K., Daley-Jones, O., & Drake, H. (1993). The South London Somatization Study I: Longitudinal course and the influence of early life experiences. *British Journal of Psychiatry, 163*, 579–588.

Cummings, N. A., & Vanden Bos, G. R. (1981). The twenty-year Kaiser-Permanente experience with psychotherapy and medical utilization: Implications for national health policy and national health insurance. *Health Policy Quarterly, 1*, 159–175.

Deanfield, J. E., Maseri, A., Selwyn, A. P., Ribeiro, P., Chierchia, S., Krikler, S., & Morgan, M. (1983). Myocardial ischemia during daily life in patients with stable angina: Its relation to symptoms and heart rate changes. *Lancet, 2*, 753–758.

Dwosh, I. L., Giles, A. R., Ford, P. M., Pater, J. L., & Anastassiades, T. P. (1983). Plasmapheresis therapy in rheumatoid arthritis. *New England Journal of Medicine, 308*, 1124–1129.

Epstein, S. D., Quyyumi, A. A., & Bonow, R. O. (1988). Current concepts. Myocardial ischemia: silent or symptomatic. *New England Journal of Medicine, 18*, 1038–1043.

Escobar, J. I., Burnham, A., Karno, M., Forsythe, A., & Golding, J. M. (1987). Somatization in the community. *Archives of General Psychiatry, 44*, 713–718.

Escobar, J. I., Golding, J. M., Hough, R. L., Karno, M., Burnham, M. A., & Wells, K. B. (1987). Somatization in the community: Relationship to disability and use of services. *American Journal of Public Health, 77,* 837–840.

Follette, W. T., & Cummings, W. A. (1968). Psychiatric services and medical utilization in a prepaid health plan setting: Part II. *Medical Care, 6,* 31–41.

Ford, C. V. (1983). *The somatizing disorders. Illness as a way of life.* New York: Elsevier.

Frimodt-Moller, P. C., Jensen, K. M., Iversen, P., Madsen, P. O., Bruskewitz, R. C. (1984). Analysis of presenting symptoms in prostatism. *Journal of Urology, 132,* 272–276.

Garfield, S. R., Collen, M. F., Feldman, R., Soghikian, K., Richart, R. H., & Duncan, J. H. (1976). Evaluation of ambulatory medical care system. *New England Journal of Medicine, 294,* 426–431.

Glazier, J. J., Chierchia, S., Brown, M. J., & Maseri, A. (1986). Importance of generalized defective perception of painful stimuli as a cause of silent myocardial ischemia in chronic stable angina pectoris. *American Journal of Cardiology, 58,* 667–672.

Goldberg, A. D., Raftery, E. B., & Cashman, P. M. (1975). Ambulatory electrocardiographic records in patients with transient cerebral attacks or palpitation. *British Medical Journal, 4,* 569–571.

Gough, H. G. (1977). Doctors' estimates of the percentage of patients whose problems do not require medical attention. *Medical Education, 11,* 380–384.

Grodman, R. S., Capone, R. J., & Most, A. S. (1979). Arrhythmia surveillance by transtelephonic monitoring. *American Heart Journal, 98,* 459–464.

Harrington, A. (1997). *The placebo effect; An interdisciplinary exploration.* Cambridge, MA: Harvard University Press.

Hasin, Y., David, D., & Rogel, S. (1976). Diagnostic and therapeutic assessment by telephone ECG monitoring of ambulatory patients. *British Journal of Medicine, 2,* 609–612.

Hilkevitch, A. (1965). Psychiatric disturbance in outpatients of a general medical outpatient clinic. *International Journal of Neuropsychiatry, 1,* 372–375.

Hussar, A. E., & Guller, E. J. (1956). Correlation of pain and the roentgenographic findings of spondylosis of the cervical and lumbar spine. *American Journal of Medical Science, 232,* 518–527.

Jamner, L. D., & Schwartz, G. E. (1986). Self-deception predicts self-report and endurance of pain. *Psychosomatic Medicine, 48,* 211–223.

Jones, G. E. (1995). Constitutional and physiological factors in heartbeat perception. In D. Vaitl & R. Schandry (Eds.), *From the heart to the brain* (pp. 173–192). Frankfurt: Peter Lang.

Kannel, W. B., & Abbott, R. D. (1984). Incidence and prognosis of unrecognized myocardial infarction: an update on the Framingham study. *New England Journal of Medicine, 311,* 1144–1147.

Katkin, E. S. (1985). Blood, sweat, and tears: Individual differences in autonomic self-perception. *Psychophysiology, 22,* 125–137.

Katon, W., Ries, R. K., & Kleinman, A. (1984). The prevalence of somatization in primary care. *Comprehensive Psychiatry, 25,* 208–215.

Keefe, F. J., Caldwell, D. S., Queen, K. T., Gil, K. M., Martinez, S., Crisson, J. E., Ogden, W., & Nunley, J. (1987). Pain coping strategies in osteoarthritis patients. *Journal of Consulting & Clinical Psychology, 55,* 208–212.

Kellner, R. (1986). *Somatization and hypochondriasis.* New York: Praeger.

Kennedy, H. L., Chandra, V., Sayther, K. L., & Caralis, D. G. (1978). Effectiveness of increasing hours of continuous ambulatory electrocardiography in detecting maximal ventricular ectopy. *American Journal of Cardiology, 42,* 925–930.

Kikuchi, Y., Okabe, S., Tamura, G., Hida, W., Homma, M., Shirato, K., & Takishima, K. (1994). Chemosensitivity and perception of dyspnea in patients with a history of near-fatal asthma. *New England Journal of Medicine, 330,* 1329–1334.

Kleinman, A., Eisenberg, L., & Good, B. J. (1978). Culture, illness, and care: Clinical lessons from anthropologic and cross-cultural research. *Annals of Internal Medicine, 88,* 251–258.

Kroenke, K., Arrington, M. E., & Mangelsdorff, A. D. (1990). The prevalence of symptoms in medical outpatients and the adequacy of therapy. *Archives of Family Medicine, 150,* 1685–1690.

Kroenke, K., & Mangelsdorff, A. D. (1989). Common symptoms in ambulatory care: Incidence, evaluation, therapy, and outcome. *American Journal of Medicine, 86,* 262–266.

Kroenke, K., Spitzer, R. L., Williams, J. B. W., Linzer, M., Hahn, S. R., deGruy, F. V., & Brody, D. (1994). Physical symptoms in primary care: Predictors of psychiatric disorders and functional impairment. *Archives of Family Medicine, 3,* 774–779.

Kunz, G., Raeder, E., & Burckhardt, D. (1977). What does the symptom "palpitation" mean? *Kardiologie, 66,* 138–141.

Lane, R. S., Barsky, A. J., & Goodson, J. D. (1988). Discomfort and disability in upper respiratory tract infection. *Journal of General Internal Medicine, 3,* 540–546.

Lipski, J., Cohen, L., Espinoza, J., Motro, M., Dack, S., & Donoso, E. (1976). Value of holter monitoring in assessing cardiac arrhythmias in symptomatic patients. *American Journal of Cardiology, 37,* 102–107.

Lustman, P. J., Clouse, R. E., & Carney, R. M. (1988). Depression and the reporting of diabetes symptoms. *International Journal of Psychiatry in Medicine, 18,* 295–303.

Macdonald, L. A., Sackett, D. L., Haynes, R. B., & Taylor, D. W. (1984). Labelling in hypertension: A review of the behavioral and psychological consequences. *Journal of Chronic Disease, 37,* 933–942.

Mahler, D. A., Matthay, R. A., Snyder, P. E., Wells, C. K., & Loke, J. (1985). Sustained-release theophylline reduces dyspnea in nonreversible obstructive airway disease. *American Review of Respiratory Disease, 131,* 22–25.

Mahler, D. A., Weinberg, D. H., Wells, C. K., & Feinstein, A. R. (1984). The measurement of dyspnea: Contents interobserver agreement, and physiologic correlates of two new clinical indexes. *Chest, 85,* 751–758.

Mechanic, D. (1974). *Politics, medicine, and social science.* New York: Wiley.

Morahan, J. P., Denes, P., & Rosen, K. M. (1975). Portable ECG monitoring. *Archives of Internal Medicine, 135,* 1188–1194.

Pennebaker, J. W. (1982). *The psychology of physical symptoms.* New York: Springer-Verlag.

Pennebaker, J. W. (1995). Beyond laboratory-based cardiac perception: Ecological introception. In R. Schandry & D. Vaitl (Eds.), *From the heart to the brain* (pp. 389–406). Frankfurt, Germany: Peter Lang.

Pennebaker, J. W., Gonder-Frederick, L., Cox, D. J., & Hoover, C. W. (1985). The perception of general vs. specific visceral activity and the regulation of health-related behavior. In E. S. Katkin & S. B. Manuck (Eds.), *Advances in behavioral medicine* (pp. 165–198). Greenwich, CT: JAI.

Pennebaker, J. W., & Watson, D. (1988). Blood pressure estimation and beliefs among normotensives and hypertensives. *Health Psychology, 7,* 309–328.

Peterson, W. L., Sturdevant, R. A. L., Frankl, H. D., Richardson, C. T., Isenberg, J. I., Elashoff, J. D., Sones, J. Q., Gross, R. A., McCallum, R. W., & Fordtran, J. S. (1977). Healing of duodenal ulcer with an antacid regimen. *New England Journal of Medicine, 297,* 341–345.

Pilowsky, I., Smith, Q. P., & Katsikitis, M. (1987). Illness behavior and general practice utilization: A prospective study. *Journal of Psychosomatic Research, 31,* 177–183.

Quyyumi, A. A., Wright, C. M., Mockus, L. J., & Fox, K. M. (1985). How important is a history of chest pain in determining the degree of ischaemia in patients with angina pectoris? *British Heart Journal, 54,* 22–26.

Rubinfeld, A. R., & Pain, M. C. F. (1976). Perception of asthma. *Lancet, 1,* 882–884.

Schandry, R. (1981). Heart beat perception and emotional experience. *Psychophysiology, 18,* 483–488.

Sternbach, R. A. (1974). *Pain patients: Traits and treatments.* New York: Academic Press.

Summers, M. N., Haley, W. E., Reveille, J. D., & Alarcón, G. S. (1988). Radiographic assessment and psychologic variables as predictors of pain and functional impairment in osteoarthritis of the knee or hip. *Arthritis & Rheumatism, 31,* 204–209.

Tyrer, P., Lee, I., & Alexander, J. (1980). Awareness of cardiac function in anxious, phobic and hypochondriacal patients. *Psychological Medicine, 10,* 171–174.

van der Gagg, J., & van de Ven, W. (1978). The demand for primary health care. *Medical Care, 26,* 299–312.

Watson, D., & Pennebaker, J. W. (1989). Health complaints, stress and distress: Exploring the central role of negative affectivity. *Psychological Review, 96,* 234–254.

Whitehead, W. E., Drescher, V. M., Heiman, P., & Blackwell, B. (1977). Relation of heart rate control to heartbeat perception. *Biofeedback Self-Regulation, 2,* 371–392.

Wiesel, S. W., Tsourmas, N., Feffer, H. L., Citris, C. M., & Patronas, N. (1984). A study of computer-assisted tomography, I: The incidence of positive CAT scans in an asymptomatic group of patients. *Spine, 9,* 549–551.

Winkle, R. A., Derrington, D. C., & Schroeder, J. S. (1977). Characteristics of ventricular tachycardia in ambulatory patients. *American Journal of Cardiology, 39,* 487–492.

Wood, M. M., & Elwood, P. C. (1966). Symptoms of iron deficiency anaemia. A community survey. *British Journal of Preventive & Social Medicine, 20,* 117–121.

Yates, A. J., Jones, K. E., Marie, G. V., & Hogben, J. H. (1985). Detection of the heartbeat and events in the cardiac cycle. *Psychophysiology, 22,* 561–567.

Zeldis, S. M., Levine, B. J., Michelson, E. L., & Morganroth, J. (1980). Cardiovascular complaints; correlation with cardiac arrhythmias on 24-hour ECG monitoring. *Chest, 78,* 456–462.

Author Index

365

Subject Index